GERIATRICS

Edited by **Craig S. Atwood**

Geriatrics
Edited by Craig S. Atwood

Published by InTech
Janeza Trdine 9, 51000 Rijeka, Croatia

Publishing Process Manager Marina Jozipovic

Technical Editor Teodora Smiljanic

Cover Designer InTech Design Team

Additional hard copies can be obtained from orders@intechopen.com

Geriatrics, Edited by Craig S. Atwood
p. cm.
ISBN 978-953-51-0080-5

For EU product safety concerns:
IN TECH d.o.o., Prolaz Marije Krucifikse Kozulić 3, 51000 Rijeka, Croatia,
info@intechopen.com or visit our website at intechopen.com.

Meet the editor

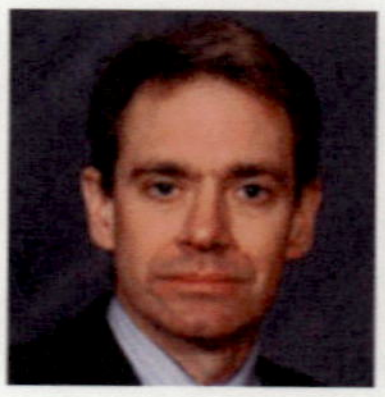

Craig S. Atwood, PhD is an Associate Professor of Medicine at the University of Wisconsin and a Health Science Specialist with the Geriatric Research, Education and Clinical Center at the William S. Middleton Memorial Veterans Administration Hospital in Madison. Dr. Atwood completed his PhD in Biochemistry at the University of Western Australia in Perth, Australia prior to post-doctoral fellowships at the National Cancer Institute, NIH, Bethesda, and Massachusetts General Hospital, Boston. He has held faculty positions at Harvard Medical School and Case Western Reserve University prior to his current position where he directs the research program of the Laboratory for Endocrinology, Aging and Disease. Dr. Atwood has broad research interests related to the endocrinology of aging as elaborated upon in 'The Reproductive-Cell Cycle Theory of Aging'. He has published over 200 scientific articles, has served on numerous review boards and is an Editor of more than 20 scientific journals including the Journal of Biological Chemistry. In 2006 he received the Zenith Fellows Award from the Alzheimer's Association in recognition of his research.

Contents

Preface

The decline in physical and mental functionality with aging has been attributed to the endocrine dyscrasia, associated with the loss of the reproductive function with aging (Bowen and Atwood, 2004; 2011). These biomolecular changes result in the dysfunction and/or death of cells, and ultimately the loss of tissue function, that presents clinically as conditions of aging (e.g. osteoporosis, arthritis) or as disease (e.g. coronary heart disease, dementia). This book addresses a broad range of issues related to geriatrics, including: 1) characterizing functional loss in the geriatric patient 2) preventive strategies for the maintenance of health in the geriatric population, and 3) end of life issues for geriatric patients that range from legal issues to patient education.

The first section of this book – 'Functional Loss Associated with Aging' addresses the physical and mental decline in function associated with aging. The first chapter by Hairi et al addresses the age-related changes in physical functioning from the perspective of demographics, interventions and the further research required to guide public health practitioners and clinicians as to the most appropriate interventions to improve and maximize a person's function. Hairi et al follow up this first chapter with an examination of sarcopenia as a major cause of the decline in physical function with age. As noted by the author, current research has shown promising results in the assessment of sarcopenia, although further work is required in the management of sarcopenic patients, in terms of prevention as well as treatment. The next two chapters focus on specific changes in functional decline in the elderly, namely the cognitive decline associated with vascular dementia (Ozbabalik et al.) and swallowing difficulties (Lacoste-Ferre). Ozbabalik examine the epidemiology of vascular dementia including the risk factors for the development of this form of dementia. Lacoste-Ferre present new data, suggesting that disrupted mastication appears to be a factor favoring dysphagia in the elderly, and that the preservation of dental status is a good objective to prevent dysphagia in the institutionalized frail and dependent elderly. Finally, Takata et al report on how lower fitness levels, for various muscle strength tests is associated with increases in all-cause mortality as well as disease-specific mortality in an 80-year-old community-dwelling population. This data fits well with previous literature indicating a lower level of physical activity, physical fitness, or muscle strength is associated with a higher total mortality in an elderly population.

In the next section of the book - 'Preventative Strategies for Maintenance of Health and Extending Longevity' we move from an appreciation of functional decline in the elderly to strategies of preventing frailty and extend longevity. In the first chapter of this section, Hunkyung reviews risk factors for geriatric syndrome prior to elaborating on treatments for frailty and falls prevention involving nutrition and exercise strategies. Yamauchi follows by also reviewing the importance of exercise (resistance training) as a countermeasure against sarcopenia and loss of muscle function. Indeed, resistance training at home or in a community center (without the need for strength training equipment) allows for important improvements in muscle function for the elderly. In a similar vein, in the next chapter Yamada et al highlight the importance of tailoring fall prevention programs to the elderly adult's level of physical well-being. Kojimahara advocate the benefits of annual immunization with influenza vaccine and 23-valent pneumococcal polysaccharide vaccine (PPV23) in the elderly with and without chronic obstructive pulmonary disease. Decreasing the risk of heart disease, the major killer in western society, by attenuating post-prandial hyperglycemia is the topic of the next chapter by Mori et al. In this paper, intestinal glucose absorption after fermented milk ingestion was shown to be attenuated experimentally in mice as well as clinically in humans. Thus, the use of 'Caspian Sea Yogurt' such as used by long-living populations in Georgia is suggested to reduce cardiovascular risk and to contribute to the longevity. The final chapter in this section by Kececi and Bulduk examines healthcare personnel attitudes towards the ability of the elderly to understand and learn new information. The authors discuss the need for healthcare professionals to be more in tune with the elderly, and to understand the physical, psychological and socio-cultural changes that might impact learning in the elderly in order to develop more efficient strategies to improve health promotion and wellness.

The final section of the book examines end of life care. The first chapter by Kahana et al advocate for educational interventions to help older patients marshal responsive care during the extended period of service needs during the final years. As indicated by the authors, effective advocacy by patients and families is an important determinant upon making the final period of life more comfortable and livable. Schelp addresses the attitudes toward autonomy and legal instruments at the end of life, and discusses the multidimensional nature of the medical, social, cultural, religious, and economic aspects involved in end of life decision making and care. The final chapter by Ratcliffe et al discusses the challenges and opportunities of health economics with respect of geriatric care. These authors discuss the methods for assessing the cost effectiveness of new health care technologies and models of aged care service delivery, as well as the methods adopted by health economists for measuring and valuing patient or consumer preferences in health care.

It is hoped that the papers and reviews described here will help to update the geriatrics research and clinical community on recent advances in identifying and quantitating functional loss experienced by the elderly, strategies to maintain function and longevity, and finally the complex issues surrounding the end of life care of the patient.

Craig S. Atwood
Geriatric Research, Education and Clinical Center,
Veterans Administration Hospital,
Department of Medicine,
University of Wisconsin,Madison,
USA,
School of Exercise, Biomedical and Health Sciences
Edith Cowan University
Joondalup,
Australia

References

Bowen, R.L. and Atwood, C.S. (2004). Living and Dying for Sex: A theory of aging based on the modulation of cell cycle signaling by reproductive hormones. Gerontology, 50(5), 265-290.

Atwood C.S. and Bowen R.L. (2011). The reproductive-cell cycle theory of aging: An update. Experimental Gerontology, 46(2-3), 100-107.

Part 1

Functional Loss Associated with Aging

1

Physical Function in Older People

Noran N. Hairi[1,2], Tee Guat Hiong[3],
Awang Bulgiba[1,2] and Izzuna Mudla[4]
[1]*Department of Social and Preventive Medicine,*
Faculty of Medicine, University of Malaya, Kuala Lumpur,
[2]*JCUM, Centre for Clinical Epidemiology and Evidence-Based Medicine,*
Faculty of Medicine, University of Malaya, Kuala Lumpur,
[3]*Institute for Public Health, National Institutes of Health, Ministry of Health,*
[4]*Ministry of Health,*
Malaysia

1. Introduction

Aging is a natural process. Improved maternal and infant health, better survival in infancy, childhood and early adult life, has led to increase life expectancy of older people. As of 2008, 7% (506 million) of the world's population was aged 65 years and older, an increased of 10.4 million since 2007 (Kinsella K and Wan He 2009). The current pace of population aging varies widely. While developed countries have relatively high proportions of people aged 65 years and over, the most rapid increases in older people are in the developing world. As of 2008, 62% (313 million) of the world's population aged 65 and over lived in developing countries (Kinsella K and Wan He 2009). Many developing countries will be experiencing a sudden rise in the proportion of older people within a single generation, with far less well developed infrastructure. In contrast, most developed countries have had decades to adjust to the changing age structure and this change has been supported by relative economic prosperity.

2. Theories of population health change

The implications of longer life mean increased risk of poor physical function as expounded by the theories of population health change. Four theories have been proposed in discussing the consequences of increased life expectancy in older people.

The expansion of Morbidity/Disability Theory (Gruenberg EM 1977), suggests that the gain in life expectancy in older people is mainly due to technological advances and secondary prevention strategies that have extended the life of older people with disability and underlying illness. This results in living with non-fatal diseases such as vision loss, arthritis, chronic pain and other diseases of old age, therefore living longer means living with more years of disability.

The opposing theory is called the Compression of Morbidity/Disability Theory(Fries 1980; Fries 2005). He suggested that primary prevention strategies modify risk factors for mortality that delays the age-at-onset and progression of disabling diseases. Assuming that maximum life expectancy is fixed, this will result in the time live with disability and disease being compressed into a shorter period before death.

Manton offered a third perspective called the "Dynamic Equilibrium Theory" that combines elements from both the expansion and compression theories (Manton KG 1982). Manton proposes that economic, medical and technical progress reduces mortality as well as having an influence on morbidity/disability. Decrease in mortality rates are accompanied by declines in the incidence and progression of chronic diseases. As a result, years of life gained are assumed to be achieved through a combination of postponement of disease onset, reduction in severity of disease and disease progression due to improvement in clinical management of diseases.

A recent theory takes into consideration the country's position in the demographic transition phase (Robine Jean-Marie and Michel Jean-Pierre 2004). Their "General Theory of Population Aging" encompasses all the three previous theories and relies on a cyclical movement. Firstly, there is an increase in the survival rates of sick people supporting the "expansion of morbidity theory". Second, medical improvements take place, slowing down the progression of chronic condition and achieving certain equilibrium with mortality decline, supporting the "dynamic equilibrium theory". The third phase is improvement in health status and health behaviours of new cohorts of older people, supporting the "compression of morbidity theory". Eventually there will be an emergence of very old and frail populations, which brings back to the starting point, that is, to a new "expansion of morbidity".

3. The language of physical function

Before further discussion regarding the subject of physical function and its relevance, some definitions are necessary. The definition of the term "disability" and "functional limitation" in this chapter follows the Nagi Disablement Model (Nagi 1976). This model has proven useful as a language used by researchers to delineate the consequences of disease and injury at the levels of body systems, the person and society. The definition of disability encompasses various aspects; pathology, impairment, and limitation are terms that are directly associated with the concept of disability.

According to the classification scheme provided by Nagi, *impairment* refers to a loss or abnormality at the tissue, organ and body system level. At the level of the individual, Nagi uses the term *functional limitations* that represent limitations in performance of specific tasks by a person. The term *disability*, as defined by Nagi, refers to limitations in performing socially defined roles and tasks expected of an individual within a socio-cultural and physical environment. Both impairment and functional limitation involve function. However, for impairment, the reference is to the levels of tissues, organs and systems while for functional limitation, the reference is to the level of the person as a whole. In differentiating functional limitation from disability, functional limitation refers to organismic performance; in contrast disability refers to social performance.

The term physical disability is often used to refer to restrictions in the ability to perform a set of common, everyday tasks, performance of which is required for personal self care and independent living. This includes the basic activities of daily living (ADL) and instrumental activities of daily living (IADL). These are the most widely used measurements of physical disability in the literature. Basic ADLs are self-care tasks such as bathing, dressing, grooming and eating (Fried LP and Guralnik 1997). The IADL's are tasks that are physically and cognitively more complicated and difficult but are necessary for independent living in the community such as getting groceries, preparing meals, performing everyday household chores. ADL and IADL are measures of disability that reflect how an individual's limitation interacts with the demands of the environment.

The evaluation of mobility refers to the individual's locomotor system. Mobility disability is a critical component of activities of daily living (Fried LP and Guralnik 1997). Mobility disability is defined as difficulty or dependency in functioning due to decreased walking ability, manoeuvrability and speed.

The building blocks of restrictions in performing ADLs are termed functional limitations (Guralnik and Luigi 2003). Functional limitations are measures independent of environmental influences, and may explain the changes in functional aspects of health. Functional limitation refers to restriction in physical performance of tasks required for independent living, such as walking, balancing and standing.

Physical function is a general term that reflects one's ability to perform mobility tasks, ADLs and IADLs. Throughout this chapter "poor physical function" is used as a general term to refer to physical disability, mobility disability and functional limitation.

4. The disablement process

To discuss poor physical function in older people, it is important to have an understanding of the progression that ends with loss of physical function, or the disablement process. The disablement process describes how chronic and acute conditions affect functioning in specific body systems, basic human performance, and people's functioning in necessary, usual, expected, and personally desired roles in society (Verbrugge and Jette 1994). It also describes how personal and environmental factors speed up or slow down this process. There are two major models describing disability and related concepts. This chapter will describe both models. – the Nagi Model (Nagi 1976) and the International Classification of Impairments, Disabilities and Handicaps (ICIDH) (World Health Organization 1980) and its current version, the International Classification of Functioning, Disability and Health (ICF) (World Health Organization 2001) developed by the World Health Organization (WHO).

4.1 The Nagi disablement model

The pathway proposed by Nagi in 1965 to describe progression from disease to disability is shown in Figure.1. Nagi's disability model is based on four related components that described the sequential steps in the theoretical pathway from disease to disability(Nagi 1976). In the Nagi pathway, *pathology* (e.g. sarcopenia) first leads to *impairment* (e.g. lower extremity weakness) (Steven M Albert and Vicki A Freedman 2010). When lower extremity weakness crosses a certain threshold, *functional limitation* (e.g. slow gait speed) becomes evident (Steven M Albert and Vicki A Freedman 2010). When this happens, a person has a *disability* (e.g. difficulty or needing help with walking across a small room).

According to this pathway, *pathology* refers to biochemical and physiological abnormalities that are medically labeled as disease, injury or congenital/developmental conditions (Ferrucci, et al. 2007; Nagi 1976; Verbrugge and Jette 1994). *Impairment* is the consequence and degree of pathology (Nagi 1976; Verbrugge and Jette 1994). *Functional limitations* are limitations in performance at the level of the whole organism or person (Ferrucci, et al. 2007). By contrast, *disability* is defined as limitation in performance of socially defined roles and tasks within a socio-cultural and physical environment(Ferrucci, et al. 2007). Disability can also refer to the expression of functional limitation in a social context. An important advantage of utilizing different definitions for functional limitation and disability, as proposed by Nagi, is that they can be considered as sequential steps on the pathway from disease to disability. The validity of this theoretical pathway is supported by a large body of literature (Ferrucci, et al. 2007; Fried and Guralnik 1997; Steven M Albert and Vicki A Freedman 2010). Practical issues of care and prevention can be addressed by utilizing this pathway.

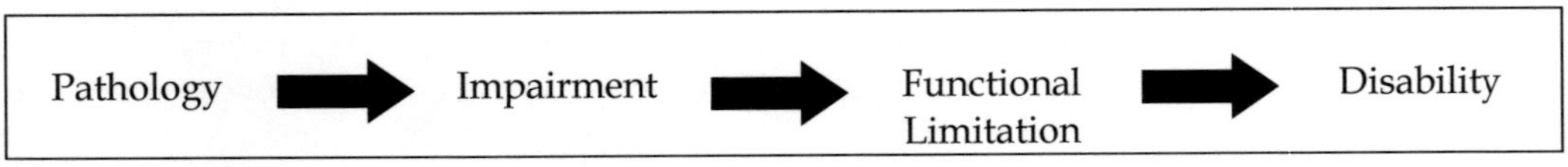

Source: Nagi S. An epidemiology of disability among adults in the United States. The Milbank Memorial Fund Quarterly. Health and Society. 1976; 54: 439-467

Fig. 1. Theoretical pathway from disease to disability proposed by Nagi (1965)

Nagi's model was extended to include personal and environmental factors that influence the evolution of the disablement process (Verbrugge and Jette 1994). Verbrugge and Jette differentiate the "main pathways" of the disablement process (i.e. Nagi's original concepts) with factors hypothesized or known to influence the ongoing process of disablement (Figure 2). This model emphasizes that predisposing risk factors, intra-individual and extra-individual factors may modify the relationship of the four components in the main pathway(Ferrucci, et al. 2007; Guralnik and Luigi 2003; Steven M Albert and Vicki A Freedman 2010; Verbrugge and Jette 1994). Risk factors are predisposing phenomena that are present prior to the onset of a disabling event that can affect the presence and/or severity of the disablement process. Intra-individual factors are those that operate within a person such as lifestyle and behavioural changes, psychosocial attributes and coping skills. Extra-individual factors are those that perform outside or external to the person. Nagi's definition of disability and the elaboration by Verbrugge and Jette also operationalizes disability as a broad range of role behaviours that are relevant to daily activities. This includes basic ADL, IADL, paid and unpaid role activities, such as occupation, social activities and leisure activities.

4.2 World Health Organization's models of disablement

In 1980, the World Health Organization (WHO) proposed a theoretical framework to describe the sequence from disease/disorder to impairment, disability and handicap named the International Classification of Impairments, Disabilities and Handicaps (ICIDH) (World Health Organization 1980)(Figure 3). At the foundation of the pathway is pathology, which is defined as any abnormality of macroscopic, microscopic or biochemical structure or function affecting an organ or organ system (Ferrucci, et al. 2007; Verbrugge and Jette 1994). The second step is impairment, defined as any abnormality of structure or function at the whole organism level, independent of any specific environment, symptom, or sign (Ferrucci, et al. 2007; Verbrugge and Jette 1994). At the third step is disability, which derives from the

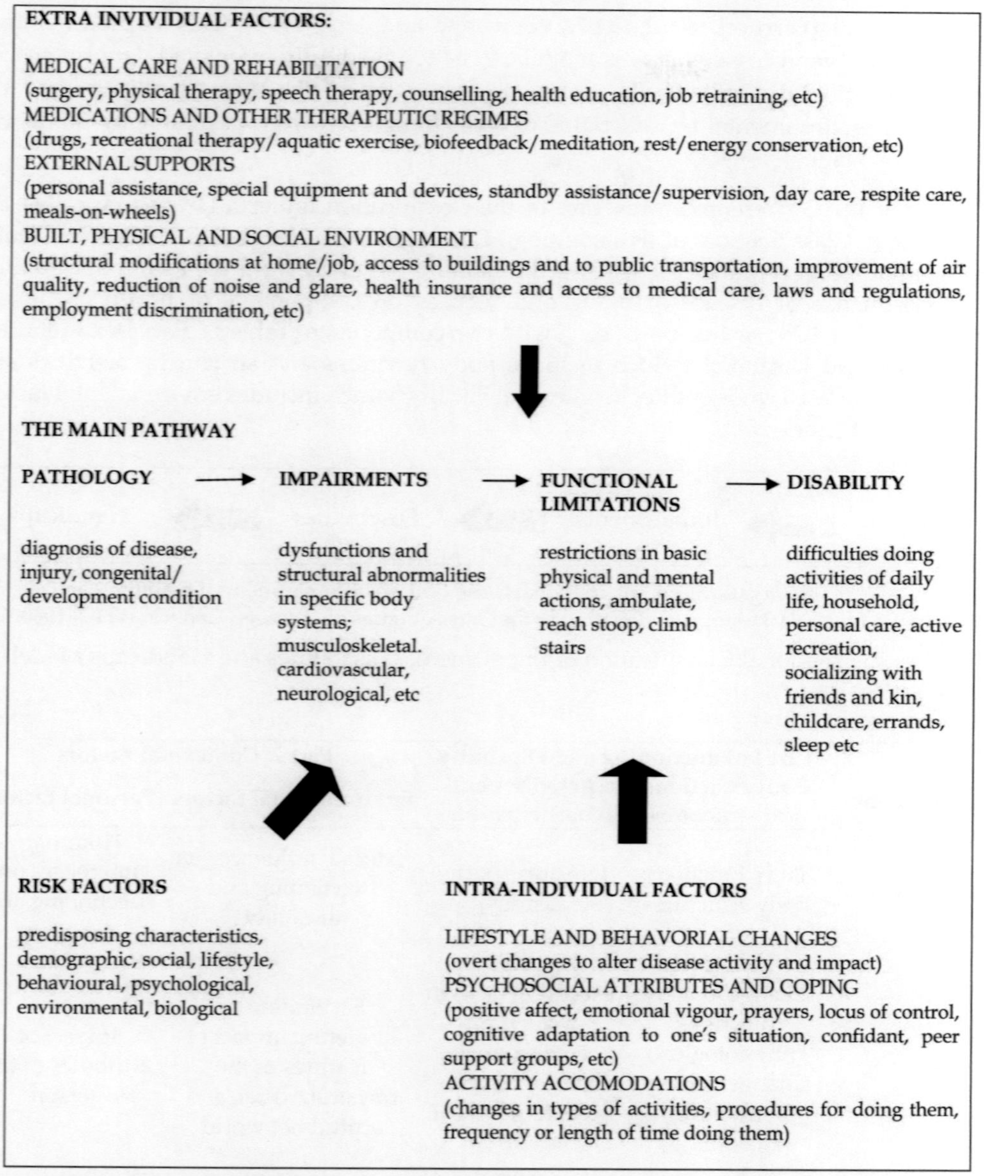

Source: Verbrugge LM, Jette AM. The disablement process. Social Science and Medicine; 1994: 38(1): 1-14

Fig. 2. The Disablement Process (1994)

interaction between the organism and the environment and is defined as any change or restriction in an individual's goal-directed behaviour (Ferrucci, et al. 2007; Verbrugge and Jette 1994). Finally, handicap is defined as any alteration in a person's status in society, including alterations in roles. Each level of the pathway should be considered as independent and may or may not be determined by the previous level and/or cause the successive level (Ferrucci, et al. 2007; Verbrugge and Jette 1994). This approach raised criticisms for several reasons: it was thought to be too medically-orientated, ignoring social and psychological dimensions; the negative connotation of the term 'handicap'; and the omission of environmental factors. Some of these limitations were overcome by the model proposed by Nagi.

In 2001, the WHO presented a revision of the classification under a new name called the International Classification of Functioning, Disability and Health (ICF) (World Health Organization 2001) (Figure 4). The revised model moves away from the idea that disability is a consequence of disease or aging and focuses on components of health as human functioning. The ICF has two parts, each with two components (Table 1). Part One is entitled Functioning and Disability (which includes body functions and structures, activities and participation). Part Two is entitled Contextual Factors, which includes environmental factors and personal factors.

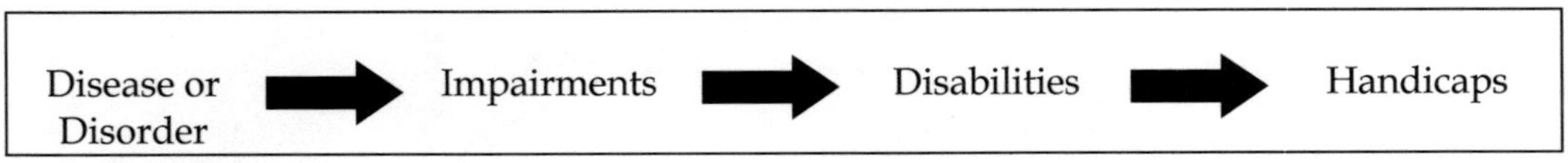

Source: World Health Organization. International Classification of Impairments, Disabilities and Handicaps: A Manual Classification Relating to the Consequences of Diseases. Geneva. WHO, 1980.

Fig. 3. The International Classification of Impairments, Disabilities and Handicaps Model (ICIDH), 1980

	Part 1 : Functioning and Disability		**Part 2: Contextual Factors**	
Component	**Body functions and structures**	**Activities and participation**	**Environmental factors**	**Personal factors**
Domains	Body functions Body structures	Life areas (tasks, actions)	External influences on functioning and disability	Internal influences on functioning and disability
Constructs	Change in body functions (physiological) Change in body structure (anatomical)	Capacity: executing tasks in a standard environment Performance: executing tasks in the current environment	Facilitating or hindering impact of features of the physical, social, and attitudinal world	Impact of attributes of the person
Positive aspect	Functional and structural integrity	Activities and Participation	Facilitators	Not applicable
Negative aspect	Impairment	Activity limitation Participation restriction	Barriers/hindrances	Not applicable

Source: World Health Organization. International Classification of Functioning, Disability and Health (ICF). Geneva. WHO, 2001.

Table 1. An overview of International Classification of Functioning, Disability and Health (ICF)

This framework starts with the concept of *health conditions,* which includes diseases, disorders, injuries and trauma. *Impairments* may occur to either body functions (e.g. reduce walking speed) or body structures (e.g. narrowing of a heart valve) (World Health Organization 2001). *Activity limitations* are difficulties an individual may have in executing activities relating to mobility, self care or domestic life (Jette AM and Keysor J 2003). *Participation restrictions* are problems an individual may experience. Disability and functioning are defined as umbrella terms (Marilyn J. Field and Alan M. Jette 2007). In the pictorial representation of the ICF (Figure 4), the terms disability and functioning do not exist. Disability and functioning are considered outcomes of interactions between health conditions and contextual factors.

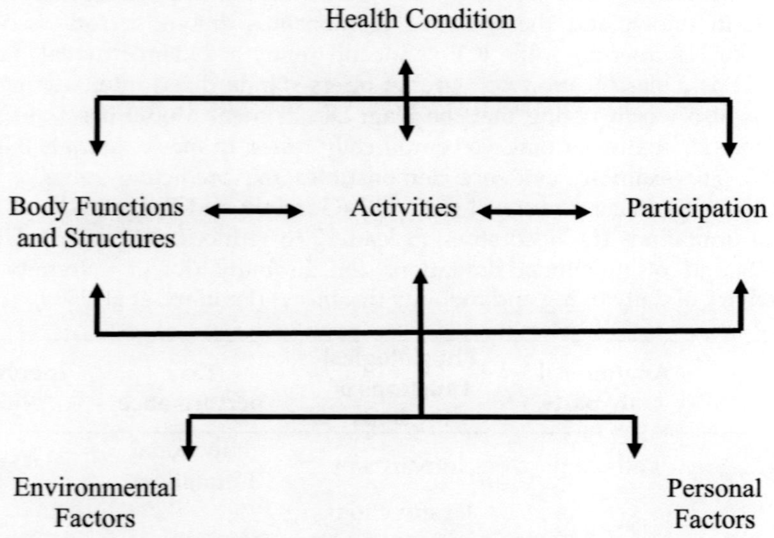

Source: World Health Organization. International Classification of Functioning, Disability and Health. Geneva. WHO, 2001.

Fig. 4. The International Classification of Functioning, Disability and Health (ICF) 2001

The first element of the ICF, the Body Functions and Structures is similar to Nagi's concept of pathology and impairment while the second component of the ICF, the Activities and Participation closely corresponds to Nagi's concept of functional limitations and disability (Jette AM and Keysor J 2003)(as shown in Table 2). The greatest limitations of the ICF is the aggregation of "activities and participation" into one domain (Guralnik and Ferrucci 2009). Using the ICF, the concepts of activity limitation and participation restriction are difficult to separate, unlike Nagi's concept of functional limitations and disability. The ICF currently does not offer crisp distinction between activity and participation, although there is an increasing movement towards defining "activities" and "participation". The Institute of Medicine (IOM) discussed this concern in its report entitled Future of Disability in America (Marilyn J. Field and Alan M. Jette 2007). Some sections of the report cited verbatim are as shown below:

"A first and well recognized aspect of the ICF that needs further development involves the interpretation and categorization of the concepts of activity and participation (page 42)"

"Several researchers have criticised the lack of clear operational differentiation between the concepts of activity and participation in the ICF as theoretically confusing and a step backward from earlier disability frameworks. Operational differentiation among concepts and the ability to measure each concept precisely and distinctly is important for clear communication, monitoring and research. (page 43)"

"Although this committee does not endorse any particular approach to resolving the problem, it believes that the lack of operational differentiation between the concepts of activity and participation is a significant deficit in the ICF. (page 44)"

Since the ICF's distinction between activity and participation is still in the developmental stage, many studies have used the Nagi Disablement Model as a conceptual framework in their research to understand the dynamic relationships among factors associated with physical function. Furthermore, the ICF is not inherently a dynamic model, similar to the ICD-10, the ICF is a classification system that offers standardized internationally accepted language. It is also worth noting that the Nagi Disablement Model has been successfully used as a theoretical pathway that was empirically tested in many datasets (Guralnik and Ferrucci 2009). For example, evidence demonstrates the predictive value of disease for impairment (arthritis causing reduced strength) (Guralnik and Luigi 2003), of impairment for functional limitations (reduced strength leading to reduced gait speed) (Guralnik and Ferrucci 2009) and of functional limitations for disability (lower extremity limitations leading to activity of daily living and mobility disability) (Penninx, et al. 2000).

	Anatomical body parts	**Physiological functions of the body**	**Task performance**	**Involvement in life roles**
Disablement Model	Pathology	Impairment	Functional Limitations	Disability
	Disease, injury, congenital condition	Dysfunctions and structural abnormalities in specific body systems	Restrictions in basic physical actions	The expression of a physical limitation in a social context
ICF	Body Functions and Structures Physiological functions of body systems and anatomical parts of body		Activities and Participation Activity : Execution of a tasks or action Participation: Involvement in a life situation	

Source: Jette AM, Keysor J. Disability Models: Implications for Arthritis Exercise and Physical Activity Interventions. Arthritis and Rheumatisn (Arthris Care and Research), 2003: 49; 114-120.

Table 2. The Disablement Model and the International Classification of Functioning, Disability and Health (ICF) frameworks.

5. Physical function measurement tools

Poor physical function can be assessed by using instruments based on self-report and by objective measurements or performance based tests. In the domain of physical and mobility disability, self report and proxy report of difficulty or inability to perform ADLs and IADLs and mobility questionnaires have been the standard assessment tools (Guralnik and Luigi 2003; Kovar and Lawton 1994). There are more than 100 published basic ADL or IADL scales, with considerable variations in the number of questions, item content, and scoring method. Examples of some of the instruments used to measure disability include Katz ADL, The Barthel Index, Instrumental Activities of Daily Living Scale (IADL), and The Health Assessment Questionnaire (HAQ) Disability Scale. The comparison of the quality of the physical disability and mobility disability tools is as shown in Table 3. Objective measurements of disability are also available but are rarely used (Cress ME 1996; Kuriansky JB 1976). Recently, Cress *et al* have created the Continuous Scale-Physical Functional Performance (CS-PFP) test, a directly observed disability test battery done in a home and neighbourhood-like setting that includes items such as transferring clothes from a washer to a dryer, vacuuming, making a bed and loading and carrying groceries.

Similarly, functional limitation may be accessed through self-report, proxy report or through performance based tests. A large number of physical performance measures, either individual tests or batteries of tests, have been developed and many of them assess different aspects of functional limitation. Some examples of performance tests commonly used are the Tinetti Performance Oriented Mobility Assessment Tool, Walking Speed, Functional Independence Measure and Timed Up and Go (TUG) test. The comparison of the quality of the functional limitation tools is as shown in Table 4.

All in all, poor physical function has been assessed with a wide variety of instruments. There is no single best way to perform an assessment and there is no single instrument that is ideal. The lack of standardization that results from the use of multiple instruments makes it difficult to compare findings across studies (Jette 1994; Kovar and Lawton 1994; Wiener, et al. 1990).

6. Prevalence of poor physical function

6.1 Prevalence of physical disability, mobility disability and functional limitation in developed countries

Several studies in developed countries have sought to gauge the prevalence of physical disability, mobility disability and functional limitation among older people.

The basic set of either the six-item ADL or the five-item ADL has been found to be most useful for valid comparison across studies. Using the six-item ADL, the prevalence of disability from the National Long-Term Care Survey in the United States ranges from 12.4% to 13.2 % from 1982 to 2005 (Lafortune 2007). Disability surveys that capture five-item ADL show lower prevalence of disability:- 6% in Canada, 10% in France and 11% in Sweden (Lafortune 2007). Using the five-item ADL, significant variations in disability have been reported between populations in the United States, China and Singapore (Chen, et al. 1995; Ng, et al. 2006; Wiener, et al. 1990; Zhe, et al. 1999). In the United States, the prevalence of five-item ADL among older people aged 65 years and over was 8.1% in the 1987 National Medical Expenditure Survey, 5.8% in the 1984 Survey on Income and Program Participation and 5.0% in the Supplement on Ageing Survey. In Asia, the prevalence of five-item ADL among older people aged 65 years and over was: 8.3% among Shanghai Chinese in the 1987 Shanghai Survey of Alzheimer's Disease and Dementia, and 6.6% among Singaporeans in the 2003 National Mental Health Survey of the Elderly.

	Instrument tool	Purpose	Description	Studies Using Method	Reliability	Validity
1.	Barthel Index	The Barthel Index measures functional independence in personal care and mobility.	It takes two to five minutes to complete. Two main versions exist: the original ten-item version and an expanded 15-item version proposed by Granger, called the Modified Barthel Index. Each item is rated in terms of whether the patient can perform the task independently, with some assistance, or is dependent on help (McDowell 2006).	Many	Ten-item version Collin *et al* studied agreement among four ways of administering the scale: self report, assessment by health care based on clinical impression, assessment by a nurse and testing by a physiotherapist. Kendall's coefficient of concordance among the four rating methods was 0.93 (McDowell 2006).	Wade and Hewer reported correlations between 0.73 and 0.77 with an index of mobility ability for 976 patients. A factor analysis identified two factors which approximate the mobility and personal care groupings of the items (McDowell 2006). Evidence for a hierarchical structure in the scale in terms of the order of recovery functions was also provided(McDowell 2006). Predictive validity has also been assessed. In studies of stroke patients, the percentage of those who died within six months of admission fell significantly ($p<0.001$) as Barthel scores at admission rose. Among survivors, admission scores also predicted the length of stay(McDowell 2006).
2.	Katz Index of ADL	The Index of ADL was developed to measure the physical functioning of elderly.	The Index of ADL assesses independence in six activities: bathing, dressing, using the toilet, transferring from bed to chair, continence and feeding. The six activities included in the index were found to	Many	Katz *et al* assessed inter-rater reliability and found differences between observers occurred once in 20 evaluations or less frequently(McDowell 2006). Guttman analyses on 100 patients in Sweden yielded coefficients of scalability ranging from 0.74 to 0.88, suggesting that the index forms a successful cumulative scale (McDowell 2006)	At a two year follow-up, Katz found that the Index of ADL predicted long term outcomes as well as or better than selected measured of physical or mental function(McDowell 2006). Brorsson and Asberg reported that 32 of 44 patients rated as independent at admission to hospital were living at home one year later whereas eight had died(McDowell 2006). By contrast 23 of 42 patients initially rated as dependent had died and only eight

	Instrument tool	Purpose	Description	Studies Using Method	Reliability	Validity
			lie in a hierarchical order of this type whereas other items (e.g. mobility, walking, stair climbing) did not fit the pattern and were excluded.			were living in their homes(McDowell 2006). Asberg also examined the ability of the scale to predict length of hospital stay, likelihood of discharge home and death (n=129). In predicting mortality, sensitivity was 73% and specificity was 80%; in predicting discharge, sensitivity was 90% and specificity, 63%(McDowell 2006).
3.	Physical Self-Maintenance Scale	The Physical Self Maintenance Scale is a measure of disability for elderly people living in the community or institution.	Brody and Lawton developed two scales: the six ADL items and an eight-item IADL scale. This scale can be administered separately or together. (Total no of items = 14).	Many	The six ADL items fell on a Guttman scale. The order of items was feeding (77% independent), toilet (66% independent), dressing (56%independent), and bathing (43% independent), grooming (42%independent) and ambulation (27% independent). A Guttman reproducibility coefficient of 0.96 was reported (n=265)(McDowell 2006). The IADL items formed a Gutman scale for women but not men, owing to gender bias in the housekeeping, cooking, and laundry items; the reproducibility coefficient was 0.93(McDowell 2006). A Pearson correlation of 0.87 was obtained between pairs of nurses who rated 36 patients; the agreement between two research assistants who independently rated 14 patients was 0.91(McDowell 2006).	The PSMS correlated 0.62 with a physician's rating of functional health (n=130)(McDowell 2006). Roskwood *et al* found the PSMS ADL questions to be less responsive (standardized response mean 0.10) than the Barthel Index (SRM 1.13) in evaluating the impact of comprehensive geriatric intervention programs (McDowell 2006) The IADL questions were slightly better than the ADL but still not useful in detecting change.

	Instrument tool	Purpose	Description	Studies Using Method	Reliability	Validity
					Very high six-month test retest reliability has been reported: 0.94 for the ADL scale (item range, 0.84-0.96) and 0.88 for the IADL scale (item range 0.80 -0.99)(McDowell 2006).	
4.	Organization for Economic Cooperation and Development (OECD)Disability Questionnaire	The OECD questionnaire is a survey instrument that summarizes the impact of ill health on essential daily activities. It was intended to facilitate international comparisons of disability and, through repeated surveys, to monitor changes in disability over time.	Of the 16 questions, ten can be used as an abbreviated instrument and represent a core set of items for international comparisons.	Several	Wilson and McNeil used 11 of the 16 questions with slight modification in interviews that were repeated after a two-week delay (n=233)(McDowell 2006). The agreement between interviews was low, ranging from 30% to 70% for the 11 items. Considering the scale as a whole, less than two thirds of those who reported disabilities on either interview reported them on both(McDowell 2006).	Twelve of the OECD questions were included in a Switzerland survey for the elderly (aged 65 years and over) (n=1600). Sensitivity ranged from 61% to 85% for different medical conditions, highest for those with hearing, vision and speech problems. Specificity was 76%(McDowell 2006).
5.	Rapid Disability Rating Scale	The Rapid Disability Rating Scale was developed as a research tool for summarising the functional capacity and mental status of elderly. It may be used with hospitalised patients and with	This scale has 18 items, covering physical, (communication, hearing, sight, diet, confined in bed, incontinence and medication),mental functioning (mental confusion, uncooperativeness, depression) and	Several	Inter-rater reliability of the 18 item version with two nurses independently rated 100 patients and items corrections ranged from 0.62 to 0.98; the three lowest correlations were for the mental status items. Test-retest reliability on 50 patients after an interval of three days produced correlations between 0.58 and 0.96(McDowell 2006).	Ratings of 845 men (mean age 68 years) were used to predict subsequent mortality using multiple regression and discriminant function analysis. Twenty percent of the variance in mortality was explained; the item correctly identified 72% of patients who died(McDowell 2006).

	Instrument tool	Purpose	Description	Studies Using Method	Reliability	Validity
		people living in the community.	independence in self-care (eating, walking, mobility, bathing, dressing, toileting, grooming and adaptive tasks) This rating scale is administered by a nurse or a person familiar with the patient			
6.	Health Assessment Questionnaire (HAQ)	The Stanford Health Assessment Questionnaire measures difficulty in performing activities of daily living.	The full HAQ instrument covers five dimensions, but development work has concentrated on two most commonly used dimensions; the disability and discomfort dimensions. They are referred to as "Short or 2-page HAQ" The disability dimension includes 20 items on daily functioning during the past week (dressing and	Many	The Spearman correlation for the disability index was 0.85, whereas correlations for individual sections ranged from 0.56 (IADL activities and hygiene) to 0.85 (eating). Two week test re-test reliability of the disability section was investigated with 37 patients with rheumatoid arthritis, showing no significance difference by t-test and a Spearman correlation of 0.87(McDowell 2006). Fries *et al* administered the HAQ on successive occasions and obtained a test-retest correlation of 0.98 after 6 months(McDowell 2006).	Principle component analysis has broadly confirmed the dimensions originally postulated by Fries. The eight disability subscales are substantially correlated with each other; with a median correlation of 0.44 (McDowell 2006). Fries compared self administered HAQ responses to performance made during house visit (n=25). The Spearman correlation for the overall score was 0.88, whereas correlations for component scores ranged from 0.47 (arising) to 0.88 (walking)(McDowell 2006).

	Instrument tool	Purpose	Description	Studies Using Method	Reliability	Validity
			grooming, arising, eating, walking, hygiene, reach, grip and outdoor activities)			
8.	Medical Outcomes Study Physical Functioning Measure	The Medical Outcome Study Physical Functioning Measure offers an extended ADL scale, suitable for use in health surveys and outcome assessment for outpatient care.	The Medical Outcome Study Physical Functioning Measure includes ten items on functioning, one on satisfaction with physical activity and three on mobility (Total no of items = 14).	Few	Eight of ten physical function items correlated 0.70 or greater with the overall physical scale score; the vigorous activity item correlated 0.62 and the bathing or dressing item showed a lower correlation of 0.48. Internal consistency for the functioning score was 0.92; and 0.71 for the mobility scale(McDowell 2006).	The physical functioning scale scores correlated 0.58 with the mobility scores and 0.63 with the satisfaction scores(McDowell 2006).

Table 3. Comparison of the physical disability and mobility disability assessment tools

	Instrument tool	Purpose	Description	Studies Using Method	Reliability	Validity
1.	Tinetti Performance Oriented Mobility Test	The Tinetti Test has been recommended and widely used in the elderly to assess mobility, balance and gait, as well as predicting falls.	The performance test of balance and gait during manoeuvres in normal daily activities. The Tinetti test takes about 10 minutes to administer.	Many	Berg *et al* found that the inter-rater reliability is 85% (Berg, et al. 1992).	With the Berg scale, r = 0.91, with stride length, r = 0.62 to 0.68 and with single leg stance, r = 0.59 to 0.64 (Berg, et al. 1992).
2. 2.1	Walking Speed Tests 6 meter walking speed	Walking speed tests are the most frequently used objective physical performance test to evaluate functional limitations of the lower limbs.	The test performed over 2.44 meters, 4 meters and 6 meters at usual gait speed	Many	Test-retest reliability on 97 patients after one day (among hospital inpatient sample) and one week (among community dweller sample) produced inter class correlation (ICC) of 0.94 (Sherrington and Lord 2005) One study reported excellent inter-rater reliability (ICC 0.99) , n=20 (Rehm-Gelin, et al. 1997).	Predictive validity has been assessed. In studies of elderly, the < 1m/s RR of mortality and hospitalization was 1.64 and 1.48 respectively during one year of follow up (Cesari, et al. 2005). Predictive validity has been assessed for risk of hip fracture where the RR for 1 SD decrease is 1.4 during a mean follow-up of 1.94 years (Dargent-Molina, et al. 2002).
2.2	2.44 meter walking speed				Test-retest reliability on 136 patients after an interval of three weeks produced inter class correlation of 0.72 (Ostchega, et al. 2000). One study reported adequate inter-rater reliability (ICC 0.52) , n=256 (Ostchega, et al. 2000)	Predictive validity assessed for mortality showed OR of 3.64 (Quartile 1: slowest), 2.57 (Quartile 2) and 2.16 (Quartile 3) compared to Quartile 4 (fastest) over a 2 year period(Markides, et al. 2001).
2.3	4 meter walking speed				Test-retest reliability after an interval of one week produced inter class correlation of 0.84 (Studenski, et al. 2003).	Predictive validity assessed for mortality showed HR 2.23, 95 % CI 1.44 – 3.64, within 5 years (Perera, et al. 2005).

3.	Functional Independence Measure	The Functional Independence Measure scale assesses physical and cognitive disability in terms of level of care required.	The Functional Independence Measure includes 18 items covering independence in self care, sphincter control, mobility, locomotion, communication and cognition. Items are scored on the level of assistance required for an individual to perform these activities. It takes half an hour to score the scale for each patient.	Many	Kappa coefficient of agreement for the 18 item is 0.54 (McDowell 2006).	Content validity was performed and factor analyses have identified three factors: handicap, disability and lower limb problems (McDowell 2006).
4.	Timed Up and Go Test	The purpose of Timed Up and Go Test is to assess basic mobility skills of elderly populations(McDowell 2006)	The Timed Up and Go test involves timing a person as they rise from a chair, walk three meters, turn and return to the chair. It takes approximately 2 minutes to complete.	Several	Three studies reported excellent inter-rater reliability (ICC 0.98 to 0.99)and excellent intra-rater reliability (ICC 0.97 to 0.99)(McDowell 2006).	Six studies reported fair to moderate correlations of the Timed Up and Go Test with Berg Balance Scale (r = 0.47), Tinetti Performance Oriented Mobility Assessment (r=0.55), Clinical Test of Sensory Interaction and Balance (r=0.44) and Multi-Directional Reach Test (r=0.26-0.42)(McDowell 2006).

Table 4. Comparison of the functional limitation assessment tools.

Mobility disability is very common among older people. Results from a United States National Prevalence Survey of Disability revealed that among older people aged 65 years and over, 30% had difficulty with mobility (Nordstrom, et al. 2007). In the United Kingdom, the Hertfordshire Cohort Study found that 32% of men and 46% of women aged 59 years and over reported that their health limited them in performing mobility activities (Syddall, et al. 2009). Data from the Netherlands National Health Survey showed that approximately 18% and 37% of older Dutch people aged 65 to 74 years and 75 years and over respectively reported mobility disability (Picavet and Hoeymans 2002).

Assessing functional limitation adds valuable information about the steps in the disability pathway. Gait speed, often termed walking speed has been regarded as the best single measure to evaluate functional limitation (Guralnik and Luigi 2003). It has also shown to be a strong and consistent predictor of adverse outcomes in older people. In a pooled analysis of individual data from nine major cohorts, gait speed has been shown to be a predictor of mortality in older people (Studenski, et al. 2011). In the same study, Studenski standardized the method to assess gait speed from different lengths (8 feet, 4 meters, or 6 meters) to a 4-meter-long track starting from a still, standing position. Using a recommended cut-off point of 0.8 meter/second as increased likelihood of poor health and function, the percentages of older people with poor mobility were : 44.2% in the Cardiovascular Health Study, 40.8% in the Established Populations for Epidemiologic Studies of the Elderly (EPESE), 84.1% in the Hispanic EPESE, 69.4% in the National Health and Nutrition Examination Survey III (NHANES III), 34.6% in the Predicting Early Performance Study and 21% in the InCHIANTI Study (Invecchiare in Chianti Study) (Studenski, et al. 2011).

6.2 Prevalence of physical disability, mobility disability and functional limitation in developing countries

The burden of poor physical function has been studied extensively in developed countries but there is little data available for older people in developing countries. Comparison of physical disability, mobility disability and functional limitation distribution between countries is difficult due to methodological differences in definition and measurements used. Surveys from around the world used different approaches in measuring disability. Different instruments within the same country often report different rates. Across countries the variation is even more cumbersome. Nevertheless, the studies discussed below used comparable methods to a certain extent.

Prevalence studies on the five-item ADL disability among older people had been carried out in several low income developing countries. The Cambodian study in 2004 showed a prevalence of 23.7% among older people aged 60 years and over (Zimmer 2008); the 1998 Housing and Population Census of the Ethiopian Government reported a prevalence of 28.6% among Ethiopians adults aged 55 years and above (Teferra 2005). In addition, two studies were conducted in Nepal among older people aged 60 years and above with prevalence of 8.8% in Kathmandu city, 2005 and a much higher prevalence of 55.8% in rural Chitwan Valley, 1998 (Shrestha 2004).

Studies on the five-item ADL disability among older people in lower middle income developing countries reported varied prevalence: 10% and 9% among older people aged 65 years and over in Sri Lanka (Nugegoda and Balasuriya 1995) and urban Chinese in Shanghai

(Chen, et al. 1995)respectively. Whereas, among older people aged 60 years and over, the prevalence were: 12% in Indians(Shantibala, et al. 2007), 10.9% and 14.7% in Filipinos in the years 1996 and 2001 respectively (Ofstedal et al), 6.5% in Beijing Chinese (Zhe, et al. 1999), 18.7% in Indonesian men and 12.1% in Indonesian women (Evi Nurvidya Arifin 2009).

Several studies in lower middle income countries have used six-item ADL scales. In the WHO Collaborative Study on Social and Health Aspects of Aging in 1990, the prevalence of six item ADL disability among older people age 60 and over was: 22.4% in Egyptian men, 28.5% in Egyptian women, 32.0% in Tunisian men and 46.8% in Tunisian women (Yount and Agree 2005). The Ibadan Study of Aging in Nigeria in 2004 reported the prevalence of six-item ADL disability at only 3% among Nigerians aged 65 years and over(Oye Gureje, et al. 2006). The prevalence of disability among Nigerians is low because of the difference in criterion definition used. In the Ibadan Study of Aging, disability is based on difficulty experience with four levels of responses. This resulted in a more restrictive definition of disability, as compared to studies that defined disability based on any level of difficulty.

Many studies on the prevalence of physical disability were conducted in upper middle income countries. From the Survey on Health and Well-Being of Elders. Palloni *et al* reported that the prevalence of six-item ADL disability among older people were: 19% in Argentina, 14% in Barbados, 24% in Brazil, 26% in Chile, 21% in Cuba, 19% in Mexico and 17% in Uruguay (Palloni and McEniry 2007). The prevalence of six-item ADL disability among older people aged 60 years and over in Puerto Rico in a 2003 study was 20%(Palloni, et al. 2005).

The epidemiology of poor physical function among older people in developing countries is incompletely understood with many unanswered questions.

7. Risk factors for poor physical function

Several factors have been identified as risk factors for disability and functional limitation. These include non-modifiable risk factors (e.g. gender, ethnicity and genetics) and modifiable risk factors, which include both individual factors (such as sedentary lifestyle, unhealthy behaviours) as well as characteristics of the environment (e.g. household hazards, disadvantaged neighbourhood conditions, common forms of transportation).

7.1 Gender, ethnic group, socioeconomic and health-related factors

Poor physical function had been reported to be associated with increasing age(Tas, et al. 2007a), being female(Tas, et al. 2007a), lower socioeconomic status(Tas, et al. 2007a), chronic diseases(Tas, et al. 2007a), depression (Tas, et al. 2007a), visual impairment(Ng, et al. 2006), cognitive impairment(Ng, et al. 2006), poor self rated health(Ng, et al. 2006), fewer social support(Tas, et al. 2007b), living alone(Ng, et al. 2006) and lack of exercise(Wu, et al. 1999).

The association between female gender and poor physical function is consistently reported in many studies. Some studies have shown that the higher prevalence of poor physical function in female is unexplainable by known differences in sociodemographic and health related factors(Auxiliadora Graciani, et al. 2004; Dunlop, et al. 1997).

There are few reports of ethnic differences in frequency of poor physical function. How differences in sociodemographic and health-related factors explain the ethnic differences in poor physical function is still unclear. Older black and Hispanic Americans have a higher prevalence of poor physical function than their white counterparts (Kelly-Moore and Ferraro 2004). Other studies from the United States have found that African-American have higher disability rates compared to the Whites even after adjustment for education (Liao, et al. 1999) and chronic disease (Kingston and Smith 1997), although one study reported that social and health factors explained these differences(Kelly-Moore and Ferraro 2004). Ng *et al* showed that Indians and Malays in Singapore have higher risk of disability than Singaporean Chinese (Ng, et al. 2006).

Older people in less advantaged socioeconomic positions report more physical disability, mobility disability and functional limitation. Lower level of education tends to be associated with a higher prevalence of poor physical function at all ages(Lafortune 2007). A lower level of education is often associated with lower income, lower standards of living, higher risk of work-related injuries, and adoption of less healthy behaviours. The "education" effect has been shown to be a proxy for broader "socioeconomic status".

Changes in the prevalence of chronic diseases play a dominant role in explaining the prevalence of poor physical function among older people. However, not all diseases are associated with poor physical function and some are more strongly associated than others. Diseases with large effects on poor physical function include stroke and other neurological diseases, diabetes, heart diseases, depression, arthritis and other musculoskeletal diseases(Avlund 2004). It has also been reported that the presence of more than one chronic disease in an individual, often called co-morbidity is associated with poor physical function(Guralnik, et al. 1993; Schmitz, et al. 2007). Guralnik *et al* showed that the presence of a single chronic disease is a significant predictor of poor physical function, with the risk increasing incrementally up to the presence of four or more chronic diseases(Guralnik, et al. 1993).

There is also some evidence of association between smoking, heavy alcohol consumption and lack of physical activity with poor physical function(Tas, et al. 2007b).

The majority of studies on risk factors for poor physical function have focused on chronic diseases and lifestyle behaviours. There are a number of health-related factors that have rarely been investigated. These include the co-existence of depression and visual impairment; chronic pain; and the role of muscle strength, muscle mass (sarcopenia) and muscle quality.

7.2 Co-existing depressive symptoms and visual impairment as risk factors of poor physical function

The accumulation of deficits across more than one health domain, including physiological, sensory, cognitive and psychological domain, is likely to explain the development of poor physical function better than decline in just one single health domain. Whitson *et a*l showed that individuals with co-existing visual impairment and cognitive impairment are at high risk of disability(Whitson, et al. 2007). Lin *et al* showed that that the burden of having both vision and hearing impairment is greater than the sum of each single impairment(Lin, et al. 2004). Rantanen *at al* reported that the odds of severe mobility disability were ten times greater among those who had both strength and balance impairments compared to those with just one or other impairment (Taina Rantanen, et al. 2001). Thus, it appears that certain pairs of co-existing conditions have a strong effect on physical function risk.

Depression and visual impairment are common conditions among older people and are also modifiable to a certain degree; depression can be treated and visual impairment can be corrected. However, it is unclear whether there is a synergistic effect of depressive symptoms (psychological health domain) and visual impairment (sensory domain) on the risk of poor physical function among older people.

7.3 Chronic pain and poor physical function

There are gender-based differences in mortality and morbidity; with men experiencing higher mortality rates and women generally having higher levels of morbidity (Steven M Albert and Vicki A Freedman 2010). In the pain literature, a robust and common finding is that women reported more pain, have lower pain thresholds and tolerance, and show different attitudes in coping with pain as compared to men (Roger, et al. 2009; Unruh 1996). Longitudinal and cross sectional population based studies have shown that the impact of pain goes beyond physical distress (Keogh, et al. 2006). The presence of pain is also associated with poor physical function (Duong, et al. 2005).

In contrast to gender differences in pain, the evidence about gender differences in pain outcomes, such as poor physical function, remains inconclusive. Cunningham *et al* found no difference in musculoskeletal pain related restriction in daily activities between genders(Cunningham and Kelsey 1984). The Health, Aging and Body Composition (ABC) Study also found no gender differences in the relationship between low back pain and physical function(Weiner, et al. 2003). However, studies that used pain-related disabilities items as an outcome found there were gender differences in reporting pain-related disabilities (Keefe, et al. 2000; Réthelyi, et al. 2001; Stubbs, et al. 2010).

7.4 Sarcopenia as risk factors for poor physical function

It is well established that the aging process in humans is associated with loss of muscle mass and strength (Doherty 2003; Y Rolland 2008). Age-related decline in muscle mass has been documented by lean body mass measurements with dual X-ray absorptiometry (DXA) and muscle cross sectional areas quantified by imaging methods such as X-ray computed tomography (CT) and magnetic resonance imaging (MRI). The age-related loss of muscle mass results from loss of both slow and fast motor units, with an accelerated loss of fast motor units. These changes in muscle morphology results in sharp age-related changes in muscle strength and muscle function(Lang, et al. 2010). Muscle quality is an indicator of muscle function, quantified by strength per unit muscle mass. Another morphological aspect of aging skeletal muscle is the infiltration of muscle tissue components by lipids. The aging process is thought to result in increased frequency of fat cells within muscle tissue(Anne B. Newman, et al. 2003).

Age-related loss of muscle mass, strength and quality is called "sarcopenia". Recent longitudinal studies have demonstrated that age-related loss of muscle strength increases the risk of poor physical function among older people (Giampaoli, et al. 1999; Taina

Rantanen, et al. 2001). Perhaps because of the various operational definitions used, the relationship between age-related muscle mass (sarcopenia) and poor physical function has not been consistent (I Janssen 2006; MJ. Delmonico, et al. 2007).

8. Conclusion

In summary, poor physical function – physical disability, mobility disability and functional limitation is developing as the population ages. Poor physical functions are complex processes with multiple risk factors at work (Steven M Albert and Vicki A Freedman 2010). As such, multifactor interventions are needed to improve and maximize older people's physical functions. Identifying the appropriate target population and window of time for targeting an intervention is critical to its success. Furthermore, the issue of sustainability and adherence to these interventions are also important for long term success (Steven M Albert and Vicki A Freedman 2010). Research up to date is still incomplete in guiding public health practitioners and clinicians as to which interventions will improve and maximize older people's physical function in the long run.

9. Acknowledgements

This work was supported by the Fundamental Research Grant Scheme (FRGS), form the Ministry of Higher Education, Malaysia. Dr. Noran N Hairi's work was supported by the University Malaya / Ministry of Higher Education (UM/MOHE) High Impact Research Grant E000014-20001.

10. References

Anne B. Newman, et al. 2003 Strength and Muscle Quality in a Well-Functioning Cohort of Older Adults: The Health, Aging and Body Composition Study. Journal of the American Geriatrics Society 51(3):323-330.

Auxiliadora Graciani, et al. 2004 Prevalence of disability and associated social and health-related factors among the elderly in Spain: a population-based study. Maturitas 48(4):381-392.

Avlund, Kirsten 2004 Disability in old age. Longitudinal population-based studies of the disablement process. Danish Medical Bulletin 51:315-349.

Berg, K. O., et al. 1992 Clinical and laboratory measures of postural balance in an elderly population. Arch Phys Med Rehabil 73(11):1073-80.

Cesari, M., et al. 2005 Prognostic value of usual gait speed in well-functioning older people results from the Health, Aging and Body Composition Study. Journal of the American Geriatrics Society 53(10):1675-80.

Chen, P, ES Yu, and M Zhang 1995 ADL dependence and medical conditions in Chinese older persons: a population-based survey in Shanghai, China. Journal of the American Geriatrics Society 43:378 - 383.

Cress ME, Buchner DM, Questad KA, Esselman PC, deLateur BJ, Schwartz RS 1996 Continous-scale physical functional performance in healthy older adults: a validation study. Archives of Physical Medicine and Rehabilitation 77:1243-1250.

Cunningham, L S, and J L Kelsey 1984 Epidemiology of musculoskeletal impairments and associated disability. Am J Public Health 74(6):574-579.

Dargent-Molina, P., et al. 2002 Use of clinical risk factors in elderly women with low bone mineral density to identify women at higher risk of hip fracture: The EPIDOS prospective study. Osteoporos International 13(7):593-9.

Doherty, T J. 2003 Aging and Sarcopenia. Journal of Applied Physiology 95:1717 - 1727.

Dunlop, D D, S L Hughes, and L M Manheim 1997 Disability in activities of daily living: patterns of change and a hierarchy of disability. Americam Journal of Public Health 87(3):378-383.

Duong, Bao D., et al. 2005 Identifying the Activities Affected by Chronic Nonmalignant Pain in Older Veterans Receiving Primary Care. Journal of the American Geriatrics Society 53(4):687-694.

Evi Nurvidya Arifin 2009 Are older women in Southeast Asia more vulnerable than the men? United Nations Economic and Social Comission for Asia and the Pacific, ed. Bangkok: UN ESCAP.

Ferrucci, L, et al. 2007 Disability, Functional Status and Activities of Daily Living. *In* Encyclopedia of Gerontology. J.E. Birren, ed. Pp. 427 -436, Vol. 1: Amsterdam; Boston: Academic Press.

Fried LP, and Jack M Guralnik 1997 Disability in older adults: evidence regarding significance, etiology, and risk. Journal of the American Geriatrics Society 45:92-100.

Fried, LP, and JM Guralnik 1997 Disability in older adults: evidence regarding significance, etiology, and risk. Journal of the American Geriatrics Society 45:92 - 100.

Fries, James F. 1980 Aging, Natural Death, and the Compression of Morbidity. New England Journal of Medicine 303(3):130-135. 2005 The Compression of Morbidity. Milbank Quarterly 83(4):801-823.

Giampaoli, S, et al. 1999 Hand-grip strength predicts incident disability in non-disabled older men. Age Ageing 28(3):283-288.

Gruenberg EM 1977 The failure of success. Milbank Q 55:3-24.

Guralnik, Jack M., and Luigi Ferrucci 2009 The Challenge of Understanding the Disablement Process in Older Persons. The Journals of Gerontology Series A: Biological Sciences and Medical Sciences 64A(11):1169-1171.

Guralnik, Jack M., et al. 1993 Maintaining Mobility in Late Life. I. Demographic Characteristics and Chronic Conditions. American Journal of Epidemiology 137(8):845-857.

Guralnik, JM, and F Luigi 2003 Assessing the building blocks of function: Utilizing measures of functional limitation. American Journal of Preventive Medicine 25(3):112-121.

I Janssen 2006 Influence of Sarcopenia on the Development of Physical Disability: The Cardiovascular Health Study. Journal of the American Geriatrics Society 54(1):56-62.

Jette, Alan M. 1994 How measurement techniques influence estimates of disability in older populations. Social Science & Medicine 38(7):937-942.

Jette AM, and Keysor J 2003 Disability Models: Implications for Arthritis Exercise and Physical Activity Interventions. Arthritis and Rheumatism 49(1):114-120.

Keefe, Francis J., et al. 2000 The relationship of gender to pain, pain behavior, and disability in osteoarthritis patients: the role of catastrophizing. Pain 87(3):325-334.

Kelly-Moore, JA, and KF Ferraro 2004 The black/white disability gap: Persistent inequality in later life? The Journals of Gerontology Series B: Psychological Sciences and Social Sciences 59B:534 - 543.

Keogh, Edmund, Lance M. McCracken, and Christopher Eccleston 2006 Gender moderates the association between depression and disability in chronic pain patients. European Journal of Pain 10(5):413-422.

Kingston, RS, and JP Smith 1997 Socioeconomic status and racial and ethnic differences in function status associated with chronic diseases. American Journal of Public Health 87:805-810.

Kinsella K, and Wan He 2009 U.S. Census Bureau. International Population Reports, P95/09-1, An Aging World 2008. *In* U.S. Government Printing Office. Washington DC,.

Kovar, Mary G., and M. Powell Lawton 1994 Functional Disability: Activities and Instrumental Activities of Daily Living. *In* Annual Review of Gerontology and Geriatrics: Focus on Assessment Techniques. M.P. Lawton and J.A. Teresi, eds. Pp. 57-75. New York: Springer Publishing Company.

Kuriansky JB, Gurland BJ, Fleiss JL 1976 The assesment of self-care capacity in geriatric psychiatric patients by objective and subjective methods. Journal of Clinical Psychology 32:95-102.

Lafortune, G. G. Balestat 2007 Trends in Severe Disability Among Elderly People: Assessing the Evidence in 12 OECD Countries and the Future Implications. OECD Health Working Papers, No 26, OECD Publishing.

Lang, T., et al. 2010 Sarcopenia: etiology, clinical consequences, intervention, and assessment Osteoporosis International 21:543 - 559.

Liao, Y, et al. 1999 Black-white differences in disability and morbidity in the last years of life. American Journal of Epidemiology 149:1097 - 1103.

Lin, M. Y., et al. 2004 Vision Impairment and Combined Vision and Hearing Impairment Predict Cognitive and Functional Decline in Older Women. Journal of the American Geriatrics Society 52(12):1996 - 2002.

Manton KG 1982 Changing concepts of morbidity and mortality in the elderly population. Milbank Q 60:183-244.

Marilyn J. Field, and Alan M. Jette 2007 The Future of Disability in America. Washington, DC: National Academic Press.

Markides, Kyriakos S., et al. 2001 Lower Body Function and Mortality in Mexican American Elderly People. The Journals of Gerontology Series A: Biological Sciences and Medical Sciences 56(4):M243-M247.

McDowell, Ian 2006 Measuring health: a guide to rating scales and questionnaire. New York: Oxford University Press, Inc.

MJ. Delmonico, et al. 2007 Alternative Definitions of Sarcopenia, Lower Extremity Performance, and Functional Impairment with Aging in Older Men and Women. Journal of the American Geriatrics Society 55(5):769-774.

Nagi, SZ 1976 An epidemiology of disability among adults in the United States. The Milbank Memorial Fund Quarterly. Health and Society. 54:439 - 467.

Ng, Tze-Pin, et al. 2006 Prevalence and Correlates of Functional Disability in Multiethnic Elderly Singaporeans. Journal of the American Geriatrics Society 54(1):21-29.

Nordstrom, CK, et al. 2007 Socioeconomic position and incident mobility impairment in the Cardiovascular Health Study. BMC Geriatrics 7:11.

Nugegoda, D. B., and S. Balasuriya 1995 Health and social status of an elderly urban population in Sri Lanka. Social Science & Medicine 40(4):437-442.

Ostchega, Y., et al. 2000 Reliability and prevalence of physical performance examination assessing mobility and balance in older persons in the US: data from the Third National Health and Nutrition Examination Survey. Journal of the American Geriatrics Society 48(9):1136-41.

Oye Gureje, et al. 2006 Functional Disability in Elderly Nigerians: Results from the Ibadan Study of Aging. Journal of the American Geriatrics Society 54(11):1784-1789.

Palloni, A., et al. 2005 The influence of early conditions on health status among elderly Puerto Ricans. Social Biology 52(3-4):132-63.

Palloni, Alberto, and Mary McEniry 2007 Aging and Health Status of Elderly in Latin America and the Caribbean: Preliminary Findings. Journal of Cross-Cultural Gerontology 22(3):263-285.

Penninx, Brenda W.J.H., et al. 2000 Lower Extremity Performance in Nondisabled Older Persons as a Predictor of Subsequent Hospitalization. The Journals of Gerontology Series A: Biological Sciences and Medical Sciences 55(11):M691-M697.

Perera, S., et al. 2005 Magnitude and patterns of decline in health and function in 1 year affect subsequent 5-year survival. Journal of Gerontology Series A: Biological Sciences and Medical Sciences 60(7):894-900.

Picavet, H. S. J., and N. Hoeymans 2002 Physical disability in The Netherlands: Prevalence, risk groups and time trends. Public Health 116(4):231-237.

Rehm-Gelin, Stephanie L., Kathye E. Light, and Jane E. Freund 1997 Reliability of Timed-Functional Movements for Clinical Assessment of a Frail Elderly Population. Physical & Occupational Therapy in Geriatrics 15(1):1-19.

Réthelyi, János M., Rita Berghammer, and Mária S. Kopp 2001 Comorbidity of pain-associated disability and depressive symptoms in connection with sociodemographic variables: results from a cross-sectional epidemiological survey in Hungary. Pain 93(2):115-121.

Robine Jean-Marie, and Michel Jean-Pierre 2004 Looking Forward to a General Theory on Population Aging. The Journals of Gerontology Series A: Biological Sciences and Medical Sciences 59(6):M590-597.

Roger, B. Fillingim, et al. 2009 Sex, Gender, and Pain: A Review of Recent Clinical and Experimental Findings. The Journal of Pain 10(5):447-485.

Schmitz, Norbert, et al. 2007 Joint Effect of Depression and Chronic Conditions on Disability: Results From a Population-Based Study. Psychosomatic Medcine 69(4):332-338.

Shantibala, K, et al. 2007 Disability in ADL Among the Elderly in an Urban Area of Manipur. Indian Journal of Physical Medicine and Rehabilitation 18(2):41-43.

Sherrington, C., and S. R. Lord 2005 Reliability of simple portable tests of physical performance in older people after hip fracture. Clinical Rehabilitation 19(5):496-504.

Shrestha, Sujan Lal 2004 Validating the Centre for Epidemiological Studies Depression Scale (CES-D) for use among older adults in Nepal, Graduate School of the University of Florida, University of Florida.

Steven M Albert, and Vicki A Freedman 2010 Public Health and Aging. Maximizing Function and Well-being. New York: Springer Publishing Company.

Stubbs, D., et al. 2010 Sex Differences in Pain and Pain-Related Disability among Primary Care Patients with Chronic Musculoskeletal Pain. Pain Medicine 11(2):232-239.

Studenski, S., et al. 2003 Physical performance measures in the clinical setting. Journal of the American Geriatrics Society 51(3):314-22.

Studenski, Stephanie, et al. 2011 Gait Speed and Survival in Older Adults. The Journal of the American Medical Association 305(1):50-58.

Syddall, H., et al. 2009 The SF-36: A simple, effective measure of mobility-disability for epidemiological studies. The Journal of Nutrition, Health & Aging 13(1):57-62.

Taina Rantanen, et al. 2001 Coimpairments as Predictors of Severe Walking Disability in Older Women. Journal of the American Geriatrics Society 49(1):21-27.

Tas, U, et al. 2007a Incidence and risk factor of disability in the elderly: the Rotterdam Study. Preventive Medicine 44(3):272 - 278. 2007b Prognostic factors of disability in older people: a systematic review. The British Journal of General Practice 57(537):319 - 323.

Teferra, Tirussew 2005 Contextualizing Disability: Ethopian Case. *In* Disability in Ethopia: Issues and Implications. Ethopia: Addis Ababa University Printing Press.

Unruh, Anita M. 1996 Gender variations in clinical pain experience. Pain 65(2-3):123-167.

Verbrugge, Lois M., and Alan M. Jette 1994 The disablement process. Social Science & Medicine 38(1):1-14.

Weiner, D. K., et al. 2003 How Does Low Back Pain Impact Physical Function in Independent, Well-Functioning Older Adults? Evidence from the Health ABC Cohort and Implications for the Future. Pain Medicine 4(4):311-320.

Whitson, H. E., et al. 2007 The Combined Effect of Visual Impairment and Cognitive Impairment on Disability in Older People. Journal of the American Geriatrics Society 55(6):885-891.

Wiener, Joshua M., et al. 1990 Measuring the Activities of Daily Living: Comparisons Across National Surveys. Journal of Gerontology 45(6):S229-S237.

World Health Organization 1980 International Classification of Impairments, Disabilities, and Handicaps: A Manual of Classification Relating to the Consequences of Disease. Geneva: World Health Organization.2001 International Classification of Functioning, Disability and Health. Geneva, Switzerland: World Health Organization.

Wu, S. C., S. Y. Leu, and C. Y. Li 1999 Incidence of and predictors for chronic disability in activities of daily living among older people in Taiwan. Journal of the American Geriatrics Society 47(9):1082-6.

Y Rolland, S Czerwinski, G Abellan Van Kan, J E Morley, M Cesari, G Onder, J Woo, R Baumgartner, F Pillard, Y Boirie, W M C Chumlea, B Vellas. 2008 Sarcopenia: Its assesment, etiology, pathogenesis, consequences and future perspectives. The Journal of Nutrition, Health & Aging. 12(7):433-50.

Yount, Kathryn M., and Emily M. Agree 2005 Differences in Disability among Older Women and Men in Egypt and Tunisia. Demography 42:169-187.

Zhe, Tang, et al. 1999 The prevalence of functional disability in activities of daily living and instrumental activities of daily living among elderly Beijing Chinese. Archives of Gerontology and Geriatrics 29(2):115-125.

Zimmer, Zachary 2008 Poverty, wealth inequality and health among older adults in rural Cambodia. Social Science & Medicine 66(1):57-71.

2

Sarcopenia in Older People

Noran N. Hairi[1,2], Awang Bulgiba[1,2],
Tee Guat Hiong[3] and Izzuna Mudla[4]
[1]Department of Social and Preventive Medicine,
Faculty of Medicine, University of Malaya, Kuala Lumpur,
[2]JCUM, Centre for Clinical Epidemiology and Evidence-Based Medicine,
Faculty of Medicine, University of Malaya, Kuala Lumpur,
[3]Institute for Public Health, National Institutes of Health,
Ministry of Health,
[4]Ministry of Health,
Malaysia

1. Introduction

It is well established that the aging process is associated with numerous changes in the human body. One of the most significant age-related anatomical changes is that which happens to the skeletal muscle mass. Aging process is associated with loss of muscle mass and strength. The term "sarcopenia" is used to indicate progressive reduction in muscle mass, muscle strength and function that affects older people. Sarcopenia is derived from the Greek word "sarx" for flesh and "penia" for loss (M.S. John Pathy 2006). This term was first used by Rosenberg in 1988 at a symposium on nutritional status and body composition to bring awareness and draw attention to this significant but then understudied problem of aging (M.S. John Pathy 2006). Sarcopenia is now acknowledged as an important geriatric syndrome and is considered one of the hallmarks of aging process (Cruz-Jentoft, et al. 2010b). Research on the process, causes, consequences, management and treatment of age-related muscle loss (mass, strength and quality) have exploded since the 1990's (Janssen 2010; Schranger M 2003).

Sarcopenia results in unfavourable and detrimental effects on an older person's physical function. Muscle mass decrease is probably the single most frequent cause of late-life disability among older people. It is directly responsible for functional impairment with loss of strength, and increased likelihood of falls and fractures (Y Rolland 2008). As muscles account for 60% of the body protein stores, the reduction in lean body mass has other health effects independent of its functional consequences (Y Rolland 2008). A number of physiological functions that take place within the muscle tissues have an essential role in human metabolism. For example, muscles are important body protein reserves and energy that can be used in extreme conditions such as stress or malnutrition; amino-acids can be mobilised during acute infections and are also used as building blocks for antibodies while hormones are produced and catabolised within the muscle tissue (M.S. John Pathy 2006). In other words, reduction in muscle mass has an adverse impact on metabolic adaptation and immunological response to disease. Nevertheless, there remains considerable unexplained variation in muscle mass and strength among older people which may partly be explained by the observation that muscle mass and strength in later life reflect not only the rate of loss but also the peak attained earlier in life (A A Sayer 2008; M.S. John Pathy 2006). Thus, a life course model of sarcopenia will enable us to understand sarcopenia, its influences and develop effective interventions (A A Sayer 2008). This is shown in Figure 1.

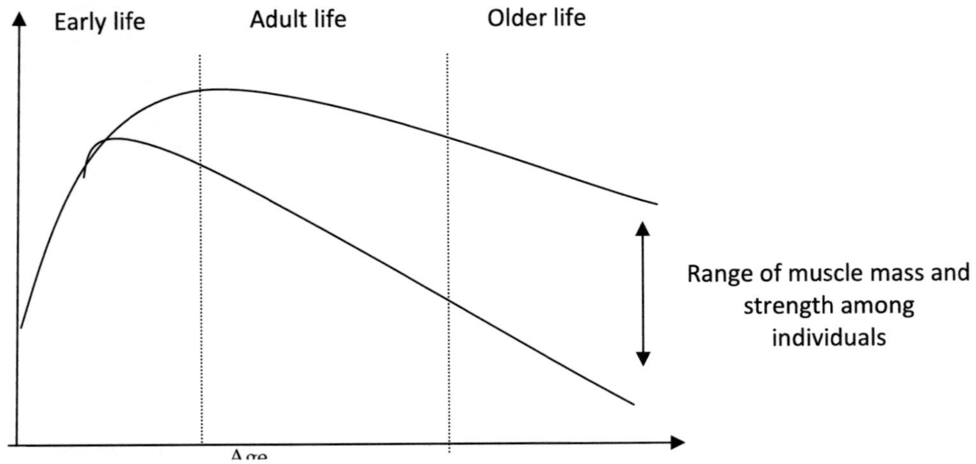

Fig. 1. A life course model of sarcopenia.

Taking all these into account, sarcopenia is now one of the main focal points in aging research; drawing attention to its epidemiology, causes, consequences as well as health care costs. Increasing awareness of sarcopenia and promoting health enhancing strategies to overcome sarcopenia offers numerous benefits. This chapter provides an overview of the current literature on sarcopenia in older people.

2. Definition of sarcopenia

Sarcopenia is now defined as a geriatric syndrome characterised by progressive and generalised loss of skeletal muscle mass, strength and quality associated with ageing (Cruz-Jentoft, et al. 2010b). Sarcopenia is also associated with multiple contributing risk factors through a common and complex path, with a risk of adverse outcomes such as increased frailty and physical and mobility disability leading to loss of dependence, poor quality of life, increased healthcare costs and ultimately death (Cruz-Jentoft, et al. 2010b; M.S. John Pathy 2006; Y Rolland 2008).

Despite agreement in the conceptual definition of sarcopenia, the consensus on the operational definition of sarcopenia has yet to be reached. The definition of sarcopenia has been thoroughly discussed and the pooled consensus is that sarcopenia is mainly, but not only an age-related condition defined by the combined presence of reduced muscle mass and muscle function (Cruz-Jentoft, et al. 2010a; Muscaritoli, et al. 2010).

The European Working Group on Sarcopenia in Older People (EWGSOP) developed a practical clinical definition and consensus diagnostic criteria for age-related sarcopenia

(Cruz-Jentoft, et al. 2010a). The EWGSOP included representatives from four participant organisations i.e. the European Union Geriatric Medicine Society (EUGMS), the European Society for Clinical Nutrition and Metabolism (ESPEN), the International Associations of Gerontology and Geriatrics -European Region (IAGG-ER) and the International Association of Nutrition and Aging (Valderrama-Gama, et al.). The EWGSOP recommends using the presence of both low muscle mass and low muscle function (strength or performance) for the diagnosis of sarcopenia (Cruz-Jentoft, et al. 2010a). The diagnosis requires the presence of criterion 1 and the presence of either criterion 2 or 3 (see Table 1).

Diagnosis is based on documentation of criterion 1 plus (criterion 2 or criterion 3)	
1.	Low muscle mass
2.	Low muscle strength
3.	Low physical performance

Source: Report of the EWGSOP. Sarcopenia: European consensus on definition and diagnosis. Age and Ageing, 2010: 39: 412-423.

Table 1. Criteria for the diagnosis of sarcopenia

The EWGSOP report argues that the rationale in using two criteria is that muscle strength does not depend solely on muscle mass and the relationship between strength and mass is not linear (Cruz-Jentoft, et al. 2010a). Furthermore, defining sarcopenia in terms of muscle mass alone is too narrow and may be of limited clinical value. The EWGSOP report also categorised sarcopenia into three staging that reflects the severity of the condition: - a presarcopenia stage (characterised by low muscle mass without impact on muscle strength or physical performance), sarcopenia stage (characterised by low muscle mass and low muscle strength or low physical performance) and severe sarcopenia (characterised by low muscle mass, low muscle strength and low physical performance) (Cruz-Jentoft, et al. 2010a).

2.1 Measuring sarcopenia – The quantitative approach

The measurement variables include muscle mass, strength and physical performance. Age-related decline in muscle mass has been documented by lean body mass measurements with dual X-ray absorptiometry (DXA), muscle cross sectional areas quantified by bioimaging methods such as X-ray computed tomography (CT) and magnetic resonance imaging (MRI), estimation of the volume of fat and lean body mass using bioimpedance analysis (BIA) and finally anthropometric measurements (i.e. calculations based on mid-upper arm circumference and skin-fold thickness) (M.S. John Pathy 2006). DXA is a better method for measuring muscle mass than bioelectric impedance and anthropometric measurements. DXA has the advantage of providing precise estimates of skeletal lean mass and being non-invasive compared to other accurate laboratory-based methods such as neutron activation and ^{40}K counting (M.S. John Pathy 2006). However, DXA is not portable and cannot be used in large-scale epidemiological studies. BIA may be considered as a portable alternative to DXA (Cruz-Jentoft, et al. 2010a). Muscle strength can be measured using isometric hand grip. Muscle strength alone has been shown to be the most useful indicator of age-related changes in muscle for use in clinical practice (Hairi NN 2010). Grip strength is a good simple measure of muscle strength and correlates with leg strength (Cruz-Jentoft, et al. 2010a). Other measures of muscle strength include knee flexion /extension and peak expiratory flow (PEF) (Cruz-Jentoft, et al. 2010a). With regards to physical performance, a wide range of tests are available including Tinetti Performance Oriented Mobility Test, Gait Speed, Functional Independence Measure and the Timed Get-Up-and-Go (TGUG) test (Guralnik and Luigi 2003). Cut-off points depend upon the measurement technique chosen and on the availability of reference studies. The EWGSOP recommends the use of normative (healthy young adult) rather than other predictive reference populations (Cruz-Jentoft, et al. 2010a).

To date, sarcopenia has not been included in common classifications of disease (i.e. International Classification of Diseases), although some recent initiatives are trying to move in this direction.

3. Aetiology and pathogenesis of sarcopenia

The aetiology of sarcopenia is multifactorial (Cruz-Jentoft, et al. 2010b; Lang, et al. 2010; Y Rolland 2008). Multiple risk factors contribute to the development and progression of sarcopenia. These risk factors can be grouped into several categories such as constitutional factors, the aging process, certain life habits such as decreased protein intake, disuse or poor physical activity including lack of exercise, the use of tobacco and alcohol intake, changes in living conditions such as prolonged bed rest and immobility and chronic health conditions (Cruz-Jentoft, et al. 2010b). Table 2 shows the risk factors of sarcopenia.

The pathogenesis of sarcopenia is part of a complex process of age-related changes in musculoskeletal cellular as well as tissue structure and function (Doherty 2003; Lang, et al. 2010). Social and lifestyle behaviours such as physical inactivity, smoking, poor diet, being obese, as well as age-related hormonal, neurological, immunological and metabolic factors are important risk factors (M.S. John Pathy 2006). Genetic susceptibility also plays a role in sarcopenia formation(Muscaritoli, et al. 2010). The putative causes of sarcopenia have been catergorised into "intrinsic" and "extrinsic" factors (M.S. John Pathy 2006; Muscaritoli, et al. 2010). Reductions in anabolic hormones (testosterone, estrogens, growth hormones, insulin like growth factor-1), increases of apoptotic activities in the myofibers, increases of proinflammatory cytokines (e.g. TNF-α, IL-6), oxidative stress due to accumulation of free radicals, changes of the mitochondrial function of muscle cells and a decline in the number of α-motoneurons are some of the intrinsic factors involved (Lang, et al. 2010; Muscaritoli, et al. 2010). Deficient intake of energy and protein, reduced intake of vitamin D, acute and chronic co-morbidities and reduced physical activity are some of the extrinsic conditions leading to sarcopenia (Cruz-Jentoft, et al. 2010b; Muscaritoli, et al. 2010). Figure 2 shows the factors contributing to sarcopenia and its consequences.

What is not known is which factors or pathways are relatively more or less important with regards to the severity and rate of development of sarcopenia components; muscle mass, strength and quality. Each factor potentially contributes differently to the loss of muscle mass, strength and quality and it is likely that there is considerable individual variability in the interactions of these factors (M.S. John Pathy 2006).

FACTORS	AGING PROCESS	CHRONIC HEALTH CONDITIONS
Constitutional Female Low birth weight Genetic susceptibility	*Increase muscle turnover* ↑Catabolic stimuli ↑ Protein degradation Low grade inflammation ↓Anabolic stimuli ↓Protein synthesis	Cognitive impairment Mood disturbances Diabetes Mellitus Heart Failure Liver Failure Renal Failure Respiratory Failure Osteoarthritis Chronic Pain
Lifestyle Malnutrition Low protein intake Alcohol abuse Smoking Physical inactivity	*Reduced number of muscle cells* ↑Myostatin (↓ recruitment) ↑ Apoptosis	Obesity Catabolic effects of drugs
Living conditions Starvation Bed rest Immobility deconditioning Weightlessness	*Hormonal deregulation* ↓ Testosterone, DHEA production ↓Oestrogen production ↓ 1-25 $(OH)_2$ vitamin D ↑ Thyroid Function ↓ Growth hormone, IGF-1 ↑ Insulin resistance	
	Changes in neuromuscular system ↓ CNS input (loss of α- motor neurons) Neuromuscular disjunction ↓ Cilliary neurotrophic factor ↓ Motor unit firing rate	Cancer ? Chronic inflammatory Disease?
	Mitochondrial dysfunction ↓ Peripheral vascular flow	

Source: Cruz-Jentoft AJ, Landi F, Topinkova E *et al*. Understanding sarcopenia as a geriatric syndrome. Current Opinion in Clinical Nutrition and Metabolic Care. 2010; 13: 1-7

Table 2. Risk factors of sarcopenia

4. Functional consequences of sarcopenia

Age-related loss of muscle mass and strength result in decreased functional limitation and physical disability among older people. Using the Nagi Model of Disablement pathology (e.g. sarcopenia) first leads to impairment such as lower extremity weakness (Steven M Albert and Vicki A Freedman 2010). When this crosses some threshold, functional impairment begins to show (which is measurable via gait speed below age-sex appropriate norm) and this in turn will lead to physical disability, e.g. needing help to cross the street (Steven M Albert and Vicki A Freedman 2010). This is as shown in Figure 3.

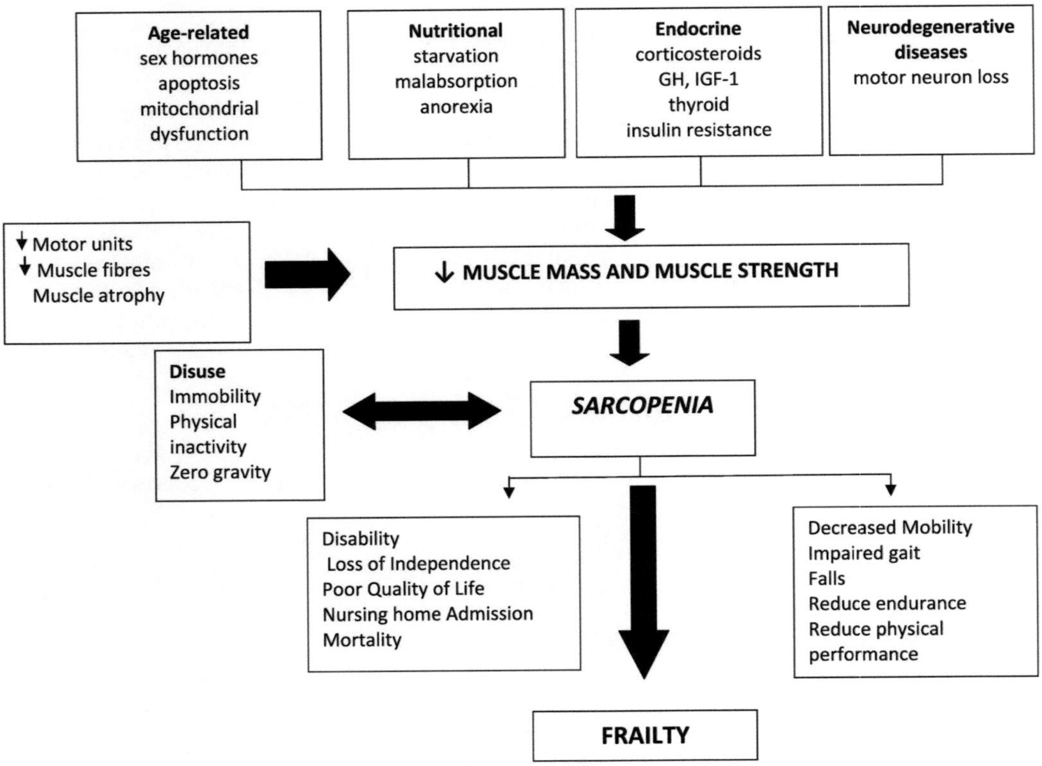

Sources: M Muscaritoli, S.D Anker, J. Argiles *et al.* Consensus definition of sarcopenia, cachexia and pre-chaexia: Joint document elaborated by Special Interest Groups (SIG) "cachexia-anorexia in chronic wasting diseases" and "nutrition in geriatrics". Clinical Nutrition; 2010 (29): 154 – 159 and Doherty T. Aging and Sarcopenia. J. Appl Physiol. 2003 (95): 1717-1727 and Cruz-Jentoft AJ, Landi F, Topinkova E *et al.* Understanding sarcopenia as a geriatric syndrome. Current Opinion in Clinical Nutrition and Metabolic Care. 2010; 13: 1-7

Fig. 2. Factors contributing to sarcopenia and its consequences

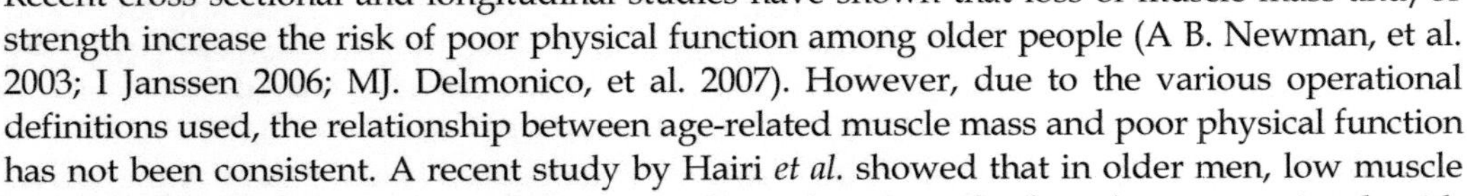

Fig. 3. Sarcopenia leading to disability following the Nagi Model of Disablement

Recent cross sectional and longitudinal studies have shown that loss of muscle mass and/or strength increase the risk of poor physical function among older people (A B. Newman, et al. 2003; I Janssen 2006; MJ. Delmonico, et al. 2007). However, due to the various operational definitions used, the relationship between age-related muscle mass and poor physical function has not been consistent. A recent study by Hairi *et al.* showed that in older men, low muscle strength, low muscle mass and low muscle quality (specific forces) are associated with physical disability in basic Activities of Daily Living (ADLs)(Hairi NN 2010) (Table 3).

	Crude	Age adjusted	Multivariable adjusted*
		Prevalence Ratio (95 % CI)	
		Physical disability (ADL)	
Grip strength§	2.83 (1.91, 4.20)	1.79 (1.17, 2.74)	1.09 (0.72, 1.65)
Quadriceps strength§	4.48 (2.43, 8.27)	3.24 (1.68, 6.23)	2.07 (1.14, 3.78)
aLM/height+	1.89 (1.25, 2.86)	1.29 (0.84, 1.99)	1.41 (0.88, 2.26)
aLM/fat mass≠	2.99 (2.05, 4.38)	2.79 (1.93, 4.05)	2.08 (1.37, 3.15)
residuals	2.95 (2.00, 4.36)	2.18 (1.43, 3.32)	1.75 (1.10, 2.78)
Upper extremity specific force §, ¶	1.95 (1.26, 3.03)	1.63 (1.07, 2.49)	1.19 (0.77, 1.85)
Lower extremity specific force §, #	3.38 (1.82, 6.30)	2.71 (1.44, 5.08)	2.01 (1.05, 3.83)

*Adjusted for country of birth, age group, education level, PASE score, co-morbidity, stroke, arthritis, depressive symptoms.

+Additionally adjusted for obesity.

≠Additionally adjusted for height.

§ Additionally adjusted for pain.

I Ratio of grip strength (measured in kg of force) to arm lean mass

Ratio of quadriceps strength (measured in kg of force) to leg lean mass.

Source: Hairi NN, Cumming R, Naganathan V *et al.* Loss of Muscle Strength, Mass (Sarcopenia), and Quality (Specific Force) and Its Relationship with Functional Limitation and Physical Disability: The Concord Health and Ageing in Men Project. Journal of the American Geriatrics Society. 2010: 58: 2055-2062

Table 3. Prevalence ratios for low muscle strength, muscle mass and muscle quality and physical disability, CHAMP Study.

The relationship between age-related muscle changes and poor physical function is complex. Muhlberg and Siber described three possible "vicious loops" that involve feedback from physiological and behavioural systems. The "vicious loops" are the immobilization loop, the nutritional loop and the metabolic loop (M.S. John Pathy 2006). The vicious loop between sarcopenia and immobilization is described as: sarcopenia → neuromuscular impairment → falls and fractures → immobilization → sarcopenia. The second loop is the "nutritional" vicious loop between sarcopenia and malnutrition: sarcopenia → immobilization → decline of nutrition skills (empty refrigerator) → malnutrition impaired protein synthesis → sarcopenia. Finally, the "metabolic" vicious loop between sarcopenia and the decline of protein reserve in the body: sarcopenia → decline of protein reserve of the body → diminished capacity to meet the extra demand of protein synthesis associated disease and injury → sarcopenia.

5. Prevention and treatments for sarcopenia

As sarcopenia (loss of muscle strength, muscle mass and quality) was found to be associated with poor physical function, improvements in muscle strength would prevent immobilization and break the cycle. Physical activity, especially resistance exercise attenuates and may reverse age associated decreases in muscle strength as well as improve physical agility. Other interventions such as combinations of exercise with dietary supplements, hormone replacement, anti-inflammatory and other pharmacological treatments are still being investigated.

5.1 The role of exercise and increased physical activity

Exercise stimulates the release of growth hormones that promotes healthy muscle mass (M.S. John Pathy 2006). Although any exercise is better than no exercise at all, in terms of preventing loss of lean muscle mass, resistance exercise is preferred (Y Rolland 2008). Resistance exercise increases muscle protein synthesis rate over proteolysis and results in a net increase in contractile protein mass and hypertrophy of muscle fibres. Strength training being part of resistance exercise remains highly effective in maintaining muscular strength throughout life (Mühlberg and Sieber 2004). However, in older people, strength levels fall far more rapidly, independent of training (Y Rolland 2008). This is due to the changes in hormones such as testosterone and growth hormones which decline more rapidly and dramatically after the age of 60 years. Reduction in the circulation of these hormones will result in a shift in the balance between muscle protein synthesis and protein breakdown (Borst 2004). The vast majority of the literature on prevention and treatment of sarcopenia is related to the effects of exercise. These studies have demonstrated that progressive resistance training in older people results in substantial improvements in muscle strength and mass (Borst 2004). The improvements in muscle strength are smaller in absolute terms but similar in relative terms, compared to the younger population. What remains unclear are issues such as optimal duration, frequency and type of resistive exercise, combinations of resistive and aerobic training, compliance and long term maintenance, adjuvant nutritional supplementation and/or pharmacologic treatment. **A recent review by Borst SE suggested that resistance training is an effective intervention fo**r increasing muscle mass and strength in older people (Borst 2004).

Additional benefits of resistance exercise include normalisation of blood pressure, improved insulin sensitivity, decreased total and abdominal fat, increased metabolic rate, prevention of bone loss, reduction of risk for falls, reduced pain and improved physical function. Other forms of exercise, such as aerobic exercises have well-established benefits on cardiovascular fitness, improving lipid profile and flexibility (M.S. John Pathy 2006). Therefore, engaging in some form of resistance training is essential to preserve and increase muscle mass and strength.

5.2 Nutritional strategies for prevention and treatment of sarcopenia

Aging is associated with a progressive reduction in food intake, which predisposes to energy-protein malnutrition. In other words, aging is associated with physiological anorexia, decrease in caloric intake and weight loss (Marcell 2003). The decline in food intake that happens even in healthy older people has been termed "anorexia of ageing" (M.S. John Pathy 2006). Studies have shown that low dietary energy intake is common among healthy older people. Other factors that influence food intake in older people include psychological state (e.g. depression or depressive symptoms), social support and network (e.g. loneliness) and physical change (poor dentition, impaired taste and smell). Changes in food preferences with an increased liking for sweet and protein-poor foods have also been reported among older people. Dietary factors that contribute to sarcopenia include inadequate protein intake, insufficient calorie intake and low level metabolic acidosis (Paddon-Jones, et al. 2008). Metabolic efficiency in older people has been shown to be lower. Older people have a higher rate of protein catabolism and needing a higher requirement for dietary protein than their younger counterparts (Paddon-Jones, et al. 2008). There are research findings to support the ability of dietary protein to stimulate protein synthesis in older people. A review paper by Borst concludes that there is insufficient research to define an optimal value for protein ingestion (moderate intake or high intake)(Borst 2004). There are also uncertainties linking high protein intake to increased risk of impaired kidney function in healthy older people. This is further complicated by the fact that renal function decreases with age.

Older people have reduced food intake and increased protein requirements. Therefore, older people should strive to ensure adequate intake of protein (leucine-enriched amino acids and possibly creatine) from a variety of sources, accompanied by an increase in fruits and vegetables.

5.3 Hormone replacement and management of sarcopenia

Aging is accompanied by declining levels of many essentials hormones in the body, especially growth hormone (GH) and testosterone. The Reproductive-Cell Cycle Theory of Aging is a new theory explaining the process of aging (Bowen and Atwood 2004). This theory proposes that the rate of aging is synonymous with the rate of change. The rate of change/aging is most rapidly seen during the fetal period. Reproductive hormones are known to regulate mitogenesis (process by which a cell divides to form two daughter cells), and differentiation (process by which a cell becomes specialised to perform unique functions), hence aging is primarily regulated by these hormones (Bowen and Atwood 2004). In other words, the Reproductive-Cell Cycle Theory of Aging proposes that the hormones that regulate reproduction, promote growth and development early in life but in later life become dysregulated and drive senescence (Bowen and Atwood 2004).

Loss of testosterone is associated with loss of muscle mass and strength and decreased bone mineral density, thus increasing the risk of functional limitation, disability, fracture and falls (Lang, et al. 2010). Menopause is associated with loss of bone mass and also muscle strength (M.S. John Pathy 2006). GH stimulates growth during early life and is required for maintenance of muscle and bone in adulthood. GH exerts most of its action through insulin like growth factor (IGF-I). These are critical hormones in maintaining muscle and bone mass (Borst 2004). Without adequate levels it is impossible for anyone to maintain lean body mass, regardless of how well they eat or exercise. Secretion of GH is impaired in older people.

A recent review by Borst SE suggested that testosterone replacement in elderly hypogonadal men produces only modest increases in muscle mass and strength, which are observed in some and not all studies (Borst 2004). Furthermore, higher doses have not been given for fear of accelerating prostate cancer. With regards to GH, this review shows that growth hormone replacement in older people produces a high incidence of side effects, does not increase strength and does not augment strength gains resulting from resistance training (Borst 2004).

A review on hormone (testosterone or growth hormone) replacement to the older people produces only modest increases in muscle mass and strength in some but not all studies and the risks associated with hormone replacements are still not clear (Borst 2004). To date, exercise and more importantly resistance training remains the most effective intervention for increasing muscle mass and strength in older people.

6. A diagnostic approach to sarcopenia

The EWGSOP proposed a practical approach to screen for sarcopenia in clinical practice (Cruz-Jentoft, et al. 2010a). This is as shown in Figure 4. This algorithm is based on gait speed measurement with a cut-off point of > 0.8 m/s.

7. Conclusion

Loss of muscle mass and strength with age is a slow but progressive process with undesirable consequences. The research in sarcopenia has shown that sarcopenia is linked to multiple causations: the aging process itself, genetic susceptibility, lifestyle practices, changes in living conditions and numerous chronic diseases. Sarcopenia also represents a set of unfavourable outcomes, such as the primary outcomes of loss of muscle mass, strength and quality, and secondary outcomes which cause further functional limitation, loss of mobility and increased risk of disability, falls and fractures. Current research has shown promising results on the assessment of sarcopenia and practical approach to the management of sarcopenic patients and/or patients at risk of sarcopenia in terms of prevention as well as its treatment. Sarcopenia is firmly on the agenda for research into ageing and needs to be recognised in routine clinical practice.

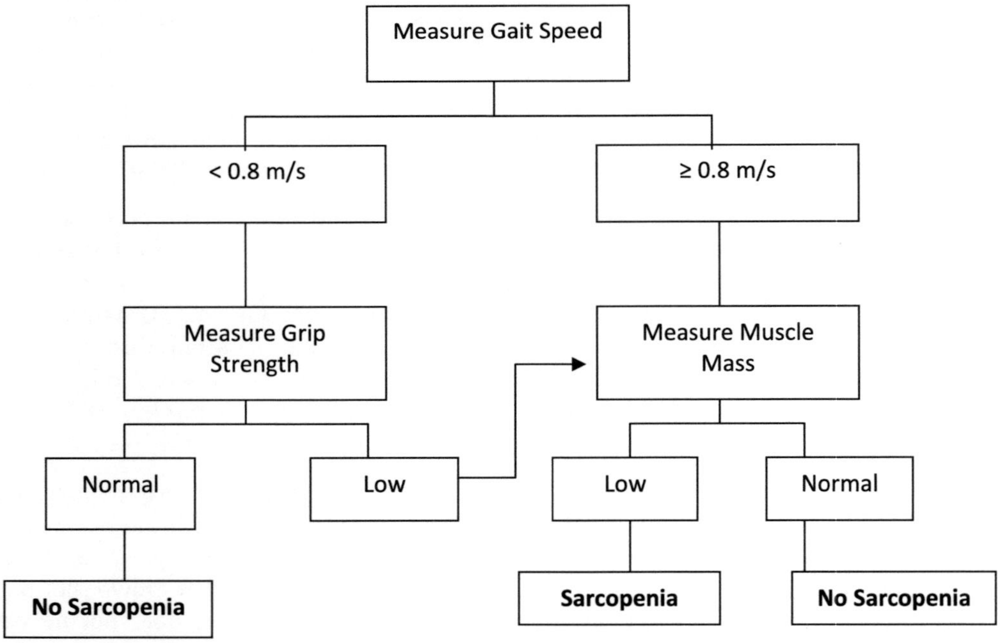

Source: Report of the EWGSOP. Sarcopenia: European consensus on definition and diagnosis. Age and Ageing, 2010: 39: 412-423.

Fig. 4. EWGSOP suggested algorithm for screening and case finding of sarcopenia

8. Acknowledgements

This work was supported by the Fundamental Research Grant Scheme (FRGS), Ministry of Higher Education, Malaysia. Dr. Noran N Hairi's work was supported by the University Malaya / Ministry of Higher Education (UM/MOHE) High Impact Research Grant E000014-20001.

9. References

A A Sayer, H Syddall, H Martin, H Patel, D Baylis, C Cooper 2008 The developmental origins of sarcopenia. The Journal of Nutrition, Health & Aging. 12(7):427-32.

A B. Newman, et al. 2003 Sarcopenia: Alternative Definitions and Associations with Lower Extremity Function. Journal of the American Geriatrics Society 51(11):1602-1609.

Borst, Stephen E. 2004 Interventions for sarcopenia and muscle weakness in older people. Age and Ageing 33(6):548-555.

Bowen, R. L., and C. S. Atwood 2004 Living and Dying for Sex. Gerontology 50(5):265-290.

Cruz-Jentoft, Alfonso J., et al. 2010aSarcopenia: European consensus on definition and diagnosis. Age and Ageing 39(4):412-423. 2010b Understanding sarcopenia as a geriatric syndrome. Current Opinion in Clinical Nutrition & Metabolic Care 13(1):1- 7.

Doherty, T J. 2003Aging and Sarcopenia. Journal of Applied Physiology 95:1717 - 1727.

Guralnik, JM, and F Luigi 2003 Assessing the building blocks of function: Utilizing measures of functional limitation. American Journal of Preventive Medicine 25(3):112-121.

Hairi NN, Cumming R, Naganathan V, Hendelsman D, Le Couteur D, Creasey H, Waite L, Seibel M, Sambrook P 2010 Loss of Muscle Strength, Mass (Sarcopenia), and Quality (Specific Force) and Its Relationship with Functional Limitation and Physical Disability: The Concord Health and Aging in Men Project. Journal of the American Geriatrics Society 58(11).

I Janssen 2006 Influence of Sarcopenia on the Development of Physical Disability: The Cardiovascular Health Study. Journal of the American Geriatrics Society 54(1):56-62.

Janssen, Ian 2010 Evolution of sarcopenia research. Applied Physiology, Nutrition, and Metabolism 35(5):707-712.

Lang, T., et al. 2010 Sarcopenia: etiology, clinical consequences, intervention, and assessment Osteoporosis International 21:543 - 559.

M.S. John Pathy, Alan J Sinclair, John E Morley., ed. 2006 Principles and Practice of Geriatric Medicine. Volume 2: John Wiley and Sons, Ltd.

Marcell, Taylor J. 2003 Review Article: Sarcopenia: Causes, Consequences, and Preventions. J Gerontol A Biol Sci Med Sci 58(10):M911-916.

MJ. Delmonico, et al. 2007 Alternative Definitions of Sarcopenia, Lower Extremity Performance, and Functional Impairment with Aging in Older Men and Women. Journal of the American Geriatrics Society 55(5):769-774.

Mühlberg, W., and C. Sieber 2004 Sarcopenia and frailty in geriatric patients: Implications for training and prevention. Zeitschrift für Gerontologie und Geriatrie 37(1):2-8.

Muscaritoli, M., et al. 2010 Consensus definition of sarcopenia, cachexia and pre-cachexia: Joint document elaborated by Special Interest Groups (SIG) "cachexia-anorexia in chronic wasting diseases" and "nutrition in geriatrics" . Clinical Nutrition 29(2):154-159.

Paddon-Jones, Douglas, et al. 2008 Role of dietary protein in the sarcopenia of aging. The American Journal of Clinical Nutrition 87(5):1562S-1566S.

Schranger M, Bandinelli S, Maggi S, Ferrucci L, 2003 Sarcopenia: Twenty Open Questions for a Research Agenda. Basic Appl Myol 13(4):203-208.

Steven M Albert, and Vicki A Freedman 2010 Public Health and Aging. Maximizing Function and Well-being. New York: Springer Publishing Company.

Valderrama-Gama, Emiliana, et al. 2002 Chronic Disease, Functional Status, and Self-Ascribed Causes of Disabilities Among Noninstitutionalized Older People in Spain. J Gerontol A Biol Sci Med Sci 57(11):M716-721.

Y Rolland, S Czerwinski, G Abellan Van Kan, J E Morley, M Cesari, G Onder, J Woo, R Baumgartner, F Pillard, Y Boirie, W M C Chumlea, B Vellas. 2008 Sarcopenia: Its assesment, etiology, pathogenesis, consequences and future perspectives. The Journal of Nutrition, Health & Aging. 12(7):433-50.

3

The Epidemiology of Vascular Dementia

Demet Ozbabalık[1], Didem Arslantaş[1] and Nese Tuncer Elmacı[3]
[1]*Eskisehir Osmangazi University, Medical Faculty, Department of Neurology, Eskisehir,*
[2]*Marmara University, Medical Faculty, Department of Neurology, Istanbul,*
[3]*Eskisehir Osmangazi University, Medical Faculty, Department of Public Health, Eskisehir, Turkey*

1. Introduction

Average life expectancy in the world is getting longer in the developing countries as well as developed countries. This means that we will encounter some of the diseases more than diseases which are only seen in elderly, in the coming years. Dementia is one of the most important health problems of the elderly population today, up to the developed countries is seen as a major threat in developing countries. WHO projections suggest that by 2025, about three-quarters of the estimated 1·2 billion people aged 60 years and older will reside in developing countries (1). Thus, by 2040, if growth in the older population continues, 71% of 81·1 million dementia cases will be in the developing world (Figure 1) (2).

Epidemiology is the study of health-event patterns in a society (3). It is the cornerstone method of public health research, and helps inform evidence-based medicine for identifying risk factors for disease and determining optimal treatment approaches to clinical practice and for preventive medicine. Epidemiologic measures are named as two types; incidence and prevalence. Whereas incidence deals with what is new, prevalence deals with what exists. By definition, prevalence is the number of cases of a given disease that exists in a defined population at a specified time. Incidence represents new event.

Dementia is actually a syndrome. It may be caused by various underlying diseases, each characterized by specific clinical features and neuropathology. Alzheimer disease (AD) which is a neurodegenerative is the most prevalent cause of dementia. The neuropathology of disease include in neuritic plaques and neurofibrillary tangle in the brain. Vascular dementia (VaD), describing impairments in cognitive function caused by problems in cerebral or cardiac blood vessels, is the second most common cause of dementia after Alzheimer disease in the aging population (Figure 2) (4). It comprises 10-20 % of all dementia. A meta-analysis of the European studies on incidence of dementia showed that VaD constitute 17.6 % of all dementia (5). In Europe and North America, AD is more common than VaD in a 2:1 ratio; in contrast in Japan and China VaD accounts for almost 50 % of all dementia (6, 13).

Vascular dementia is a complex disease and a common complication resulting from a blocked blood vessel causing a stroke. The most common mechanisms underlying VaD are multiple large-vessel infarcts, a single strategically placed infarct (angular gyrus, thalamus, basal forebrain, posterior cerebral artery or anterior cerebral artery), multiple basal ganglia and white matter lacunes, or extensive periventricular white-matter lesions. The most commonly encountered subtype of VaD is extensive periventricular white-matter lesions. Multiple large vessel infarcts and others follow up them (14).

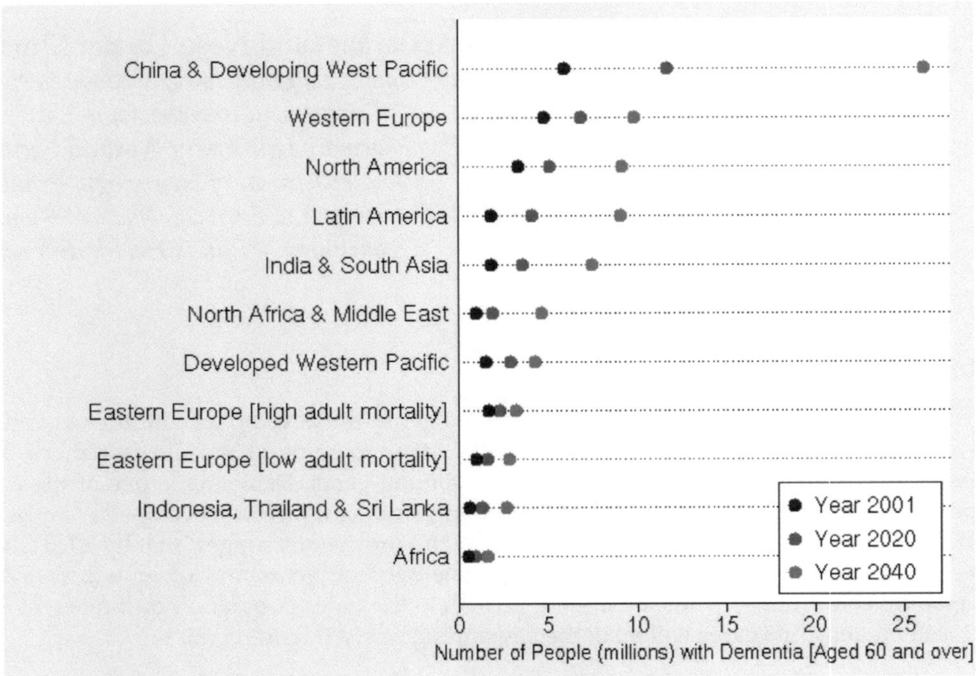

Fig. 1. Dementia prevalence 2001, 2020, 2040 by WHO Region Source: Ferri et al. (2005).

Vascular dementia is historically reflected by the diagnoses of "dementia with stroke" or "multi-infarct dementia," although these terms have been replaced with the broader concepts of vascular dementia and vascular cognitive impairment, recognizing the contribution to dementia of all vascular disease. Pathological findings have shown that much dementia cannot be attributed to a single underlying cause but arises from a combination of factors among which cerebrovascular disease, including infarct and haemorrhage, is an important contributor.

Although the incidence and prevalence of dementia are increasing, determining the incidence and prevalence of dementia is difficult (15-20).

Even with the difficulties of detecting and defining to prevalence and incidence in the population, it is clear that dementia causes a substantial burden on societies. There is an urgent need to develop preventive strategies and to identify of modifiable risk factors about each type of dementia. Newer imaging techniques and neuropsychological test batteries provide an opportunity to identify subclinical manifestations of "dementias" that can be limited to the risk factors and subsequent clinical disease. Problems with diagnostic inaccuracy and insidious disease onset influence results of the epidemiologic studies (21).

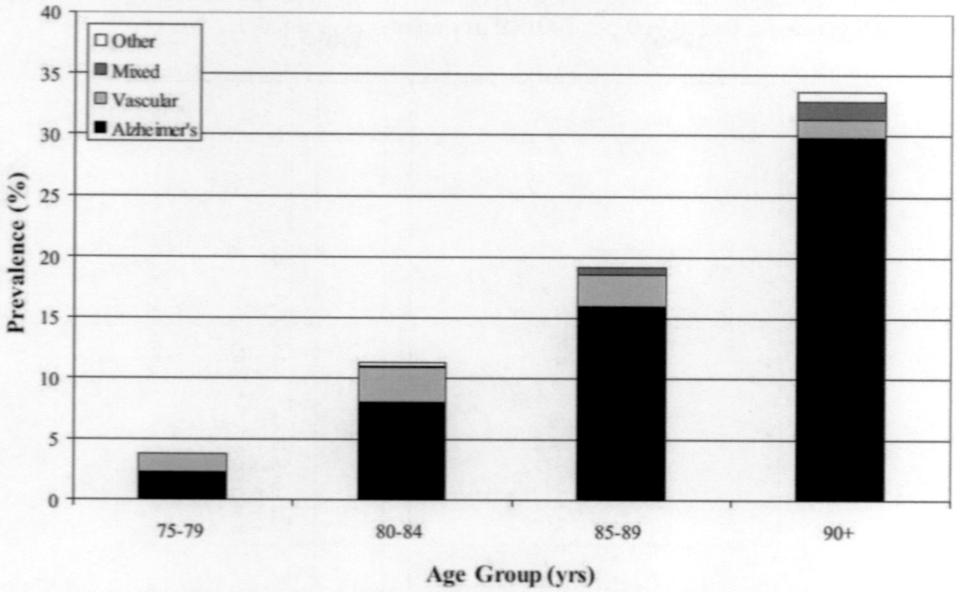

Fig. 2. Prevalence of dementia subtypes Data from the Cambridge City Over-75s Cohort Study (CC75C).

Epidemiologic studies of VaD have been also affected by variations in the definition of the disorders, the clinical criteria used and the methods. Analysis of data from 12 centres for which imaging findings were available indicates that 26% of cases of dementia fulfilled the US National Institute of Neurological Disorders and Stroke and Association Internationale pour la Recherché et l'Enseignement en Neurosciences (NINDS–AIREN) criteria for VaD (22,23).

2. Prevalence and incidence

Prevalence estimates vary highly between studies because of methodological and geographical differences (Table 1) (24). However, the prevalence of VaD ranges from one to four percent in people over the age of 65 and seems to be higher in China and Japan than in Europe and North America. While the rate is 1.5% in Western countries and in Japan is approximately 2.2%. In Japan, vascular dementia accounts for 50% of all dementias that occur in individuals older than 65 years. In Europe, vascular dementia and mixed dementia account for approximately 20% and 40% of cases, respectively (25-28).

In 2000, prevalence data from 11 European population based studies were pooled to obtain stable estimates of prevalence of dementia in the elderly (>65 years). Age standardised prevalence was 6.4% for dementia (all causes), and 1.6% for VaD (29). In clinical studies, the prevalence of VaD ranges from 4.4% and 39%, its incidence from 0.42 to 2.65, with doubling every 5 years in western memory clinical and population based series. In Asia, a number of studies on the prevalence of dementia have been published in Chinese, yielding varied results. By comparison with these studies that reported a prevalence range of VaD as 0.2 % to 2.7 %, respectively for those aged 60 years and older (30).

Data suggests that the annual incidence of VaD may range from 20-40 per 100000 between persons 60-69 years old to 200-700 per 100.000 in persons over age 80.

	Year	Criteria	Sample size (n)	Age (years)	Prevalence (95% CI)	
					All dementia	VaD
Asia						
China	2007	DSM-III, ICD-10	87 761	>65	3.1% (2.8–3.5)	0.9% (0.7–1.1)
China (Beijing, Xian,Shanghai, Chengdu)	2005	DSM-IV	34 807	>65	5.0%	1.1% (0.9–1.1)
Taiwan	1995-1998	DSM-IIIR, DSM-IV	7149	>65	3.2%	0.7% (0.1–1.3)
South Korea	1994-2005	DSM-III, DSM-IV	7096	>65	10.1% (7.3–12.9)	2.1% (1.2–2.9)
Thailan	2001	DSM-III	4048	>60	3.4% (2.8–4.0)	
India	1996-2006	DSM-III, DSM-IV	14 767	>65	2.7% (1.4–4.0)	1.1% (0.2–1.9)
Sri Lanka	2003	DSM-IV	703	>65	3.98% (2.6–5.7)	0.6%
Israel (Wadi Ara)	2002	DSM-IV	823	>65	21.1%	6.0%
Turkey	2009	DSM-IV	3100	>55	8.4%	
Africa						
Egypt	1998	DSM-IV	1366	>65	5.93%	1.25%
Nigeria	1995	DSM-III, ICD-10	2494	>65	2.3% (1.2 -3.4)	0.72%
Latin America						
Cuba	1999	DSM-IV	799	>60	8.2% (6.3–10.4)	1.9% (1.0–3.0)
Argentina	1999	DSM-IV	1900	>65	11.5%	
Brazil	2002-2008	DSM-IIIR, DSM-IV	7513	>65	5.3% (1.5–8.9)	0.9% (0.06–1.78)
Chile	1997	DSM-IIIR	2213	>65	4.3% (3.5–5.3)	
Colombia	2000	DSM-IV	1611	>65 and >75	1.8% (1.2–2.7)	
Peru	2007	DSM-IV	1532	>65	6.7% (5.5–8.0)	
Venezuela	2002	DSM-IV	2438	>55 and >65	8.0% (7.0–9.2)	4.0% (3.3–4.8)

Table; Brayne C, Cambridge City Over-75s Cohort Cc75c Study Neuropathology Collaboration. Neuropathological correlates of dementia in over-80-year-old brain donors from the population-based Cambridge city over-75s cohort (CC75C) study. J Alzheimers Dis. 2009 (The Turkish data was added).

Table 1.

3. Age and gender

Studies show that the occurrence of VaD exponentially increases with age from 65 to 85 years. The prevalence of dementia of all causes increases between the seventh and tenth decade from 0.8 to 28.5% that of vascular dementia (VD) (15.8% of total) from 0.3 to 5.2% or from 0.2 to 16% over age 80. In 2030, nearly 70 million patients with dementia is expected in 65 and older populations, without any substantial difference between men and women. Under eighty-five years of age the prevalence of VaD was higher in men compared to women and thereafter the prevalence was higher in women (29). In a longitudinal community survey of Japanese American men (Honolulu Asia Aging Study), 23% of vascular dementia was attributed. to large-vessel, 50% to small-vessel, and 16% to mixed-vessel disease (31).

The age-standardized prevalence of VaD was 1.6% and also increased with age. However, contrary to AD, the difference in prevalence between men and women was age dependent. This finding might also be attributed to differences in survival between men and women. However, it may also reflect changes in incidence pattern.

4. Variation across region

There are differences amongst cultural, demographic and ethnic variability in incidence and prevalence studies. The proportion of AD and VaD dementia was different from that in Europe and other Asian countries. For example, VD tends to be more common than AD in Japan and Russia (31-32). Even, a marked geographical dissociation in Europe between the north and south, linked to differences in vascular risk factors has been proposed to account for the higher incidence rates in the oldest-old of north-western countries (Finland, Sweden, Denmark, the Netherlands, and the United Kingdom) compared to southern countries (France and Spain). This difference is further supported by north–South regional findings of differences in MRI-detected white matter lesion (WML) pathology. Greater WML pathology linked to progression of dementia has been observed in southern Europe relative to northern and central European countries (33,35).

Few studies reported the differences in the distribution of dementia subtypes between rural and urban areas. Interestingly, they found that there was a significantly higher prevalence of Alzheimer disease in the rural area than the urban area. And on the contrary, there was a higher prevalence of vascular dementia in the urban area than the rural area. It may be owing to the differences in education levels, socioeconomic status, obesity and body mass index, diet, and life style between the two areas. If the future studies continue to report the higher prevalence of vascular dementia in urban areas, it means that there will be increased demands on healthcare system particularly among urban populations (36-40).

5. Family history and genetic

Dementia risk can increase two- to four-fold among individuals who have at least one first degree relative with dementia. Genetic factors play an important role in the aetiology of VaD. However, there is less epidemiological evidence for a genetic component of risk factors of VaD like cardio embolic stroke. Two known genetic disease can be thought that VaD have genetic characteristics. These are cerebral autosomal dominant arteriopathy with subcortical infarcts and leucoencephalopathy (CADASIL: a subcortical small vessel disease accompanied by lacunars' strokes, migraine, and dementia) and hereditary cerebral haemorrhage with amyloidosis- Dutch type (HCHWA-D) (41).

The CADASIL condition is a heritable small-vessel disease caused by mutations in NOTCH3 gene which is normally expressed in vascular smooth muscle cells and pericytes (including those of the cerebral vasculature) and that encodes a cell-surface receptor, which has a role in arterial development and is expressed on vascular smooth-muscle cells. About 95% of patients have missense mutations that cluster in exons 3, but the pathogenic mechanism is still unknown. With regard to HCHWA-D (a syndrome of primarily hemorrhagic strokes and dementia), it is caused by a mutation in the gene for amyloid precursor protein (APP) that causes abnormal deposition of amyloid in the walls of leptomeningeal arteries and cortical arterioles, it is known as cerebral amyloid angiopathy [CAA] (42).

The studies using the candidate gene approaches has identified a number of genetic variants possibly involved in risk factor development. They can contribute to conventional risk factors such as hypertension, diabetes, or homocysteine concentrations. Recently, APO E4 was studied in VaD after AD as risk factors. As authors, VaD risk also increases with the number of alleles: homozygous carriers are at a greater risk than heterozygous carries or those who do not carry the E4 variant (43, 44).

A study showed that MAPT (microtubule-associated protein tau) was associated with VaD and since MAPT is a gene playing an important role in AD. Moreover, G allele of rs1467967 is the risk allele, which is the major allele in Chinese population (45).

6. Hypertention and other vascular risk factors

Mid-life hypertension (high blood pressure) has been associated with impaired cognitive function even in otherwise healthy individuals (46). Traditionally VaD has been considered affected by hypertension and the alleviation of it. In a Japan study, the age- and sex-adjusted incidence of VaD significantly increased with elevated late-life blood pressure levels whereas no such association was observed for Alzheimer disease. The current meta-analysis highlights the potential importance of rigorous treatment of hypertension as a key measure to help prevent the development of VaD (47).

Except hypertension, histories of diabetes, metabolic syndrome, hyperlipidemia, myocardial infarction/cardiac decomposition, heavy smoking, obesity and a history of stroke are other risk factors for VaD. The Cardiovascular Health Cognition Study developed a late-life dementia risk index that included older age, worse cognitive test performance, lower body mass index (BMI), APOE _4 allele, MRI findings of white matter disease or ventricular enlargement, internal carotid artery thickening on ultrasound, history of bypass surgery, slower physical performance, and lack of alcohol consumption (48).

7. Lifestyle

Risk finding for alcohol is not consistent. Alcohol has been found to have a protective effect in moderate drinkers with a five-fold increase in dementia in both abstainers and those who drink heavily. A study found a link between increasing alcohol consumption and VaD (49).

In some studies alcohol and smoking are neither strongly protective nor predictive (50). In some studies were informed that high educational attainment, eating fish or shellfish, physical exercise, use of supplementary antioxidants like beta-carotene, omega-3, Vitamins E and C, use of Vitamin B12, Mediterranean diet might be potential protective factors for VaD (51,53).

8. Conclusion remarks

1. Vascular dementia (VaD) is the second most common cause of dementia after Alzheimer disease in the aging population.
2. Prevalence estimates vary highly between studies because of methodological and geographical differences.
3. Prevalence rate is 1.5% in Western countries and in Japan is approximately 2.2%.
4. Annual incidence of VaD may range from 20-40 per 100000 between persons 60-69 years old to 200-700 per 100.000 in persons over age 80.
5. There are differences amongst cultural, demographic and ethnic variability in incidence and prevalence studies.
6. Sex patterns remain unclear for prevalence and incidence.
7. Dementia risk can increase two- to four-fold among individuals who have at least one first degree relative with dementia.
8. Hypertension, histories of diabetes, metabolic syndrome, hyperlipidemia, myocardial infarction/cardiac decomposition, heavy smoking, obesity and a history of stroke are other risk factors for VaD.
9. Finally, about epidemiology of VaD is not clear as well as AD. We need more studies in the world.

9. References

[1] WHO. Active Ageing: a policy framework, 2002 Health Report. Geneva: world health organization, 2002.

[2] Ferri CP, Prince M, Brayne c. Global prevalence of dementia: a delphi consensus study. Lancet 2005; 366: 2112–17

[3] Rothman K, Greenland S. Modern epidemiology, 2nd ed. Philadelphia: Lippincott-Raven, 1998

[4] Brayne C, Richardson K, Matthews FE, Fleming J, Hunter S, Xuereb JH, Paykel E,Mukaetova-Ladinska EB, Huppert FA, O'Sullivan A, Dening T; Cambridge City Over-75s Cohort Cc75c Study Neuropathology Collaboration. Neuropathological correlates of dementia in over-80-year-old brain donors from the population-based Cambridge city over-75s cohort (CC75C) study. J Alzheimers Dis. 2009;18(3):645-58.

[5] Rocca WA, Hofman A, Brayne C. Frequency and distribution of alzheimer's disease in Europe: a collaborative study of 1980–1990 prevalence findings. The EURODEM prevalence research group. Ann neurol 1991; 30: 381–90

[6] From the Centers for Disease Control and Prevention. Public health and aging: trends in aging--United States and worldwide. JAMA. 2003,19;289(11):1371-3.

[7] Wimo A, Winblad B, Agu¨ Ero-Torres H, Von Strauss E. The magnitude of dementia occurrence in the world. Alzheimer Dis Assoc Disord 2003; 17: 63–67.

[8] Yamada t, Hattori H, Miura A, Prevalence of Alzheimer's disease, vascular dementia and dementia with lewy bodies in a japanese population. Psychiatry Clin Neurosci. 2001;55:21–25.

[9] Dong MJ, Peng B, Lin XT, Zhao J, Yan-Rong Zhou YR, Wang RH. The prevalence of dementia in the people's republic of china: a systematic analysis of 1980–2004 studies. Age and Ageing 2007; 36: 619–624.

[10] Gorelick PB, Roman G, Mangone CA (1994) Vascular Dementia. In: Gorelick PB, Alter MA (eds) handbook of Neuroepidemiology. Mecel Dekker, New York, pp 197–214

[11] Hachinski VC, Lassen MA, Marshall J Multi-infarct dementia. A cause of mental deterioration in elderly. Lancet 1974,2:207–210

[12] Roman GC, Sachdev P, Royall DR, Vascular cognitive disorder: a new diagnostic category updating vascular cognitive impairment and vascular dementia. Neurol Sci, 2004, 226:81–87

[13] Sachdev P, Vascular cognitive disorder. Int J Geriatr Psychiatry, 1999, 14: 402–403

[14] Nizam Z, Hyer L, Vascular cognitive impairment: perspective and review The Journal of Psychiatry , 2007 325-325

[15] O'brien JT, Erkinjuntti T, Reisberg B , Vascular cognitive impairment. Lancet Neurol, 2003, 2:89–98

[16] Cagnin A, Battistin l (2007) vascular dementia. In: Readerer Battistin (ed) handbook of neurochemistry and molecular neurobiology. Springer-Verlag, 253–265

[17] Cowan LD., Leviton A., Dammann O. New Research Directions In neuroepidemiology. Epidemiology review, 2000, 22: 18–23.

[18] Dartigues JF., Letenneur, L., Joly, P., Helmer, C., Orgogozo,J. Age specific risk of dementia according to gender, education and wine consumption. Neurobiology of Aging, 2000, 21: 64.

[19] Fratiglioni L, De Ronchi D, Agüero-Torres H. Worldwide prevalence and incidence of dementia. Drugs Aging 1999;15:365–75.

[20] Fratiglioni L, Roccaw. Epidemiology of dementia. In: Boller F, Cappa SF, editors. Handbook of Neuropsychology: Aging and dementia. Amsterdam: elsevier sc publ; 2001. P. 193–215.

[21] Fratiglioni L, Launer LJ, Andersen K, Breteler MM, Copeland JR, Dartigues JF, Incidence of dementia and major subtypes in Europe: a collaborative study of population-based cohorts. Neurologic diseases in the elderly research group. Neurology 2000;54(suppl 5):s10–5.

[22] Román GC. Vascular dementia revisited: diagnosis, pathogenesis, treatment, and prevention. Med Clin North Am. 2002;86:477–499.

[23] Roman GC, Tatemichi TK, Erkinjuntti T, Vascular dementia: diagnostic criteria for research studies: report of the NINDSAIREN international workshop. Neurology 1993; 43: 250–60

[24] Zhang ZX, Zahner GE, Roman GC. Dementia subtypes in China: Prevalence in Beijing, Xian, Shanghai, and Shengdu. Arch Neurol 2005; 62: 447–53

[25] Yang B. Meta prevalence estimates: generating combined prevalence estimates from separate population surveys. Centre for epidemiology and research, nsw department of health (australia). Http://www.health.nsw.gov.au

[26] Kalaria RN, Maestre GE, Arizaga R, Friedland RP, Galasko D, Hall K, Luchsinger JA, Ogunniyi A, Perry EK, Potocnik F, Prince M, Stewart R, Wimo A, Zhang ZX,

Antuono P; World Federation of Neurology Dementia Research Group. Alzheimer's disease and vascular dementia in developing countries: prevalence, management,and risk factors. Lancet Neurol. 2008 Sep;7(9):812-26

[27] Plassman BL, Langa KM, Fisher GG, Heeringa SG, Weir DR, Ofstedal MB, Burke JR,Hurd MD, Potter GG, Rodgers WL, Steffens DC, Willis RJ, Wallace RB. Prevalence of dementia in the United States: the aging, demographics, and memory study.Neuroepidemiology. 2007;29(1-2):125-32.

[28] Lobo A, Launer LJ, Fratiglioni L, Andersen K, Di Carlo A, Breteler MM, Copeland JR, Dartigues JF, Jagger C, Martinez-Lage J, Soininen H, Hofman A. Prevalence of dementia and major subtypes in Europe: A collaborative study of population-based cohorts. Neurologic Diseases in the Elderly Research Group. Neurology. 2000;54(11 Suppl 5):S4-9

[29] Dong MJ, Peng B, Lin XT, Zhao J, Zhou YR, Wang RH. The prevalence of dementia in the People's Republic of China: a systematic analysis of 1980-2004 studies. Age Ageing. 2007 Nov;36(6):619-24.

[30] Harvey RJ, Skelton-Robinson M, Rossor MN. The prevalence and causes of dementia in people under the age of 65 years. J Neurol Neurosurg Psychiatry. 2003 ;74(9):1206-9.

[31] Launer LJ, Ross GW, Petrovitch H, Masaki K, Foley D, White LR, Havlik RJ.Midlife blood pressure and dementia: the Honolulu-Asia aging study. Neurobiol Aging. 2000;21(1):49-55

[32] Karasawa A, Homma A. Recent changes in the prevalence of dementia in the Tokyo Metropolis. In: Hasegawa K, Homma A, eds. Psychogeriatrics:Bbiomedical and Social Advances, Vol. 1, Amsterdam Excerpta Medica 1990; 24–9. 37.

[33] Ikeda M, Hokoishi K, Maki N, Nebu A, Tachibana N, Komori K, Shigenobu K, Fukuhara R, Tanabe H. Increased prevalence of vascular dementia in Japan: a community-based epidemiological study. Neurology. 2001 Sep 11;57(5):839-44.

[34] Fratiglioni L, Launer LJ, Andersen K, Breteler MM, Copeland JR, Dartigues JF, Lobo A, Martinez-Lage J, Soininen H, Hofman A. Incidence of dementia and major subtypes in Europe: A collaborative study of population-based cohorts. Neurologic Diseases in the Elderly Research Group. Neurology. 2000;54(11 Suppl 5):S10-5.

[35] Launer LJ, Berger K, Breteler MM, Dufouil C, Fuhrer R, Giampaoli S, Nilsson LG, Pajak A, de Ridder M, van Dijk EJ, Sans S, Schmidt R, Hofman A. Regional variability in the prevalence of cerebral white matter lesions: an MRI study in 9 European countries (CASCADE). Neuroepidemiology. 2006;26(1):23-9.

[36] Baiyewu O, Unverzagt FW, Ogunniyi A, Hall KS, Gureje O, Gao S, Lane KA, Hendrie HC. Cognitive impairment in community-dwelling older Nigerians: clinical correlates and stability of diagnosis. Eur J Neurol. 2002 Nov;9(6):573-80.

[37] Xu G, Meyer JS, Huang Y, Chen G, Chowdhury M, Quach M. Cross-cultural comparison of mild cognitive impairment between China and USA. Curr Alzheimer Res. 2004 Feb;1(1):55-61.

[38] Das SK, Bose P, Biswas A, Dutt A, Banerjee TK, Hazra AM, Raut DK, Chaudhuri A, Roy T. An epidemiologic study of mild cognitive impairment in Kolkata, India. Neurology. 2007 Jun 5;68(23):2019-26

[39] Lopes MA, Hototian SR, Bustamante SE, Azevedo D, Tatsch M, Bazzarella MC,Litvoc J, Bottino CM. Prevalence of cognitive and functional impairment in a community sample in Ribeirão Preto, Brazil. Int J Geriatr Psychiatry. 2007 Aug;22(8):770-6.

[40] Hototian SR, Lopes MA, Azevedo D, Tatsch M, Bazzarella MC, Bustamante SE, Litvoc J, Bottino CM. Prevalence of cognitive and functional impairment in acommunity sample from São Paulo, Brazil. Dement Geriatr Cogn Disord.2008;25(2):135-43.

[41] Hachinski V, Iadecola C, Petersen RC, Breteler MM, Nyenhuis DL, Black SE,Powers WJ, DeCarli C, Merino JG, Kalaria RN, Vinters HV, Holtzman DM, RosenbergGA, Wallin A, Dichgans M, Marler JR, Leblanc GG. National Institute ofNeurological Disorders and Stroke-Canadian Stroke Network vascular cognitive impairment harmonization standards. Stroke. 2006 Sep;37(9):2220-41.

[42] Bohlega S, Al Shubili A, Edris A, Alreshaid A, Alkhairallah T, AlSous MW,Farah S, Abu-Amero KK. CADASIL in Arabs: clinical and genetic findings. BMC Med, Genet. 2007 Nov 9;8:67.

[43] Nilsson K, Gustafson L, Nornholm M, Hultberg B. Plasma homocysteine, apolipoprotein E status and vascular disease in elderly patients with mental illness. Clin Chem Lab Med. 2010;48(1):129-35.

[44] Chuang YF, Hayden KM, Norton MC, Tschanz J, Breitner JC, Welsh-Bohmer KA, Zandi PP. Association between APOE epsilon4 allele and vascular dementia: The Cache County study. Dement Geriatr Cogn Disord. 2010;29(3):248-53.

[45] Ning M, Zhang Z, Chen Z, Zhao T, Zhang D, Zhou D, Li W, Liu Y, Yang Y, Li S,He L. Genetic evidence that vascular dementia is related to Alzheimer's disease: genetic association between tau polymorphism and vascular dementia in the Chinese population. Age Ageing. 2011;40(1):125-8

[46] Qiu C,Winblad B, Fratiglioni L. The age-dependent relation of blood pressureto cognitive function and dementia. Lancet Neurol 2005;4:487–99

[47] Ninomiya T, Ohara T, Hirakawa Y, Yoshida D, Doi Y, Hata J, Kanba S, Iwaki T, Kiyohara Y. Midlife and late-life blood pressure and dementia in Japanese elderly: the hisayama study. Hypertension. 2011;58(1):22-8

[48] Sharp SI, Aarsland D, Day S, Sønnesyn H; Alzheimer's Society Vascular Dementia Systematic Review Group, Ballard C. Hypertension is a potential risk factor for vascular dementia: systematic review. Int J Geriatr Psychiatry. 2011 ;26(7):661-9.

[49] Hajjar I, Quach L, Yang F, Chaves PH, Newman AB, Mukamal K, Longstreth W Jr,Inzitari M, Lipsitz LA. Hypertension, white matter hyperintensities, and concurrent impairments in mobility, cognition, and mood: the Cardiovascular Health Study. Circulation. 2011,1;123(8):858-65

[50] Anstey KJ, Mack HA, Cherbuin N. Alcohol consumption as a risk factor for dementia and cognitive decline: meta-analysis of prospective studies. Am J Geriatr Psychiatry. 2009 ;17(7):542-55

[51] Rusanen M, Kivipelto M, Quesenberry CP Jr, Zhou J, Whitmer RA. Heavy smoking in midlife and long-term risk of Alzheimer disease and vascular dementia. Arch Intern Med. 2011 28;171(4):333-9

[52] Frisardi V, Panza F, Seripa D, Imbimbo BP, Vendemiale G, Pilotto A, Solfrizzi V. Nutraceutical properties of Mediterranean diet and cognitive decline: possible underlying mechanisms. Review. J Alzheimers Dis. 2010, 1;22(3):715-40.

[53] Solfrizzi V, Panza F, Frisardi V, Seripa D, Logroscino G, Imbimbo BP, Pilotto A. Diet and Alzheimer's disease risk factors or prevention: the current evidence. Expert Rev Neurother. 2011;11(5):677-708.

4

Swallowing Difficulties in Elderly People: Impact of Maxillomandibular Wedging

Marie-Hélène Lacoste-Ferré[1,2],
Sophie Hermabessière[2] and Yves Rolland[2]
[1]*Faculté de Chirurgie Dentaire de Toulouse,*
Université Paul Sabatier,
[2]*Hôpital Garonne,*
France

1. Introduction

Situated in a particular anatomic zone: the aero digestive crossroad, swallowing is going to allow the transport of the food from the oral cavity toward the stomach while protecting the upper air tracts [1-2]. The first phase of swallowing is a voluntary, necessary phase: the labiooral phase. It starts with the elaboration of the bolus: food is incised (with incisors), masticated (laterally and behind with molars), and impregnated with saliva. The lips, the cheeks, the tongue and the mandible are animated by rhythmic movements; the oral cavity must remain closed. Once the bolus is prepared, it is gathered in only one entity on the back of the tongue which forms a gutter [3-5]. At this stage, the mandible takes support on the jaw by dental contact so that the bolus can be expelled towards the base of the tongue, by the action of the tongue like a piston but also the lips which lean on the superior incisors. It is impossible to swallow with the mouth open without jaw stabilization [6-8]. During the pharyngeal phase, the bolus advances towards the oesophagus. The mechanisms of protection of the upper air tracts are implemented by successive rise of the palate, the hyoid bone and the larynx. The epiglottis topples over towards the back, comes to cover the supra-glottal floor. The crossing of the air and digestive tracts imposes a narrow coordination between pharyngeal phase and respiratory activity [1, 9].

In geriatrics, swallowing difficulties are frequent and remain a problem for the medical staff [10]. They manifest themselves most often during meals by signs from the simple cough of expectoration to the systematic false passage. One of the frequent complications is pulmonary infection which can aggravate the general health of the old person and be life-threatening [11-17].

During the labiooral time, different elements are important to consider: the viscosity, the volume and the homogeneity of the bolus, the peripheral musculature (lips, tongue, cheeks), the occlusal contacts, the jaw stabilization [9, 18, 19]. In elderly people, these elements are affected by frequent difficulties.

The neuromusculoarticular coordination and the driving performances of the orofacial region appear slightly influenced by ageing. Baum and Bodner [20] pointed out a muscular impairment of lips and muscles dependent on age. The speed and the amplitude of mandibular vertical movements decrease with ageing. The study of Koshino et al [21] showed modifications of the shape and the speed of mastication cycles with age.

The neuromuscular disorders which characterize the frequent general pathologies in the elderly such as Parkinson's disease, Alzheimer's dementia, the consequences of cerebral strokes (hemiplegia), the muscular pathologies, all increase risks of dysphagia [14, 19, 22-24]. The movements of the tongue and chewing are strongly unsettled, and the ascent of the larynx and the hyoid bone are incomplete. It results in a partial persistence of the bolus in the oral cavity after swallowing, and a stagnation of particles in the pharynx [10-11].

The health status and a poor oral health of elderly people particularly in residential aged care facilities can be in origin or aggravate dysphagia [7; 24-28]. If food is not correctly crushed, not twisted and not impregnated with saliva, the bolus will been broken up, too dry, not homogeneous and can stagnate in the oral cavity without being able to be completely swallowed [8, 24, 29-32]. The adaptation of the texture of food and (mixed, smooth, thickened) drinks is the answer most usually adopted in geriatrics to resolve the problem of mastication and constitution of the bolus [10].

Moreover, an inadequate dental status (missing teeth, inadapted denture, edentulousness) prevents a correct maxillomandibular position and efficient jaw stabilization for swallowing. The occlusal contacts (with natural or prosthetic teeth) must be stable, balanced, and centered at the posterior teeth i.e molars and premolars to ensure a correct oral function [12, 16, 17, 30, 33-35].

If, during swallowing, the mandible cannot "settle" in the jaw, it will be pulled forwards, because of the architecture of the temporomandibular joint (which can be schematized as a plane tipped up forward): it is the mandibular protrusion [6, 12, 33]. The epiglottis is then pulled forwards; the hyoid bone and the larynx cannot rise correctly: the laryngeal tightness cannot be ensured and increases the risk of false passage [36]. Also, the absence of the posterior teeth (premolars and molars) is frequent among the old people. If this posterior edentulousness is not compensated with a removable denture or if the removable denture has prosthetic teeth which are inadequate (old, damaged), the patient then attains the maximum of anterior contacts to prop up his mandible and to avoid stiffness: this creates a mandibular protrusion [30]. The profile of the patient is characteristic: lower floor of the face reduced, chin positioned forward, cutaneous folds (nasogenian, labiogenian) accentuated. Among elderly people, a bad posture, a reduced muscular tonicity and an increased ligamentary laxity accentuate the subsidence of the tissues and the mandibular protrusion [37].

The purpose of this preliminary study is to assess swallowing disorders and the oral and dental status among an elderly population living in a long-term care unit.

2. Materials and methods

The study was carried out on residents of the long-term care unit of Toulouse Hospital (geriatrics university center). This unit admits patients with a high level of disability and very poor general health (mean life expectancy of 2 years). All resident of the unit were screened. To be eligible for inclusion, subjects were required not to be fed by percutaneous endoscopic gastrotomy (PEG) and to accept to participate in the study. Enrolment lasted 1 month.

Baseline age, sex, current sialoprive medication (number of medication, psychotropic treatments [anxiolytics, neuroleptics, serotonin reuptake inhibitors, and other antidepressants] and antihistaminic) were recorded.

Disability was assessed using the Katz's disability scale [38]. Each item (eating, transferring from bed to chair, walking, using the toilet, bathing, and dressing) was scored from 0 to 1 (0 = unable to perform the activity without complete help, 0.5 = able to perform the activity with little help, 1 = able to perform the activity without any help). The scoring system gave a score range from 0 to 6. The body mass index (BMI = weight (kg) /height^2 (m^2)) was calculated at baseline.

An assessment of the swallowing disorders and the oral status were carried out by a trained geriatrician and an odontologist using two observational scales. The first was a meal observation, serving for estimating dysphagia. It was elaborate and used by the Toulouse otorhinolaryngology department. The assessment was performed once, during a usual midday meal. The variables collected were listed and described in the table 1.

Variables	Description
Sitting down	Sitting position, wedged head with support head or cushion
Assistance	No assistance, complete or partial assistance
Texture of food	Normal, tender, soft, smooth or mixed texture
Texture of drinks	Liquid or thickened drinks
Type of mastication	Vertically mastication when the mandibular movements are regular and well centred on the jaw during the chewing Disrupted mastication when the mandibular movements are backward and forward horizontally.
Coughing before/ after having swallowed	Coughing before having swallowed if there is a disease of labiooral phase (explained by the bolus constituting badly or the delay of the ascent of the larynx) Coughing after having swallowed if there is a disease of pharyngeal phase (explained by a bad tightness of the larynx or the food stagnating in the epiglottis fold)

Table 1. Summary of variables used for meal observation

The second was an oral examination in order to estimate the oral status. It was elaborate and is used by the odontology department of Toulouse. The oral status is illustrated by a quantitative dental status and a functional dental status. The variables collected were listed and described in the table 2.

3. Results

Forty patients (31 women and 9 men) were recruited from 53 residents. Ten patients refused and three patients had a PEG. The mean age of the patients was of 85.2 years with range of 63-100 years for the women and of 68-87 years for the men. Patients were dependant (mean ADL score = 2,125 (mini = 0; maxi = 5)). Twenty two participants needed assistance (22,7% partial, 77,3% complete) during the meal. The patients took on average 6 different medicines per day among which 1 medicine, on average was sialoprive. Fifteen patients took no sialoprive medicine. The mean BMI was 23 (mini = 12,21; max = 36,83).

Variables	Description
Quantitative dental status	Number of maxillary or mandibular missing teeth Presence of partial or complete removable dentures
Functional units (FU)	Number of opposing natural or prosthetic tooth pairs which are going to be in contact during the chewing and during the swallowing [30]. The anterior functional units (ant FU) represent incisors and canines. The posterior functional units (post FU) represent premolars and molars. If the patients have a complete dentition, they have 8 posterior functional units, but if they are complete edentulous, they have no functional unit.
Maxillomandibular wedging	It is assured by the presence of natural or prosthetic anterior functional units (incisive or canines) and\or by the presence of natural or prosthetic posterior functional units (premolars or molars).
Vertical Dimension of Occlusion (VDO)	It is the dimension measured on the median sagittal plane between a point situated on the face and a point situated on the mandible when teeth are in intercuspidal position i.e in maximum intercuspidation. When it exists neither wedging, nor later functional units, the VDO cannot be measured. When the natural or prosthetic teeth are inadequate (worn or damaged), the VDO is decreased.
Protrusion	It is connected to a disturbance of the intermaxillary relation i.e the mandible slips forward during closing.

Table 2. Summary of variables used for quantitative and functional dental status

3.1 Installation-assistance

Wherever the meal took place (bed room or dining room), the nursing staff were careful to sit down the patient properly: sitting position for the majority of patients, with wedged head with support or cushion. One patient could not be correctly settled because he presented an inflexible bending of the head. More than half of the patients (55 %) needed a complete or partial assistance.

3.2 Texture of food and drinks

The liquid drinks where consumed by 75 % of the patients; the texture of food (7,5% tender, 10% soft, 22,5% smooth or 45% mixed) was adapted for 85 % of the patients.

3.3 Type of mastication

52 % of the patients masticated vertically.

3.4 Dysphagia

35 % of the patients coughed before and\or after swallowing: 4 patients coughed before having swallowed, 4 patients coughed after having swallowed, 6 patients coughed before

and after having swallowed during the same meal. 26 patients (65 %) did not show signs of coughing.

3.5 Quantitative dental status

On average, the studied population presented 21.7 absent teeth (on 32 teeth) of which 11.7 missing teeth in the maxilla and 10 missing teeth in the mandible. In spite of the large edentulousness (~ 21 teeth / 32 teeth), the number of patients wearing removable prosthesis was few: 25 % of the patients (7 complete dentures, 3 partial removable dentures). On 9 edentulous patients, 7 wore complete dentures.

3.6 Functional dental status

40 % of the patients (16 patients) had no maxillomandibular wedging: for them, there was no functional unit. 60 % of the patients (24 patients) had a maxillomandibular wedging: 8 patients owing to the presence of ant FU, 16 patients owing to the presence of post FU. The 6 patients who have 8 FU post i.e the maximum number of functional units are edentulous wearing complete dentures.

A vertical dimension of occlusion (VDO) exists of the patients who had a wedging, that were 60 % of the patients (24 patients). VDO is decreased at 1/3 of the patients.

37,5 % of the patients (15 patients) presented a mandibular protrusion: 3 patients wore complete dentures with a decreased VDO, 8 patients had no FU post and no wedging, 3 patients had no post FU but had a wedging owing to the presence of anterior teeth, 1 patient had 5 post FU with a correct VDO.

4. Discussion

Among 24 patients who had a maxillomandibular wedging due to the presence of anterior FU (8 patients) or posterior FU (16 patients), only 5 patients presented swallowing difficulties.

Two patients who had a posterior wedging ie posterior FU cough during the meal, they present mandibular protrusion: it can be explained by an insufficient wedging (2 to 4 FU instead of 8). Three patients, who had a wedging with anterior FU, coughed during the meal and did not chew vertically. They also presented a mandibular protrusion explained by the lack of posterior contacts.

The swallowing difficulties for these five patients can be explained by an unstable wedging: because of the mandibular protrusion, the epiglottis blocks incorrectly the upper air tracts and so these patients do not chew vertically.

All the patients who had a wedge due to natural posterior teeth chew vertically.

Six complete denture wearers did not present swallowing difficulties: these prostheses assured a reproducible and reliable wedging. Among these patients, four patients chewed vertically and two others did not chew vertically: they wore a worn complete denture, with a decreased VDO. Imaizaki et al [33] show the roles of prosthetic teeth during swallowing: particularly supporting the function of the tongue to perform skillful movements for the passage of food to the oropharynx and maintaining the mandible in a constant position near the intercuspal position i.e. without protrusion.

Among 16 patients who had no maxillomandibular wedging, 14 present swallowing difficulties and had an uncoordinated chewing.

Two patients without wedging and without dysphagia maintained a vertical chewing. They wore complete dentures, but a very recent loss of these prostheses could explain the persistence of a "reflex of chewing ".

The dental status was very poor for the patients who had no wedging: they had 14 absent teeth by arch and more than two roots, while the patients who had a maxillomandibular wedging have 4 absent teeth on average and less than one root.

All the patients who needed a partial or total assistance seemed predisposed to dysphagia: they had disrupted chewing and\or coughed before or after having swallowed and\or spat out their food. One patient who needed no assistance to eat coughed during swallowing. This could be explained by a very poor oral state and thus a bad constitution of the food bolus.

One patient had complete dentures which allowed him to make correct wedging, with a correct VDO and without protrusion. He benefited from partial help during the meals of mashed food. He absorbed no sialoprive medicine. He did not present swallowing difficulties but chewed incorrectly. This fact can be explained by the inflexible bending of the head which never allowed him to sit down properly.

It is difficult to correlate the oral status of the patients and the swallowing difficulties to textures of food and drinks. The dietician always gave his viewpoint without dental status. Also, the textures of food and drinks were not re-evaluated regularly.

It is difficult to correlate the functional status (particularly the maxillomandibular wedging) and the cough: the patients who have no FU cough sometimes before or sometimes after having swallowed during the same meal. The oral phase and the pharyngeal phase cannot be dissociated during the meal observation. But the cough is constant for these patients.

The study carried out by Kayser-Jones et al. [39] with a similar population (institutionalized old patients) observed for 6 months emphasized the crucial role of the medical staff for the sitting down of the patients, the position of the head and the help in eating to the meals but also the adaptation of the texture of food. On the other hand, no dental or prosthetic data are taken into account.

5. Conclusion

The starting of swallowing is situated in the mouth and more exactly on the dental arcades: the natural or artificial teeth incise, crush, and mix food with saliva, the tongue, the lips and the cheeks until the bolus is formed. Then, the jaw is stabilized by an efficient maxillomandibular wedging during the bolus expulsion towards the oesophagus. This description points out the importance of the maxillomandibular position during the function of masticating-swallowing.

This descriptive study shows frequent associations between the oral and dental status, the maxillomandibular wedging and the dysphagia among a representative population living in the long-term care unit i.e older patients who have a poor general health and take some medicines. Moreover, the absence of a correct wedging and particularly premolomolar wedging and also a disrupted mastication seem to be factors causing dysphagia. So, the improvement of functional oral status and the preserving of dental status seem to be good objectives to prevent dysphagia.

6. References

[1] Robert D., Giovanni A., Zanaret M. Physiologie de la déglutition. *Encycl Méd Chir* : Paris Elsevier 1996 Oto-Rhino-laryngologie, 20-801-A-10, 12 p.

[2] Chevalier D. Biomécanique de la déglutition pp 287-294 in : les troubles de la parole et de la déglutition dans la maladie de Parkinson : Marseille Ed Solal 2005.

[3] Woda A, Mishellany A, Peyron MA. The regulation of masticatory function and food bolus formation. *J Oral Rehabil* 2006; 33:840–9.

[4] Palmer JB. Integration of oral and pharyngeal bolus propulsion: a new model for the physiology of swallowing. *J Dysphagia Rehabil* 1997;1:15–30.

[5] Hiiemae KM, Palmer JB. Food transport and bolus formation during complete feeding sequences on foods of different initial consistency. *Dysphagia* 1999; 14:31–42.

[6] Tamura F., Mizukami M Ayani R. Mukai Y. Analysis of feeding function and jaw stability in bedridden elderly. *Dysphagia* 2002; 17: 235-241.

[7] Ono T, Hori K, Nokubi T. Pattern of Tongue Pressure on Hard Palate During Swallowing. *Dysphagia* 2004 ; 19:259-264.

[8] Prinz J.F., Lucas P.W. Swallow thresholds in human mastication. *Archs Oral Biol* 1995; 40 (5): 401-403.

[9] Saitoh E, Shibata S, Matsuo K, Baba M, Fujii W, Palmer JB. Chewing and Food Consistency: Effects on Bolus Transport and Swallow Initiation. *Dysphagia* 2007 ; 22:100–107.

[10] Campbell-Taylor I. Oropharyngeal dysphagia in long-term care: misperceptions of treatment efficacity. *J Am Med Dir Assoc* 2008; 9: 523–531.

[11] Boczko F. Patients' Awareness of Symptoms of Dysphagia. *J Am Med Dir Assoc* 2006; 7: 587–590

[12] Mazille M-N, Nicolas E, Veyrune J-L, Roger-Leroi V, Hennequin M. Down Syndrome: Need for Jaw Stabilization to Prevent Dysphagia . Chapter 10 In: Handbook of Dental Care, Ed Jose C. Taggart, Nova Science Publishers, Inc, 2009.

[13] Ekberg O., Hamdy S.H., Woisard V., Wuttge-Hannig A., Ortega P. Social and psychological burden of dysphagia : its impact on diagnosis and treatment. *Dysphagia* 2002; 17: 139-142.

[14] Akhtar A, Shaikh A, Funnye. Dysphagia in elderly people. *J Am Med Dir Assoc* 2002,3 (1): 16-20

[15] Gelperin A. Sudden death in the elderly population from aspiration of food. *J.Am Geriatr Soc* 1974; 22: 135-136.

[16] Kosta J C, Mitchell C A. Current procedures for diagnosing dysphagia in elderly clients. *Geriatric Nursing* 1998; 19(4), 195-200.

[17] O'Loughlin G, Shanley C. Swallowing problems in the nursing home: a novel training response. *Dysphagia* 1998; 13: 172-183.

[18] Mioche L., Bourdiol P., Monier S., Martin J.F., Cormier D. Changes in jaw muscles activity with age: effects on food bolus properties. *Physiology and Behavior* 2004; 82: 621-627.

[19] Troche MS, Sapienza CM, John C. Rosenbek JC, Effects of Bolus Consistency on Timing and Safety of Swallow in Patients with Parkinson's Disease. *Dysphagia* 2008 ; 23:26–32.

[20] Baum B.J., Bodner L. Aging and oral motor function. Evidence for altered performance among older persons. *J Dent Res* 1983; 63: 2-6.

[21] Koshino H., Hirai T., Ishijima T., Ikeda Y. Tongue motor skill and masticatory performance in adult dentates, elderly dentates, and complete denture wearers. *J Prosthet Dent* 1997; 77: 147-152.

[22] Terpenning MS, Taylor GW, Lopatin DE, Kerr CK, Dominguez BL, Loesche WJ. Aspiration pneumonia: dental and oral risk factors in an older veteran population. *J. Am Geriatr.Soc* 2001, 49:557-63.

[23] Kim I.S., Han T.R. Influence of mastication and salivation on swallowing in stroke patients. *Arch Phys Med Rehabil* 2005; 86: 1986-90.

[24] Feldman R.S., Alman J., Muench M.E., Chauncey H.H. Longitudinal stability and masticatory function of human dentition. *Gerodontology* 1984; 3: 107-113.

[25] Tramini P, Montal S, Valcarcel J: Tooth loss and associated factors in long-term institutionalised elderly patients. *Gerodontology* 2007; 24: 196-203.

[26] Gluhak C, Arnetzl GV, Kirmeier R, Jakse N ,Arnetzl G. Oral status among seniors in nine nursing homes in Styria, Austria. *Gerodontology* 2009; 27:47-52.

[27] Lamy M., Mojon Ph., Kalykakis G., Legrand R., Butz-Jorgensen E. Oral status and nutrition in the institutionalized elderly. *J Dent* 1999; 27: 443-448.

[28] Chen P-H, Golub JS, Hapner ER, Johns MM. Prevalence of Perceived Dysphagia and Quality-of-Life Impairment in a Geriatric Population. *Dysphagia* 2009 ; 24:1–6

[29] Robbins J., Hamilton J.W., Lof C.L., Kempster G.B. Oropharyngeal swallowing in normal adults of different ages. *Gastroenterol* 1992; *103*: 823-829.

[30] Hildebrandt G.H., Dominguez B.L., Schork M.A., Loesche W.J. Functional units, chewing, swallowing and food avoidance among the elderly. *J Prosthet Dent* 1997; 77: 588-595.

[31] Vissink A., Spijkervet F.K.L., Amerongen A.V.N. Aging and saliva: a review of the literature. *Special Care Dent* 1996; 16(3): 95-103.

[32] Robbins J., Levine R., Wood J., Roecker E.B., Luschei E. Age effects on lingual pressure generation as a risk factor for dysphagia. *J Gerontol* 1995; 5(5): 257-262.

[33] Imaizaki T, Nishi Y, Kaji A, Nagaoka E. Roles of the artificial tooth arch during swallowing in edentates. *Journal of Prosthodontic Research* 2010; 54: 14–23.

[34] Liedberg B, Stoltze K, Owall B. The masticatory handicap of wearing removable dentures in elderly men. *Gerodontology* 2005; 22:10–16

[35] Avci M., Aslan M. Measuring pressures under maxillary complete dentures during swallowing at various occlusal vertical dimensions. Part II: Swallowing pressures, *J. Prosth. Dent.* 1991; 65: pp 808-812.

[36] Ishida R., Palmer J.B., Hiiemae K. Hyoid motion during swallowing: factors affecting forward and upward displacement. . *Dysphagia* 2002; 17: 235-241.

[37] Martone AL. Anatomy of facial expression and its prothodontic significance. *J Prosthet Dent* 1962; 12:1020–42.

[38] Katz S, Ford AB, Moskowitz RW et al. Studies of illness in the aged; the index of ADL; a standardized measure of biological and psychosocial function. *JAMA* 1963 ; Sep 21;185:914-9.

[39] Kayser-Jones J, Pengilly K. Dysphagia among nursing home residents. *Geriatric Nursing* 1999; 20(2), 77-84.

5

Association of Disease-Specific Mortality with Fitness Measurements and Nonparticipation in an 80-Year-Old Population

Yutaka Takata et al.*
Kyushu Dental College, Kitakyushu
Japan

1. Introduction

A lower level of physical fitness and activity is known to be associated with a shorter survival rate in community-dwelling populations of adults and elderly (Blair et al., 2001; Erlichman et al., 2002; Rantanen, 2003; Mitnitski et al., 2005). Subjects' cardiorespiratory fitness level based on a cycle ergometer or treadmill was predictive of total mortality (Kampert et al., 1996; Bodegard et al., 2005; Park et al., 2009), fatal cardiac event (Laukkanen et al., 2004; Bodegard et al., 2005), or cancer mortality (Evenson et al., 2003) in adult persons. Leisure time activity and walking pace were also inversely associated with all-cause mortality and mortalities due to coronary heart disease, cardiovascular disease, respiratory disease, and cancers in middle-aged men (Kampert et al., 1996; Simith et al., 2000; Lam et al., 2004; Batty et al., 2010).

In an elderly population of 75-year-olds, poor physical activity was a predictor of mortality in women but not in men (Era and Rantanen, 1997). Increasing and maintaining physical activity could lengthen life for older women aged between 65 and 75 years (Gregg et al., 2003). Physical fitness as measured by the stepping rate of legs was also inversely related to all-cause 4-year mortality in an 80-year-old population (Takata et al., 2007). In an elderly population, poor muscle strength is related to increased mortality. Lowest tertiles of 75- and 80-year-old individuals for strength of handgrip, elbow flexion, knee extension, trunk extension, and trunk flexion had a higher total mortality than that of individuals in the highest tertiles (Portegijs et al., 2007). Handgrip strength was a predictor of all-cause mortality in the oldest elderly population (Ling et al., 2010), persons aged 65 and over (Gale et al., 2007), and persons aged 70-79 years (Newman et al., 2006).

As mentioned above, although a lower level of physical activity, physical fitness, or muscle strength is likely to be associated with a higher total mortality in an elderly population, the

---

* Toshihiro Ansai[1], Inho Soh[1], Shuji Awano[1], Yutaka Yoshitake[2], Yasuo Kimura[3], Ikuo Nakamichi[1], Sumio Akifusa[1], Kenichi Goto[1], Akihiro Yoshida[1], Ritsuko Fujisawa[1], Kazuo Sonoki[1] and Tatsuji Nishihara[1]
[1]*Kyushu Dental College, Kitakyushu, Japan*
[2]*National Institute of Fitness and Sports in Kanoya, Kanoya, Japan*
[3]*Saga University, Saga, Japan*

association between these findings and disease-specific mortality has not been investigated. Therefore, the purpose of the present study was to determine an association in physical fitness measurements including muscle strength with disease-specific mortality during a 12-year follow-up in an 80-year-old population.

2. Materials and methods

In 1998, a total of 1282 individuals who were 80 years old resided in three cities (Buzen, Yukuhashi, and Munakata), four towns (Katsuyama, Tikujo, Toyotsu, and Kanda), one village (Shinyoshitomi), and one ward (Tobata of Kikakyushu City) in Japan's Fukuoka Prefecture. These nine locations were selected randomly from urban, suburban, and rural communities with the goal of achieving a balance of living environments, including socio-demographic backgrounds, dietary habits, health behaviors, and medical treatment. Of these 1282 individuals, 694 (54.1%) (274 males and 420 females) agreed to participate in the present study, and each participant underwent both a physical examination and a laboratory blood examination. The 694 participants were followed up for 12 years after the baseline examination. Confirmation of whether the patient was living or had died was obtained by asking the family via a telephone call or home visit. The cause of death was classified according to the 10th version of the International Classification of Diseases (ICD-10). Thirty-eight subjects were lost to follow-up over the 12 years. The study was conducted according to the principles expressed in the Declaration of Helsinki and was approved by the Human Investigations Committee of Kyushu Dental College. Informed consent for study participation was obtained from all participants.

Measurements of physical fitness included hand-grip strength, one-leg standing time, leg extensor strength of a single leg, leg extensor strength of both legs, stepping rate of legs, and isokinetic leg extensor power. The numbers of subjects participating in these physical fitness tests were 642, 551, 555, 556, 567, and 547, respectively. Hand-grip strength was measured in each hand using a Smedley hand dynamometer (DM-100s; Yagami, Nagoya, Japan). The best value of two trials for each hand was taken as the score for the test. One-leg standing time was measured with the eyes open. This time represented the number of seconds until the subject had to hop, since the subject was instructed to hop as a way to avoid putting the raised foot down, until the raised foot was lowered to the floor, or until 2 min had elapsed. One trial was performed on the right and one on the left leg; the better score was used for statistical analysis. The leg extensor strength test was measured using a portable chair incorporating a strain gauge connected to a load cell. The subject sat in the chair in a vertical position with the legs hanging vertically and the knee initially bent at 90°. The trial was performed three times—once for each leg individually, and again for both legs simultaneously. The value for each side in this test was summed as the subject's score for leg extension strength of single leg. On the other hand, the value for both legs simultaneously was used as leg extension strength of both legs. The stepping rate was measured using an industrial stepping rate counter (Stepping Counter; Yagami, Nagoya, Japan); while sitting, the subject was instructed to step with each leg as rapidly as possible during 10 seconds. The stepping rate for both legs was summed as the subject's score. Isokinetic leg extensor power was determined by a dynamometer (Aneropress 3500; Combi, Tokyo, Japan). The subject sat on the seat of the instrument and was instructed to press his or her feet forward on the plate as rapidly as possible until the legs were fully extended. The body mass of the subject was applied as resistance. The best score from five trials was used for statistical analysis.

All data are reported as means ± SD. Differences in mean values between groups were assessed by analysis of variance. Categorical variables were compared using the χ^2 test. Associations between physical fitness and time to 12-year mortality were assessed using the multivariate Cox proportional hazards regression model. Gender, smoking, body mass index (BMI), and levels of total serum cholesterol and glucose were fitted as continuous variables. Comparisons of the survival rates among groups according to physical fitness measurements and participation in tests were assessed by the method of Kaplan and Meier, followed by a log-rank test to assess the significance between survival curves. All statistical analyses were performed using SPSS 16.0 (SPSS Japan, Inc., Tokyo, Japan). Results were considered statistically significant when P had a value below 0.05.

3. Results

During the follow-up period of 12 years from April 1998 to March 2010, out of 694 subjects who participated in the present study, 414 died, 242 were alive, and 38 were lost to follow-up. The follow-up rate was 94.5%. Of the 414 who died, 106 deaths were due to cardiovascular and cerebrovascular diseases, 73 to respiratory disease, 71 to cancer, 39 to senility, 18 to digestive system disease, 14 to exogenous death, 7 to neurological disease, 6 to urinary tract diseases, 12 to other diseases, and 68 to unknown reasons. The percentages of death due to all causes for men and women were 75.5% and 54.7% (χ^2=29.184, P=0.000), those of death due to cardiovascular and cerebrovascular diseases for men and women were 18.1% and 14.8% (χ^2=1.254, P=0.281), those of death due to cancers for men and women were 14.0% and 8.7% (χ^2=4.539, P=0.040), those of death due to respiratory diseases for men and women were 16.2% and 7.7% (χ^2=11.686, P=0.001), and those of death due to senility for men and women were 4.2% and 7.2% (χ^2=2.560, P=0.130), respectively. The cardiovascular cerebrovascular diseases suffered by study participants were heart failure (37), brain infarction (23), myocardial infarction (16), aortic aneurysm (9), brain bleeding (3), ischemic heart diseast (3), hypertension (2), stroke (1), pulmonary infarction (1), sick sinus syndrome (1), subdural bleeding (1), subarachnoidal bleeding (1), carotid artery aneurysm (1), angina (1), and cardiac rupture. Details were unknown in 5 cases. The respiratory diseases suffered by study participants were pneumonia (59), respiratory failure (8), bronchial asthma (1), emphysema (1), chronic bronchitis (1), and chronic obstructive lung disease (1). Details were unknown in 2 cases. The cancers suffered by study participants were lung cancer (16), gastric cancer (12), hepatic cancer (10), colon cancer (6), urinary tract cancer (5), pancreatic cancer (4), uterine cancer (4), bile duct cancer (2), ovarian cancer (1), leukemia (1), gallbladder cancer (1), multiple myeloma (1), laryngeal cancer (1), peritoneal cancer (1), chondrosarcoma (1), malignant lymphoma (1), and malignant mesothelioma (1). Details were unknown in 2 cases.

Basal characteristics at the start of study in individuals at age of 80-year who died or did not die during the following 12-year are shown in Table 1. BMI and serum level of total cholesterol were lower in non-survivors than in survivors, while serum level of glucose was higher in the former than in the latter. Systolic blood pressure (SBP) did not differ between individuals who were alive and those who died during the follow-up period. Men and smokers were more prevalent in the non-survivor than in the survivor group, whereas no difference was found in the percent of alcohol drinkers or the percent who suffered complications between the non-survivors and the survivors.

	Alive (n)	Dead (n)	P-value
SBP, mmHg	151.0±22.5 (230)	149.7±23.9 (384)	0.517
Cholesterol, mg/dL	214.4±35.3 (235)	199.6±38.2 (399)***	0.000
Glucose, mg/dL	115.0±40.7 (233)	126.1±57.5 (395)**	0.005
BMI, kg/m^2	23.2±3.1 (241)	22.4±3.4 (397)**	0.006
% Men	26.9% (242)	48.3% (414)***	0.000
% Smokers	4.6% (240)	17.7% (407)***	0.000
% Alcohol drinkers	56.7% (231)	54.8% (403)	0.648
% Complications	84.1% (232)	83.5% (401)	0.867

Table 1. Basal characteristics at the start of study in individuals at age of 80-year-old who die or did not die during the following 12-year period. *P<0.05, **P<0.01, ***P<0.001

At the start of the study, when all participants were 80 years old, 642, 551, 555, 556, 567, and 547 individuals completed the handgrip strength test, one-leg standing test, leg extension strength test of a single leg, leg extension strength test of both legs, stepping rate test of legs, and leg extension power test, respectively. Scores for each physical fitness test were compared between men (Table 2A) or women (Table 2B) who were alive and those who died from all causes, cardiovascular disease, respiratory disease, cancer, or senility during the 12-year follow-up period. Scores of handgrip strength, one-leg standing, leg extension strength of a single leg, leg extension strength of both legs, and leg extension power were higher in men who survived than in those in the all-cause mortality group, while scores of stepping rate of legs were not different. Scores for handgrip strength, leg extension strength of a single leg, leg extension strength of both legs, and leg extension power were higher in men who did not die due to respiratory disease than in those who died due to respiratory disease. Men who did not die due to senility also had a higher score of one-leg standing time than that of men who died due to senility. Similarly, in women, scores for handgrip strength, leg extension strength of a single leg, leg extension strength of both legs, stepping rate of legs, and leg extension power were higher in survivors than in non-survivors. Scores for stepping rate were slightly higher in women who did not die due to cardiovascular disease than in women who died due to cardiovascular disease. Women who did not die from respiratory disease had a higher score for leg extension power than that of women who died from respiratory disease. Women who died from cancer had a slightly higher score of leg extension strength of a single leg than that of women who did not die from cancer. Scores for handgrip strength, leg extension strength of a single leg, leg extension strength of both legs, and leg extension power were higher in women who did not die due to senility than in women who died due to senility.

A. Men

	Alive			Died			P value
	n	Mean	SD	n	Mean	SD	
Handgrip strength							
All-cause death	61	33.8	6.2	186	31.1**	6.4	0.005
Cardiovascular death	204	31.9	6.4	43	31.2	6.5	0.554
Respiratory death	207	32.3	6.4	40	29.2**	5.9	0.006
Cancer death	212	32.0	6.2	35	30.5	7.4	0.227
Senile death	237	31.7	6.5	10	32.5	5.0	0.711
One-leg standing time							
All-cause death	54	22.0	22.0	155	15.4*	18.7	0.033
Cardiovascular death	174	17.4	19.9	35	15.8	19.4	0.659
Respiratory death	180	17.3	19.8	29	15.8	20.0	0.693
Cancer death	178	17.6	20.5	31	14.5	15.1	0.428
Senile death	201	17.5	20.1	8	7.8***	2.8	0.000
Leg extension strength (right leg + left leg)							
All-cause death	59	57.3	13.2	163	51.5**	15.1	0.009
Cardiovascular death	185	52.4	14.7	37	56.2	15.2	0.147
Respiratory death	189	50.0	13.3	32	45.4**	13.7	0.001
Cancer death	190	53.3	15.1	32	51.2	13.0	0.443
Senile death	214	52.9	14.9	8	56.3	10.3	0.530
Leg extension strength (both legs)							
All-cause death	59	52.9	12.5	162	47.5**	13.7	0.009
Cardiovascular death	184	48.8	13.6	37	49.6	13.5	0.750
Respiratory death	189	50.0	13.3	32	42.8**	13.5	0.006
Cancer death	189	49.1	13.6	32	47.8	13.2	0.620
Senile death	213	48.8	13.6	8	53.9	12.8	0.295
Stepping rate of legs							
All-cause death	59	68.6	14.8	166	64.9	15.6	0.116
Cardiovascular death	187	66.4	15.8	38	63.7	13.8	0.345
Respiratory death	193	65.9	15.3	32	66.1	17.0	0.951
Cancer death	193	65.7	15.6	32	67.5	14.7	0.539
Senile death	217	65.5	15.5	8	76.4	11.7	0.051
Leg extension power							
All-cause death	59	568.2	160.2	163	461.7***	180.4	0.000
Cardiovascular death	182	493.1	177.9	40	476.1	197.1	0.593
Respiratory death	191	501.4	178.0	31	419.7*	187.5	0.019
Cancer death	191	495.3	183.8	31	457.3	163.2	0.279
Senile death	214	489.4	182.1	8	505.3	166.0	0.799

B. Women

	Alive			Died			P value
	n	Mean	SD	n	Mean	SD	
Handgrip strength							
All-cause death	166	21.8	3.3	193	20.2***	4.7	0.000
Cardiovascular death	304	20.9	4.1	55	21.1	4.7	0.743
Respiratory death	332	21.0	4.2	27	19.9	4.0	0.161
Cancer death	328	20.9	4.2	31	21.4	4.4	0.504
Senile death	336	21.1	4.1	23	18.7**	4.2	0.009
One-leg standing time							
All-cause death	150	12.2	13.4	160	10.6	11.9	0.280
Cardiovascular death	262	11.6	13.0	48	9.9	10.4	0.388
Respiratory death	288	11.2	12.8	22	13.2	10.5	0.474
Cancer death	282	11.2	12.1	28	13.2	17.6	0.427
Senile death	290	11.6	13.0	20	8.6	6.6	0.307
Leg extension strength (right leg + left leg)							
All-cause death	144	37.0	11.9	156	31.8***	12.4	0.000
Cardiovascular death	254	34.5	12.2	46	33.3	13.3	0.547
Respiratory death	278	34.5	12.4	22	31.7	11.5	0.308
Cancer death	270	33.8	12.4	30	38.6*	11.4	0.042
Senile death	282	35.0	12.2	18	23.4***	10.4	0.000
Leg extension strength (both legs)							
All-cause death	146	32.1	10.5	156	28.2**	10.7	0.001
Cardiovascular death	254	29.9	10.3	48	30.9	12.9	0.548
Respiratory death	280	30.3	10.7	22	27.2	10.9	0.202
Cancer death	273	29.8	11.0	29	32.0	8.0	0.293
Senile death	284	30.7	10.6	18	20.4***	8.9	0.000
Stepping rate of legs							
All-cause death	148	59.3	13.3	161	55.5*	13.5	0.014
Cardiovascular death	261	58.0	13.5	48	53.7*	13.2	0.042
Respiratory death	287	57.4	13.5	22	56.2	14.6	0.687
Cancer death	279	57.1	13.8	30	59.4	11.3	0.391
Senile death	290	57.3	13.6	19	58.0	13.4	0.829
Leg extension power							
All-cause death	142	273.1	103.5	150	236.1**	99.7	0.002
Cardiovascular death	247	254.4	101.8	45	252.4	110.7	0.907
Respiratory death	271	257.5	103.9	21	210.2*	81.9	0.019
Cancer death	263	250.3	102.4	29	288.3	104.8	0.059
Senile death	277	257.3	102.8	15	195.1*	92.1	0.023

Table 2. Physical fitness measurements at the start of the study in 80-year-old men (A) and women (B) who died or did not die due to all causes, cardiovascular disease, respiratory disease, cancer, or senility, during the 12-year follow-up period.. *P<0.05, **P<0.01, ***P<0.001

Overall survival curves obtained by the Kaplan-Meier method during the 12-year follow-up period in men and women who had a higher score, lower score, or did not participate in physical fitness tests such as handgrip strength (Fig. 1A), one-leg standing (Fig. 1B), leg extension strength of a single leg (Fig. 1C), leg extension strength of both legs (Fig. 1D), stepping rate of legs (Fig. 1E), and leg extension power (Fig. 1F) are shown in Figure 1. Table 3A shows the χ^2 and P with the log rank test by the Kaplan-Meier method for comparisons of the overall survival curves among groups. Men and women who had a high score on the handgrip strength test survived longer than those with a low score. Women with a high score on the handgrip test also survived longer than women who did not participate in this test (Fig 1A, Table 3A). The survival rate in the group with a high score on the one-leg standing test was better than that in men or women nonparticipants. Women with a low score on the one-leg standing time test also had a better survival rate than that of those who did not participate in this fitness test (Fig. 1B, Table 3A). Men and women with high scores for leg extension strength of a single leg, leg extension strength of both legs, or leg extension power had a better survival rate than that of those with low scores on these tests or that of those who did not participate in these tests. Men with low scores for leg extension strength of both legs also survived slightly longer than nonparticipants (Figs. 1C, 1D, 1F, Table 3A). Men or women with high scores for stepping rate had a better survival rate than those who did not participate in this test. Women with a high score for stepping rate also had a better survival rate than that of those with a low score (Fig. 1E, Table 3A).

Survival rates for men who did not die from cardiovascular diseases were better in those with a high score on the leg extension strength test of both legs and on the stepping rate test of legs than for those who did not participate in these fitness tests. Men with cardiovascular disease and with a low score on the leg extension strength test of a single leg or both legs also had a better survival rate than that of nonparticipants. Women with high score on stepping rate test also did not die from cardiovascular diseases as compared to women with low score on this test (Table 3B).

Survival curves in men and women who did not die due to respiratory disease also were compared among individuals with a high score, a low score, or nonparticipation for various fitness tests. Men and women with high score on leg extension power test had better survival rate from respiratory disease than those with low score or nonparticipation on this test. Men with low score on the leg extension power test also had a better survival rate than that of nonparticipants. Men with high score on leg extension strength test of single leg and leg extension strength test of both legs had longer survival curves from respiratory disease than men with low score or without participation on these fitness tests. Longer survival curves from respiratory disease were found in men with a high score on the handgrip test than in those with a low score. Similarly, men with a high score on the one-leg standing time test or the stepping rate test survived longer than nonparticipants. Men with a low score on the stepping rate test also survived longer than men who were nonparticipants (Table 3C).

Survival curves in men and women, who did not die from cancer, were not different among individuals with high score, low score, and nonparticipation for each fitness test (Table 3D). Men with low score for leg extension strength test of double legs or stepping rate test of leg died from senility fewer than nonparticipants. Survival rate in men who did not die from senility were longer in those with high score for leg extension power test than in those without participation. A better survival rate was found in women with high score for

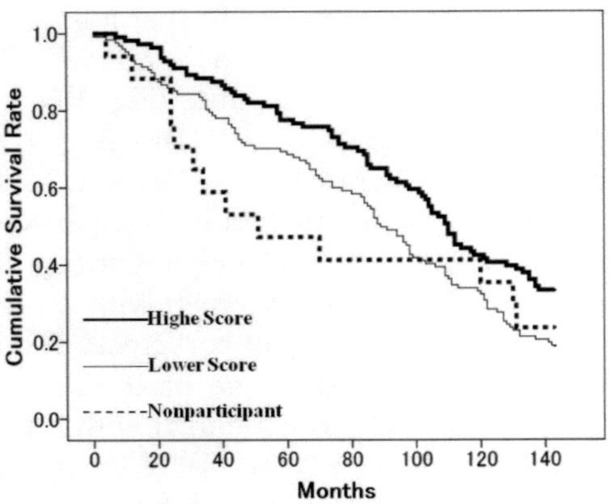

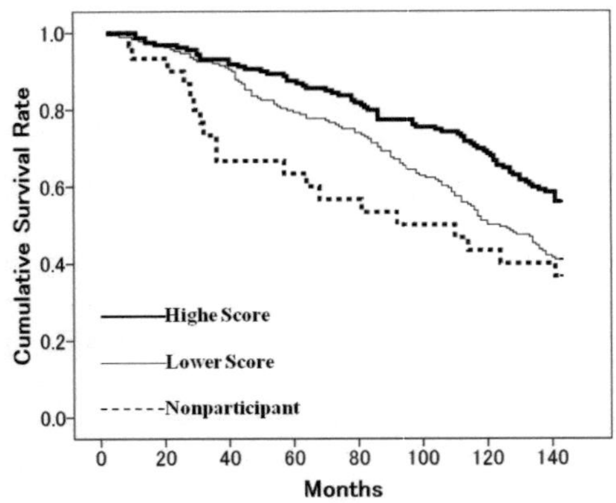

Men Women

A. Handgrip strength

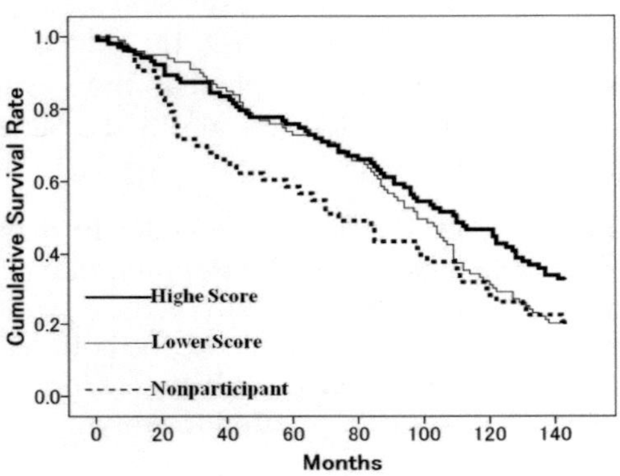

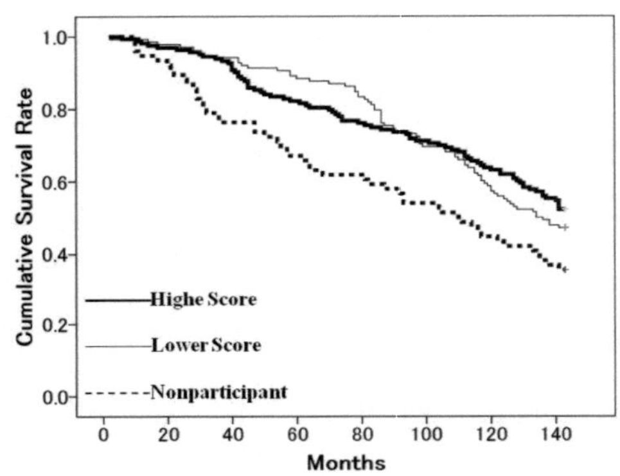

Men Women

B. One-leg standing

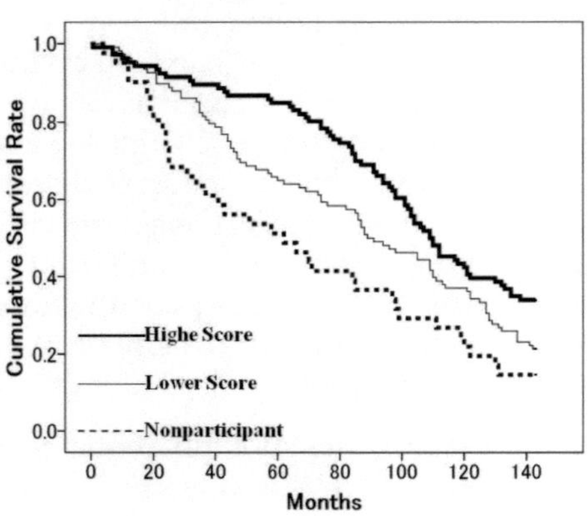

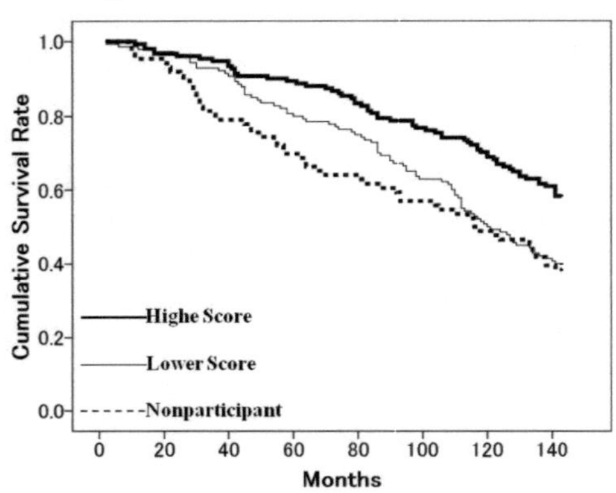

Men Women

C. Leg extension strength of a single leg (right leg + left leg)

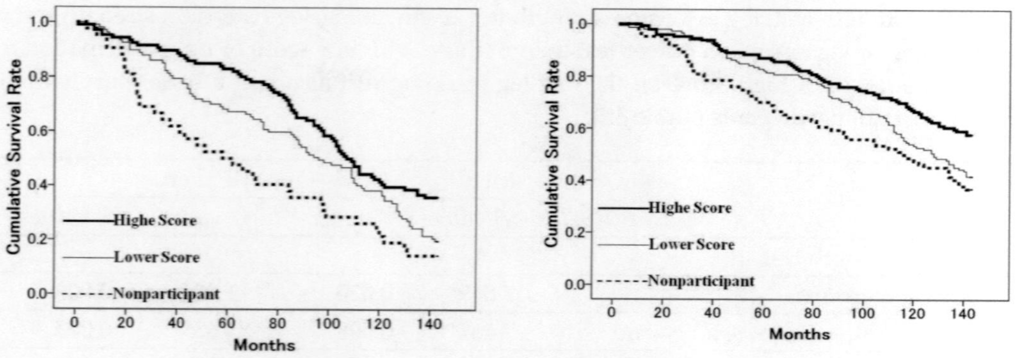

Men Women

D. Leg extension strength of both legs

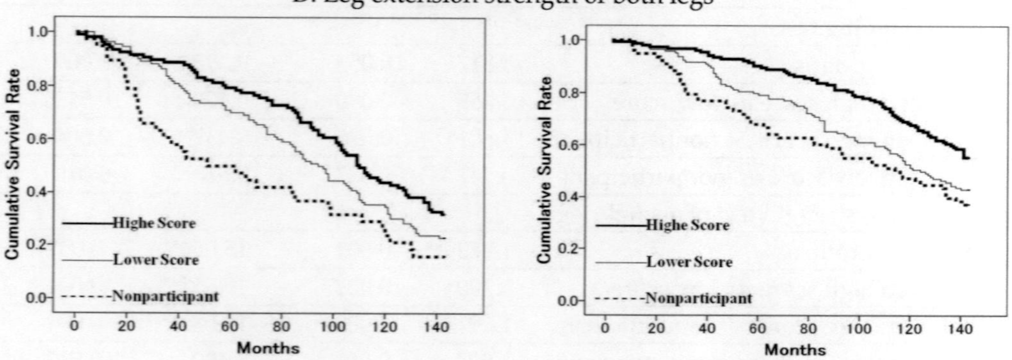

Men Women

E. Stepping rate of legs

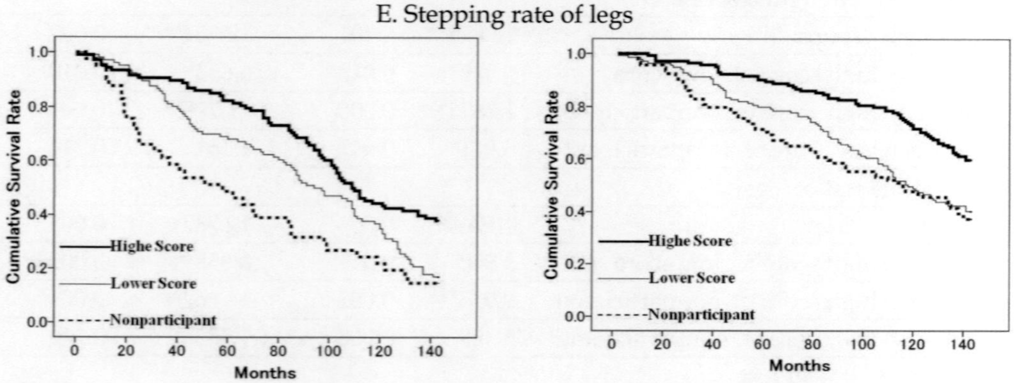

Men Women

F. Leg extension power

Fig. 1. Overall survival curve during the 12-year follow-up period in men and women who had a higher score (▬▬▬), lower score (———), or did not participate (············) in physical fitness tests such as handgrip strength (Fig. 1A), one-leg standing (Fig. 1B), leg extension strength of a single leg (Fig. 1C), leg extension strength of both legs (Fig. 1D), stepping rate of legs (Fig. 1E), and leg extension power (Fig. 1F) .

handgrip strength test, leg extension strength test of single leg, leg extension strength test of double legs, or leg extension power test than in those with low score or nonparticipation for test. Women with a high score on the one-leg standing test also had a better survival rate than that of nonparticipants (Table 3E).

	Men		Women	
	χ^2 value	P values	χ^2 value	P values
Handgrip strength test				
among 3 groups	7.849*	0.020	11.904**	0.003
between high score *vs.* low score	7.467**	0.006	8.743**	0.003
between high score *vs.* nonparticipant	2.249	0.134	7.452**	0.006
between low score *vs.* nonparticipant	0.011	0.917	1.147	0.284
One-leg standing test				
among 3 groups	5.817	0.055	9.333**	0.009
between high score *vs.* low score	3.058	0.080	0.428	0.513
between high score *vs.* nonparticipant	4.801*	0.028	8.437**	0.004
between low score *vs.* nonparticipant	0.747	0.387	5.513*	0.019
Leg extension strength test of a single leg				
among 3 groups	13.729**	0.001	15.064**	0.001
between high score *vs.* low score	5.200*	0.023	10.651**	0.001
between high score *vs.* nonparticipant	12.912***	0.000	12.088**	0.001
between low score *vs.* nonparticipant	3.500	0.061	0.430	0.512
Leg extension strength test of both legs				
among 3 groups	14.970**	0.001	12.904**	0.002
between high score *vs.* low score	5.577*	0.018	6.663*	0.010
between high score *vs.* nonparticipant	13.671***	0.000	11.709**	0.001
between low score *vs.* nonparticipant	3.941*	0.047	1.551	0.213
Stepping rate test of legs				
among 3 groups	10.760**	0.005	12.787**	0.002
between high score *vs.* low score	3.800	0.051	6.858**	0.009
between high score *vs.* nonparticipant	9.935**	0.002	11.662**	0.001
between low score *vs.* nonparticipant	3.320	0.068	1.383	0.240
Leg extension power test				
among 3 groups	19.701***	0.000	19.175***	0.000
between high score *vs.* low score	9.682**	0.002	13.530***	0.000
between high score *vs.* nonparticipant	16.706***	0.000	16.197***	0.000
between low score *vs.* nonparticipant	3.520	0.061	0.597	0.440

A. Comparisons among survival curves during the 12-year follow-up period in men or women who did not die from any cause, and had a high score, low score, or nonparticipation in the physical fitness tests listed.

	Men		Women	
	χ^2 value	P values	χ^2 value	P values
Handgrip strength test				
among 3 groups	2.724	0.256	0.801	0.670
between high score *vs.* low score	0.582	0.446	0.726	0.394
between high score *vs.* nonparticipant	2.752	0.097	0.025	0.875
between low score *vs.* nonparticipant	1.345	0.246	0.194	0.660
One-leg standing test				
among 3 groups	4.030	0.133	0.015	0.993
between high score *vs.* low score	0.917	0.338	0.000	0.996
between high score *vs.* nonparticipant	3.822	0.051	0.003	0.953
between low score *vs.* nonparticipant	1.400	0.237	0.014	0.905
Leg extension strength test of a single leg				
among 3 groups	6.730*	0.035	2.766	0.251
between high score *vs.* low score	0.317	0.573	2.800	0.094
between high score *vs.* nonparticipant	3.677	0.055	0.698	0.403
between low score *vs.* nonparticipant	6.280*	0.012	0.275	0.600
Leg extension strength test of both legs				
among 3 groups	6.223*	0.045	0.196	0.907
between high score *vs.* low score	0.000	0.992	0.051	0.821
between high score *vs.* nonparticipant	4.216*	0.040	0.195	0.659
between low score *vs.* nonparticipant	5.045*	0.025	0.065	0.798
Stepping rate test of legs				
among 3 groups	8.064*	0.018	6.648*	0.036
between high score *vs.* low score	3.448	0.063	6.678*	0.010
between high score *vs.* nonparticipant	7.440**	0.006	0.972	0.324
between low score *vs.* nonparticipant	1.809	0.179	1.014	0.314
Leg extension power test				
among 3 groups	3.411	0.182	2.391	0.302
between high score *vs.* low score	1.914	0.166	2.388	0.122
between high score *vs.* nonparticipant	2.509	0.113	0.652	0.419
between low score *vs.* nonparticipant	0.481	0.488	0.250	0.617

B. Comparisons among survival curves during the 12-year follow-up period in men or women who did not die from cardiovascular disease, and had a high score, low score, or nonparticipation in the physical fitness tests listed.

	Men		Women	
	χ^2 value	P values	χ^2 value	P values
Handgrip strength test				
among 3 groups	9.739**	0.008	3.426	0.180
between high score *vs.* low score	9.992**	0.002	2.941	0.086
between high score *vs.* nonparticipant	1.979	0.160	2.089	0.148
between low score *vs.* nonparticipant	0.110	0.740	0.131	0.718
One-leg standing test				
among 3 groups	8.307*	0.016	3.646	0.162
between high score *vs.* low score	2.035	0.154	1.681	0.195
between high score *vs.* nonparticipant	7.718**	0.005	0.747	0.388
between low score *vs.* nonparticipant	2.665	0.103	3.531	0.060
Leg extension strength test of a single leg				
among 3 groups	17.233***	0.000	4.006	0.135
between high score *vs.* low score	11.127**	0.001	3.581	0.058
between high score *vs.* nonparticipant	17.127***	0.000	2.719	0.099
between low score *vs.* nonparticipant	1.656	0.198	0.000	0.999
Leg extension strength test of both legs				
among 3 groups	16.817***	0.000	4.564	0.102
between high score *vs.* low score	11.044**	0.001	3.948*	0.047
between high score *vs.* nonparticipant	16.284***	0.000	3.383	0.066
between low score *vs.* nonparticipant	1.534	0.215	0.012	0.914
Stepping rate test of legs				
among 3 groups	9.651**	0.008	1.992	0.369
between high score *vs.* low score	0.010	0.920	0.375	0.541
between high score *vs.* nonparticipant	7.836**	0.005	2.059	0.151
between low score *vs.* nonparticipant	7.124**	0.008	0.740	0.390
Leg extension power test				
among 3 groups	17.995***	0.000	11.839**	0.003
between high score *vs.* low score	7.648**	0.006	12.360***	0.000
between high score *vs.* nonparticipant	17.326***	0.000	7.351**	0.007
between low score *vs.* nonparticipant	3.989*	0.046	0.176	0.675

C. Comparisons among survival curves during the 12-year follow-up period in men or women who did not die from respiratory disease, and had a high score, low score, or nonparticipation in the physical fitness tests listed.

	Men		Women	
	χ^2 value	P values	χ^2 value	P values
Handgrip strength test				
among 3 groups	0.374	0.830	0.385	0.825
between high score *vs.* low score	0.383	0.536	0.061	0.806
between high score *vs.* nonparticipant	0.013	0.908	0.173	0.678
between low score *vs.* nonparticipant	0.014	0.907	0.377	0.539
One-leg standing test				
among 3 groups	0.726	0.696	0.480	0.787
between high score *vs.* low score	0.713	0.398	0.473	0.492
between high score *vs.* nonparticipant	0.018	0.894	0.032	0.858
between low score *vs.* nonparticipant	0.252	0.616	0.141	0.707
Leg extension strength test of a single leg				
among 3 groups	1.181	0.554	3.132	0.209
between high score *vs.* low score	1.099	0.295	1.385	0.239
between high score *vs.* nonparticipant	0.544	0.461	2.475	0.116
between low score *vs.* nonparticipant	0.011	0.915	0.363	0.547
Leg extension strength test of both legs				
among 3 groups	0.473	0.789	1.630	0.443
between high score *vs.* low score	0.415	0.519	0.999	0.318
between high score *vs.* nonparticipant	0.286	0.592	1.120	0.290
between low score *vs.* nonparticipant	0.000	0.984	0.042	0.838
Stepping rate test of legs				
among 3 groups	0.653	0.721	0.881	0.644
between high score *vs.* low score	0.444	0.505	0.012	0.914
between high score *vs.* nonparticipant	0.474	0.491	0.890	0.346
between low score *vs.* nonparticipant	0.069	0.793	0.685	0.408
Leg extension power test				
among 3 groups	2.552	0.279	1.158	0.561
between high score *vs.* low score	1.864	0.172	0.081	0.776
between high score *vs.* nonparticipant	2.011	0.156	1.149	0.284
between low score *vs.* nonparticipant	0.111	0.739	0.574	0.449

D. Comparisons among survival curves during the 12-year follow-up period in men or women who did not die from cancer, and had a high score, low score, or nonparticipation in the physical fitness tests listed.

	Men		Women	
	χ^2 value	P values	χ^2 value	P values
Handgrip strength test				
among 3 groups	0.692	0.708	13.709**	0.001
between high score *vs.* low score	0.287	0.592	7.993**	0.005
between high score *vs.* nonparticipant	0.500	0.479	14.736***	0.000
between low score *vs.* nonparticipant	0.155	0.694	2.190	0.139
One-leg standing test				
among 3 groups	3.034	0.219	3.999	0.135
between high score *vs.* low score	2.160	0.142	0.868	0.352
between high score *vs.* nonparticipant	2.960	0.085	4.126*	0.042
between low score *vs.* nonparticipant	0.151	0.697	1.369	0.242
Leg extension strength test of a single leg				
among 3 groups	4.290	0.117	14.829**	0.001
between high score *vs.* low score	0.012	0.914	12.770***	0.000
between high score *vs.* nonparticipant	3.190	0.074	14.281***	0.000
between low score *vs.* nonparticipant	3.387	0.066	0.145	0.704
Leg extension strength test of both legs				
among 3 groups	4.901	0.086	16.023***	0.000
between high score *vs.* low score	0.830	0.362	13.538***	0.000
between high score *vs.* nonparticipant	2.192	0.139	16.511***	0.000
between low score *vs.* nonparticipant	5.041*	0.025	0.315	0.575
Stepping rate test of legs				
among 3 groups	5.060	0.080	4.525	0.104
between high score *vs.* low score	0.638	0.424	0.000	0.988
between high score *vs.* nonparticipant	2.671	0.102	3.554	0.059
between low score *vs.* nonparticipant	5.046*	0.025	3.196	0.074
Leg extension power test				
among 3 groups	4.874	0.087	15.178**	0.001
between high score *vs.* low score	0.000	0.994	6.547*	0.011
between high score *vs.* nonparticipant	3.907*	0.048	15.939***	0.000
between low score *vs.* nonparticipant	3.234	0.072	2.446	0.118

E. Comparisons among survival curves during the 12-year follow-up period in men or women who did not die from senility, and had a high score, low score, or nonparticipation in the physical fitness tests listed.

Table 3. χ^2 value and P value with the log rank test by the Kaplan-Meier method for comparisons of the survival curves among groups in men or women who had a high score, a low score, or nonparticipation in physical fitness tests during the 12-year follow-up period in subjects who did not die due to any cause (A), cardiovascular diseases (B), respiratory disease (C), cancer (D), or senility (E).

Survival curves were also compared between participants and nonparticipants. Men who participated survived longer than nonparticipants in the case of the fitness tests of single or double leg extension strength, stepping rate of legs, or leg extension power, while women who participated survived longer than nonparticipants in the case of the fitness tests for one-leg standing time, single or double leg extension strength, stepping rate of legs, or leg extension power (Table 4A). Cardiovascular deaths were more prevalent in men who did not participate than in men who participated in fitness tests of single or double leg extension strength or stepping rate of legs, while no difference in cardiovascular deaths was found between women who participated and those who did not participate in any fitness test (Table 4B). Similarly, mortality due respiratory disease was more prevalent for nonparticipating men than for participating men in the case of the fitness tests of one-leg standing time, single or double leg extension strength, stepping rate of legs, or leg extension power, while there was no difference in respiratory mortality between women who participated and those who did not participate in any fitness test (Table 4C). No difference was found in cancer mortality between nonparticipants and participants in men or women (Table 4D). Mortality due to senility was higher in women who did not participate in the handgrip strength test, single or double leg extension strength test, stepping rate test of legs, and leg extension power test, whereas senility mortality was more prevalent in nonparticipating men for tests of single or double leg extension strength, stepping rate of legs, or leg extension power (Table 4E).

	Men		Women	
	χ^2 value	P values	χ^2 value	P values
Handgrip strength test				
between participants and nonparticipants	0.629	0.428	3.664	0.056
One-leg standing test				
between participants and nonparticipants	3.087	0.079	8.955	0.003**
Leg extension strength test of a single leg				
between participants and nonparticipants	9.102	0.003**	5.609	0.018*
Leg extension strength test of both legs				
between participants and nonparticipants	9.994	0.002**	6.969	0.008**
Stepping rate test of legs				
between participants and nonparticipants	7.449	0.006**	6.759	0.009**
Leg extension power test				
between participants and nonparticipants	11.226	0.001**	7.530	0.006**

A. Comparisons among survival curves during the 12-year follow-up period in men or women who did not die from any cause, between participants and nonparticipants in the physical fitness tests listed.

	Men		Women	
	χ^2 value	P values	χ^2 value	P values
Handgrip strength test				
between participants and nonparticipants	2.228	0.136	0.096	0.757
One-leg standing test				
between participants and nonparticipants	3.287	0.070	0.014	0.904
Leg extension strength test of a single leg				
between participants and nonparticipants	6.391	0.011*	0.028	0.868
Leg extension strength test of both legs				
between participants and nonparticipants	6.220	0.013*	0.141	0.708
Stepping rate test of legs				
between participants and nonparticipants	5.256	0.022*	0.003	0.957
Leg extension power test				
between participants and nonparticipants	1.793	0.181	0.028	0.867

B. Comparisons among survival curves during the 12-year follow-up period in men or women who did not die from cardiovascular disease, between participants and nonparticipants in the physical fitness tests listed.

	Men		Women	
	χ^2 value	P values	χ^2 value	P values
Handgrip strength test				
between participants and nonparticipants	0.132	0.716	0.698	0.403
One-leg standing test				
between participants and nonparticipants	6.816	0.009**	2.163	0.141
Leg extension strength test of a single leg				
between participants and nonparticipants	8.190	0.004**	0.852	0.356
Leg extension strength test of both legs				
between participants and nonparticipants	7.829	0.005**	1.063	0.302
Stepping rate test of leg				
between participants and nonparticipants	9.650	0.002**	1.702	0.192
Leg extension power test				
between participants and nonparticipants	12.316	0.000***	1.234	0.267

C. Comparisons among survival curves during the 12-year follow-up period in men or women who did not die from respiratory disease, between participants and nonparticipants in the physical fitness tests listed.

	Men		Women	
	χ^2 value	P values	χ^2 value	P values
Handgrip strength test				
between participants and nonparticipants	0.000	0.984	0.311	0.577
One-leg standing test				
between participants and nonparticipants	0.041	0.840	0.010	0.919
Leg extension strength test of a single leg				
between participants and nonparticipants	0.083	0.773	1.480	0.224
Leg extension strength test of both legs				
between participants and nonparticipants	0.059	0.808	0.492	0.483
Stepping rate test of legs				
between participants and nonparticipants	0.220	0.639	0.857	0.355
Leg extension power test				
between participants and nonparticipants	0.819	0.365	1.031	0.310

D. Comparisons among survival curves during the 12-year follow-up period in men or women who did not die from cancer, between participants who had a high score and nonparticipants in the physical fitness tests listed.

	Men		Women	
	χ^2 value	P values	χ^2 value	P values
Handgrip strength test				
between participants and nonparticipants	0.375	0.540	6.758	0.009**
One-leg standing test				
between participants and nonparticipants	1.283	0.257	3.290	0.070
Leg extension strength test of a single leg				
between participants and nonparticipants	4.284	0.038*	4.792	0.029*
Leg extension strength test of both legs				
between participants and nonparticipants	4.284	0.038*	5.421	0.020*
Stepping rate test of leg				
between participants and nonparticipants	4.537	0.033*	4.524	0.033*
Leg extension power tests				
between participants and nonparticipants	4.874	0.027*	11.045	0.001**

E. Comparisons among survival curves during the 12-year follow-up period in men or women who did not die from senility, between participants and nonparticipants in the physical fitness tests listed.
*P<0.05, **P<0.01, ***P<0.001

Table 4. χ^2 value and P value with the log rank test by the Kaplan-Meier method for comparisons of the survival curves among groups in men or women who participated or did not participate in physical fitness tests during the 12-year follow-up period in subjects who did not die due to any cause (A), cardiovascular diseases (B), respiratory disease (C), cancer (D), or senility (E).

Associations between physical fitness measurements and mortalities due to all causes, cardiovascular diseases, respiratory diseases, cancers, or senility were assessed by multivariate Cox regression analyses adjusted for gender, serum level of total cholesterol and glucose, BMI, and smoking, being performed to calculate the risk for mortality associated with a 1 kg, 1 s, 1 step/10 s, 1 W increase (continuous analysis) in each fitness measurement (Table 5). Since all subjects were 80 years old at the start of the study, age was not included as a confounding factor in these analyses. All-cause mortality adjusted for various confounding factors fell 0.2% with 1 W increase in leg extension power. Similarly, total mortality decreased by 1-2% with 1 kg increase in single or double leg extension strength. A decrease in all-cause mortality by 3% was also found with 1 kg increase in handgrip strength. A 1% fall in all-cause mortality was found with an increase of 1 s in one-leg standing time or an increase of 1 step/10 s in stepping rate (Table 5A). Mortality due to cardiovascular diseases was decreased by 2% with a 1 step/10 s increase in stepping rate, while the mortality rate was not associated with the other fitness measurements (Table 5B). There were associations between muscle strength of leg extension or handgrip and mortality due to respiratory diseases. A 3-4% decrease in mortality due to respiratory diseases was found with a 1 kg increase in single or double leg extension strength. Similarly, mortality due to respiratory diseases was decreased by 0.3% with a 1 W increase in leg extension power. A 1 kg increase in handgrip strength was also associated with a 6% fall in mortality from respiratory diseases (Table 5C). No associations were found between mortality from cancers and physical fitness measurements (Table 5D). Mortality due to senility was associated with muscle strength. A 5-6% fall in mortality from senility was found with a 1 kg increase in single or double leg extension strength. Similarly, a 0.3% fall in mortality from senility was found with a 1 W increase in leg extension power. A 1 kg increase in handgrip strength was associated with a 9% decrease in mortality due to senility (Table 5E).

Physical fitness measurement	Hazard ratio	95% CI	P value
Hand grip strength (kg)	0.970**	0.949-0.990	0.004
One-leg standing time (s)	0.991*	0.983-0.999	0.030
Leg extension strength, single leg (kg)	0.983***	0.974-0.992	0.000
Leg extension strength, two legs (kg)	0.986**	0.976-0.997	0.009
Stepping rate (steps/10 s)	0.987**	0.980-0.995	0.001
Leg extension power (W)	0.998***	0.998-0.999	0.000

A. Mortality due to all causes

Physical fitness measurement	Hazard ratio	95% CI	P value
Hand grip strength (kg)	0.987	0.946-1.029	0.525
One-leg standing time (s)	0.989	0.973-1.006	0.194
Leg extension strength, single leg (kg)	0.996	0.979-1.013	0.649
Leg extension strength, two legs (kg)	0.999	0.980-1.018	0.916
Stepping rate (steps/10 s)	0.981**	0.966-0.995	0.008
Leg extension power (W)	0.999	0.997-1.000	0.087

B. Mortality due to cardiovascular diseases

Physical fitness measurement	Hazard ratio	95% CI	P value
Hand grip strength (kg)	0.943*	0.897-0.992	0.022
One-leg standing time (s)	0.992	0.974-1.011	0.422
Leg extension strength, single leg (kg)	0.963**	0.941-0.985	0.001
Leg extension strength, two legs (kg)	0.968*	0.944-0.993	0.012
Stepping rate (steps/10 s)	0.991	0.972-1.009	0.324
Leg extension power (W)	0.997**	0.995-0.999	0.006

C. Mortality due to respiratory diseases

Physical fitness measurement	Hazard ratio	95% CI	P value
Hand grip strength (kg)	1.001	0.953-1.051	0.965
One-leg standing time (s)	0.995	0.978-1.013	0.608
Leg extension strength, single leg (kg)	1.004	0.983-1.024	0.725
Leg extension strength, two legs (kg)	1.002	0.979-1.025	0.859
Stepping rate (steps/10 s)	1.007	0.989-1.025	0.452
Leg extension power (W)	1.000	0.998-1.002	0.765

D. Mortality due to cancers

Physical fitness measurement	Hazard ratio	95% CI	P value
Hand grip strength (kg)	0.911*	0.847-0.980	0.012
One-leg standing time (s)	0.957	0.910-1.007	0.089
Leg extension strength, single leg (kg)	0.945**	0.914-0.976	0.001
Leg extension strength, two legs (kg)	0.941**	0.906-0.978	0.002
Stepping rate (steps/10 s)	1.009	0.982-1.037	0.520
Leg extension power (W)	0.997*	0.993-1.000	0.036

E. Mortality due to senility

Note: In A through E, the analyses calculate the risk of mortality associated with a 1 kg, 1 s, 1 step/ 10 s, and 1 W increase in each fitness measurement (continuous analysis), and were adjusted for gender, serum level of total cholesterol and glucose, BMI, and smoking.

*P<0.05, **P<0.01, ***P<0.001

Table 5. Multivariate Cox analyses for mortality in total subjects (men and women) due to all causes (A), cardiovascular diseases (B), respiratory diseases (C), cancers (D), or senility (E) with physical fitness measurements at the start of study.

4. Discussion

We found an inverse association between muscle strength of leg extension or handgrip and mortalities due to all causes, respiratory disease, or senility in an 80-year-old community-dwelling Japanese population. One-leg standing time and stepping rate of legs were also inversely associated with total mortality. Mortality due to cardiovascular disease was associated only with stepping rate, and mortality due to cancers was not associated with any fitness measurement. Not only low scores but also nonparticipation for all fitness tests was related to shorter survival. Nonparticipation in tests for leg extension strength or stepping rate was partly related to cardiovascular death, while nonparticipation in tests of leg extension strength, steeping rate, leg extension power, or one-leg standing was partly related to respiratory disease death. No association was found in cancer death with nonparticipation for any fitness test. Senility death was partly related to nonparticipation for all fitness tests.

Poor muscle strength has been reported to be independently associated with mortality risk in healthy middle-aged men (Rantanen et al., 2000; Rantanen, 2003; Metter et al., 2004), people aged 20-69 years (Katzmarzyk et al., 2002), and elderly people (Era and Rantanen, 1997; Gale et al., 2006; Newman et al., 2006a; Portegijs et al., 2007; Takata et al., 2007; Ling et al., 2010). After adjusting for confounders, a significant elevation in all-cause mortality was found in the lowest tertile of handgrip strength at age 85 years, and in the lowest two tertiles of handgrip strength at age 89 years (65.0% women; Ling et al., 2010). Both handgrip strength and knee extension strength (51.6% women) were strongly related to all-cause mortality in participants aged 70-79 years (Newman et al., 2006). Similarly, the lowest tertile of handgrip, elbow flexion, knee extension, trunk extension, and trunk flexion was related to approximately twofold higher mortality from all causes in community-dwelling 75- and 80-year-old people (67.2% women; Portegijs et al., 2007). Poorer grip strength was associated with increased mortality from not only all causes but also from cardiovascular disease and from cancer in men aged 65 and over (Gale et al., 2006), while this association was not found in women. We also previously found an association between pneumonia mortality and leg extension strength of a single leg in an 80-year-old population with a 4-year follow-up period (Takata et al., 2007). The present findings that mortality due to respiratory disease or senility was higher in elderly with poor muscle strength of leg extension or handgrip indicate a new association between disease-specific mortality and muscle strength. Since there have been only a few investigations of the elderly with regard to the association between disease-specific mortality and muscle strength, further investigations are needed.

In studies of middle-aged populations, there have been several reports indicating an association in disease-specific mortality with physical activity or physical fitness. Blair and his coworkers (2001) summarized results from 67 articles and found greater longevity and reduced risk of coronary heart disease, cardiovascular disease, stroke, and colon cancer in more active individuals. They also found that men aged 20 to 82 years who maintained adequate fitness or improved their physical fitness were less likely to die from all causes and from cardiovascular disease than persistently unfit men (1995). An inverse association between exercise frequency and mortality in adults aged 35 years and over was stronger for cardiovascular than cancer deaths and was strongest in the case of respiratory mortality (Lam et al., 2004). Leisure time activity was inversely related to all-cause, cardiovascular, coronary heart disease, and noncardiovascular mortality among men aged 40 to 64 years (Batty et al., 2003). Walking pace was inversely related to mortality due to all causes, coronary heart disease, and total cancer in males aged 40 to 69 years (Batty et al., 2010). Similarly, a strong inverse association was found in individuals with an average age of 43 years between all-cause mortality and level of physical fitness in both men and women. The risk of mortality from cancer declined with increasing levels of fitness or physical activity among men, but not among women with an average age of 43 years (Kampert et al., 1996). Walking pace in men aged 40 to 64 years demonstrated inverse relations with mortality from all causes, coronary heart disease, other cardiovascular disease, all cancers, respiratory disease, colorectal cancer, and hematopoietic cancer with adjustment for confounding factors (Smith et al., 2000). Adjusted cancer mortality was lower in the most fit quintile relative to the other four quintiles for men but not for women with an average age of 46 years (Evenson et al., 2003). Peak exercise oxygen consumption with a cycle ergometer exercise test in men aged 42 to 60 years was predictive of non-fatal and fatal cardiac events among men with and without risk factors (Laukkanen et al., 2004). Both regular physical activity and a high level of fitness in middle-aged men were inversely related to all-cause, cancer, and cardiovascular mortalities (Park et al, 2009).

In a similar fashion to the middle-aged population, there are studies indicating an association between poor physical activity and disease-specific mortality in the elderly population, though there are fewer studies investigating an association between disease-specific mortality and physical fitness level of the elderly population. Women aged 65 years or over with increased walking and physical activity had lower mortality from all causes, cardiovascular disease, and cancer (Gregg et al., 2003). Inability to complete walking 400 m in participants aged 70 to 79 years was associated with a higher risk of total mortality and incident cardiovascular disease (Newman et al., 2006b).

Nonparticipation in regular exercise was associated with high mortality due to all causes and cardiovascular disease, but not cancers among women aged 40 to 70 years (Nechuta et al., 2010). In a population-based survey for 54,372 Finnish people aged 25 to 64 years, nonparticipant men had twice and nonparticipant women had 2.5-fold higher all-cause mortality than the participating men and women. Nonparticipants had also significantly higher cause-specific mortalities due to cardiovascular disease and violence, whereas no difference was found in mortality due to cancer between participants and nonparticipants (Jousilahti et al., 2005). Annual mortality among nonparticipants was twice that of the participants during a follow-up period of 11.8 years in that study. Coronary death was significantly more common among nonparticipants (Rosengren et al., 1987). In very elderly persons older than 90 years, nonparticipants for follow-up study had lower levels of physical activity and leisure activity (Fernandez-Ballesteros et al., 2010), suggesting that nonparticipants are likely to have a worse survival rate than participants. These investigations all suggest that all-cause and cardiovascular disease mortality seems higher in nonparticipants than in participants during long-term surveys or in regular exercise program. However, little is known about an association in mortality with nonparticipation in fitness tests in an elderly population. We found in the present study that 80-year-old subjects who were nonparticipants in physical fitness tests were partly associated with higher mortality from all causes, cardiovascular disease, respiratory disease, and senility as compared to participants, while no association was found between nonparticipation and cancer mortality.

A limitation of the present study is that the sample size was relatively small. Since the subject age was limited to 80 years, the association between physical fitness and mortality in very elderly individuals older than 80 years should be evaluated in a future study. It is also possible that residual confounding factors other than gender, serum level of total cholesterol and glucose, BMI, and smoking could influence the findings. However, the present findings clearly suggest that physical fitness measurements and nonparticipation in tests predict all-cause and disease-specific mortality at the age of 80 in community-dwelling adults.

5. Conclusion

In the present study, lower fitness levels for various muscle strength tests were found to be associated with increases in not only all-cause mortality but also disease-specific mortality in an 80-year-old community-dwelling population. Nonparticipation in fitness tests was also associated with increased mortalities. These findings suggest that very elderly persons could survive longer by elevating their level of physical fitness and muscle strength. Intervention study in a very elderly population is needed to clarify the effect of fitness on longevity.

6. References

Batty GD, Shipley MJ, Kivimaki M, Marmot M, Smith GD. Walking pace, leisure time physical activity, and resting heart rate in relation to disease-specific mortality in London: 40 years follow-up of the original Whitehall study. An update of our work with Professor Jerry N. Morris. Ann Epidemiol 2010: 20: 661-669.

Batty GD, Shipley MJ, Marmot MG, Smith GD. Leisure time physical activity and disease-specific mortality among men with chronic bronchitis: evidence from the Whitehall study. Am J Public Health 2003: 93: 817-821.

Blair SN, Cheng Y, Holder JS: Is physical activity or physical fitness more important in defining health benefits? Med Sci Sports Exerc 2001: 33: s379-s399.

Blair SN, Kohl III HW, Barlow CE, Paffenbarger RS, Gibbons LW, Macera CA. Changes in physical fitness and all-cause mortality. A prospective study of healthy and unhealthy men. JAMA 1995: 273: 1093-1098.

Era P, Rantanen T. Changes in physical capacity and sensory/psychomotor functions from 75 to 80 years of age and from 80 to 85 years of age – a longitudinal study. Scan J Soc Med Suppl 1997: 53: 25-43.

Erlichman J, Kerbey AL, James WPT. Physical activity and its impact on health outcomes. Paper 1: The impact of physical activity on cardiovascular disease and all-cause mortality: an historical perspective. Obesity 2002: 3: 257-271.

Evenson KR, Stevens J, Cai J, Thomas R, Thomas O. The effect of cardiorespiratory fitness and obesity on cancer mortality in women and men. Med Sci Sports Exerc 2003; 35: 270-277.

Fernandez-Ballesteros R, Zamarron MD, Diet-Nicolas J, Lopez-Bravo MD, Molina MA, Schettini R. Mortality and refusal in the longitudinal 90+ project. Arch Gerontol Geriatr 2010: 2010.09.007.

Gale GR, Martyn CN, Cooper C, Sayer AA. Grip strength, body composition, and mortality. Internat J Epidemiol 2007: 36: 228-235.

Gregg EW, Cauley JA, Stone K, Thompson TJ, Bauer DC, Cummings SR, Ensrud KE. Relationship of changes in physical activity and mortality among older women. JAMA 2003: 289: 2379-2386.

Jousilahti P, Salomaa V, Kuulasmaa K, Niemela M, Vartiainen E. Total and cause specific mortality among participants and non-participants of population based health surveys: a comprehensive follow up of 54372 Finnish men and women. J Epidemiol Community Health 2005: 59: 310-315.

Kampert JB, Blair SN, Barlow CE, Kohl III HW. Physical activity, physical fitness, and all-cause and cancer mortality: a prospective study of men and women. Ann Epidemiol 1996: 6: 452-457.

Katzmarzyk PT, Craig CL. Musculoskeletal fitness and risk of mortality. Med Sci Sports Exerc 2002: 34: 740-744.

Lam T-H, Ho S-Y, Hedley AJ, Mak K-H, Leung GM. Leisure time physical activity and mortality in Hong Kong: case-control study of all adult deaths in 1998. Ann Epidemiol 2004: 14: 391-398.

Laukkanen JA, Kuri S, Salonen R, Rauramma R, Salonen JT. The predictive value of cardiorespiratory fitness for cardiovascular events in men with various risk profiles: a prospective population-based cohort study. Eur Heart J 2004: 25: 1428-1437.

Ling CHY, Taekema D, de Craen AJM, Gussekloo J, Westendorp RGJ, Maier AB. Handgrip strength and mortality in the oldest old population: the Leiden 85-plus study. Can Med Assoc J 2010: 23: 429-435.

Metter EJ, Talbot LA, Schrager M, Conwit RA. Arm-cranking muscle power and arm isometric muscle strength are independent predictors of all-cause mortality in men. J Appl Physiol 2004: 96: 814-821.

Mitnitski A, Song X, Skoog I, Broe GA, Cox JL, Grunfeld E, Rockwood K. Relative fitness and frailty of elderly men and women in developed countries and their relationship with mortality. J Am Geriatr Soc 2005: 53: 2184-2189.

Nechuta SJ, Shu X-O, Li H-L, Yang G, Xiang Y-B, Cai H, Chow W-H, Ji B, Zhang X, Wen W, Gao Y-T, Zheng W. Combined impact of lifestyle-related factors on total and cause-specific mortality among Chinese women: prospective cohort study. Plos Med 2010: 7: e1000339.

Newman AB, Kupelian V, Visser M, Simonsick EM, Goodpaster BH, Kritchevsky SB, Tylavsky FA, Rubin SM, Harris TB. Strength, but not muscle mass, is associated with mortality in the health, aging and body composition study cohort. J Gerontol A Biol Sci Med Sci 2006a: 61: 72-77.

Newman AB, Simonsick EM, Naydeck BL, Boudreau RM, Kritchevsky SB, Nevitt MC, Pahor M, Satterfield S, Brach JS, Studenski SA, Harris TB. Association of long-distance corridor walk performance with mortality, cardiovascular disease, mobility limitation, and disability. JAMA 2006b: 295: 2018-2026.

Park M-S, Chung S-Y, Chang Y, Kim K. Physical activity and physical fitness as predictors of all-cause mortality in Korean men. J Korean Med Sci 2009; 24: 13-19.

Portegijs E, Rantanen T, Sipila S, Laukkanen P, Heikkinen E. Physical activity compensates for increased mortality risk among older people with poor muscle strength. Scand J Med Sci Sports 2007: 17: 473-479.

Rantanen T. Muscle strength, disability and mortality. Scand J Med Sci Sports 2003: 13: 3-8.

Rantanen T, Harris T, Leveille SG, Visser M, Foley D, Masaki K, Guralnik JM. Muscle strength and body mass index as long-term predictors of mortality in initially healthy men. J Gerontol A Biol Sci Med Sci 2000: 55: M168-173.

Rosengren A, Wilhelmsen L, Berglund G, Elmfeldt D. Non-participants in a general population study of men, with special reference to social and alcoholic problems. Acta Med Scand 1987: 221: 243-251.

Smith GD, Shipley MJ, Batty GD, Morris JN, Marmot M. Physical activity and cause-specific mortality in the Whitehall study. Public Health 2000: 114: 308-315.

Takata Y, Ansai T, Akifusa S, Soh I, Yoshitake Y, Kimura Y, Sonoki K, Fujisawa K, Awano S, Kagiyama S, Hamasaki T, Nakamichi I, Yoshida A, Takehara T. Physical fitness and 4-year mortality in an 80-year-old population. J Gerontol Med Sci 2007: 62A: 851-858.

Part 2

Preventative Strategies for Maintenance of Health and Extending Longevity

6

Behavioral Treatment for Geriatric Syndrome

Hunkyung Kim
Tokyo Metropolitan Institute of Gerontology, Japan

1. Introduction

Geriatric syndrome is a term used to capture complex clinical conditions such as frailty, falls and fractures, urinary incontinence, malnutrition, and declining mental health, which do not fit into discrete disease categories but are serious problems among the elderly population. They are highly prevalent in the elderly, especially in frail adults with low levels of functional capacity. These geriatric syndromes have a large effect on the development of disability, dependence, decrease in quality of life, morbidity, and mortality. Having multiple underlying factors involving impairments in multiple organ systems contribute to the occurrence of geriatric syndromes (Tinetti et al., 1995). Thus, prevention and treatment of geriatric syndromes such as frailty, falls, and urinary incontinence in its early stages are important strategies in maintaining health and independence among the elderly.

This chapter will focus on frailty, falls, and urinary incontinence, as they are the most common geriatric syndromes among community-dwelling elderly people.

1.1 Shared risk factors for distinct geriatric syndrome

A main feature of geriatric syndrome is that multiple risk factors contribute to their etiology. Research has suggested that vision and hearing impairment, anxiety, as well as upper and lower extremity impairments are associated with incontinence, falling, and occurrence of functional dependence.

The risk of each geriatric syndrome is greater with increasing number of predisposing factors possessed. Furthermore, incontinence and falling are associated with the occurrence of functional dependence. Geriatric syndromes; therefore, may contribute both indirectly, through shared risk factors, and directly to functional dependence in the elderly. One model unifying the concepts of geriatric syndromes has been proposed by Inouye et al., (2007) demonstrating that shared risk factors may lead to one or more geriatric syndromes, and eventually to frailty. Once frail, this may feedback to the development of more risk factors, which in turn may lead to other geriatric syndromes, further frailness, and ultimately disability, dependence, and even death.

Frailty can be defined as a condition in which three or more of the following criteria are present: unintentional weight loss, self-reported exhaustion, weakness, slow walking speed, and low physical activity (Fried et al., 2001). The prevalence of frailty is greater in women than men, and increases which age. Frailty status, or the presence of frailty can predict disability and adverse outcomes, where those who are frail have a significantly higher risk of further debilitation, specifically in mobility, activities of daily living (ADL) and falls, eventually leading to hospitalization and death (Fried et al., 2004) (Table 1).

	Hazard Ratios Estimated Over 3 Years
	Frail (Versus Not Frail)
Worsening mobility disability	1.50**
Worsening ADL disability	1.98**
Incident Fall	1.29**
First hospitalization	1.29**
Death	2.24**

**$p \leq .05$
ADL= activity of daily living

Table 1. Frailty status predicting disability, falls, hospitalizations, and death over 3 years. (Fried, L.P.; Ferrucci, L.; Darer, J.; Williamson, J.D. & Anderson, G. (2004). Untangling the concepts of disability, frailty, and comorbidity: implications for improved targeting and care. *The Journals of Gerontology. Series A, Biological Sciences and Medical Sciences,* Vol.59, No.3, pp. 255-263, by permission of the Gerontological Society of America.)

Falls are an especially serious problem among the elderly, as approximately 30% of community-dwelling older adults over the age of 65 experience falls every year. Falls are the leading cause of unintentional injury, functional decline, hospitalization, institutionalization, and increased healthcare costs. In order to prevent falls, a thorough understanding of the causes and risk factors for falls among the elderly is required for the development of effective preventative strategies.

Urinary incontinence, particularly in the elderly, is considered to be an important determining factor for admission into long-term care and has been associated with loss of independence, reduced quality of life, restricted social activities, increased anxiety and social isolation.

2. Risk factors

Many studies have demonstrated that geriatric syndromes are multifactorial, and shared risk factors including older age, cognitive impairment, functional impairment, and impaired mobility, are often associated with common geriatric syndromes of frailty, falls, and urinary incontinence. The identification and treatment of the risk factors that contribute to geriatric syndromes have been the focus in recent research.

2.1 Frailty

Frailty is highly prevalent in the elderly. Frailty often overlaps with (though is not synonymous with) comorbidity and disability, and is associated with several major chronic diseases such as cardiovascular disease, pulmonary disease and diabetes. Hence, treatments for frail older adults usually require specific care needs (Fried et al., 2004) (Fig. 1). With the presence of comorbid conditions, there may be competition between the treatments. The combinations of medications and treatment regiments may limit the desired effects of the treatments, or have adverse effects. Comorbidities lead to the over-use and mixing of prescription medication which is a risk factor for falls. Frailty, coupled with low bone mass is associated with increased risk of hip fractures which are a major threat to survival in the elderly. Research has shown that 17.4% of people who suffered hip fracture over the age of 65 died within 12 months of a fracture (Magaziner et al., 1989).

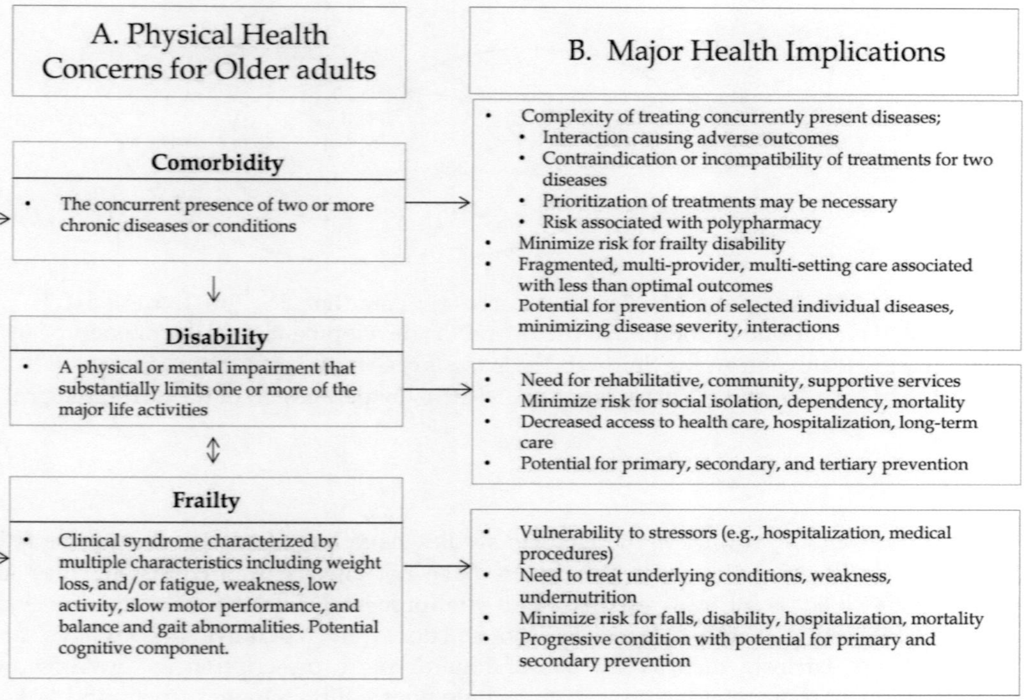

Fig. 1. Comorbidity, disability, and frailty: definitions and major health care implications. (Fried, L.P.; Ferrucci, L.; Darer, J.; Williamson, J.D. & Anderson, G. (2004). Untangling the concepts of disability, frailty, and comorbidity: implications for improved targeting and care. *The Journals of Gerontology. Series A, Biological Sciences and Medical Sciences*, Vol.59, No.3, pp. 255-263, by permission of the Gerontological Society of America.)

There are numerous factors that contribute to muscle weakness and loss of muscle mass in aging adults such as chronic disease, a sedentary lifestyle, and under-nutrition, where some factors can be reversed with lifestyle changes, and others need specific medications and cannot be reversed. Xue et al. (2008) hypothesized the cycle of frailty, as many of these factors can theoretically be unified into a cycle associated with decreasing energetics and functional reserve (Fig. 2) The core elements of this cycle, including weight loss, sarcopenia, decrease in strength and walking speed, as well as low activity, are commonly identified as clinical signs and symptoms of frailty.

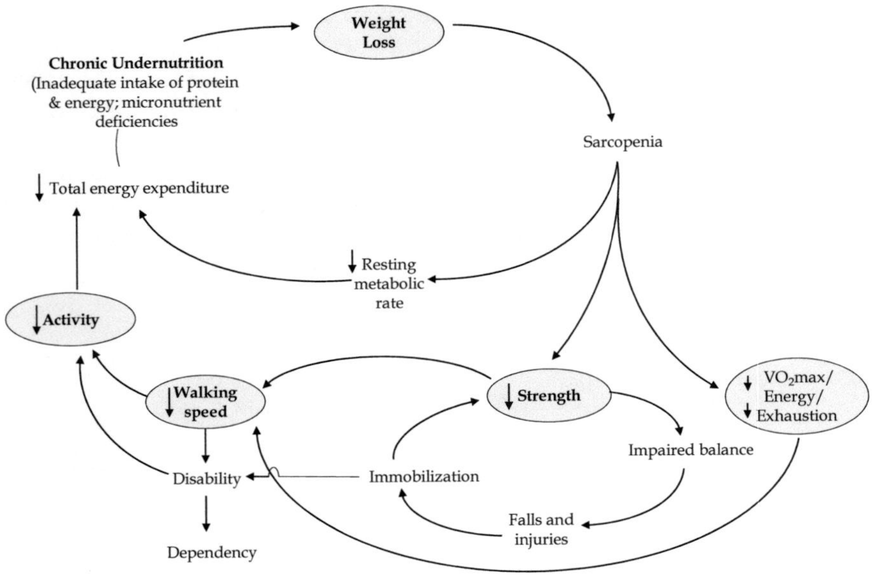

Fig. 2. Cycle of Frailty. (Xue, Q.L.; Bandeen-Roche, K.; Varadhan, R.; Zou, J. & Fried, L.P. (2008). Initial manifestations of frailty criteria and the development of frailty phenotype in the Women's Health and Aging Study II. *The Journals of Gerontology. Series A, Biological Sciences and Medical Sciences*, Vol.63, No.9, pp. 984-990, by permission of the Gerontological Society of America.)

2.2 Falls

In the recent decade, several epidemiologic studies have identified risk factors for falls. While the classifications of these risk factors have not always been consistent, they are generally classified as intrinsic, extrinsic, and environmental. Intrinsic risk factors include muscle weakness, gait and balance deficits, functional and cognitive impairments, and visual deficits, extrinsic such as the use of four or more prescription medications and bifocals, and environmental factors, which include poor lighting, loose carpets, and lack of bathroom safety equipment (American Geriatric Society et al., 2001). Low vitamin D levels are also significantly associated with a high prevalence of falls in elderly women, as well as low physical performance (Suzuki et al., 2008) (Table 2).

The most common risk factors for falls are muscle weakness, history of falls, gait deficit, balance deficit, use of assistive device, visual deficit, arthritis, impaired ADL, depression, cognitive impairment, and older age (over 80 years old) (American Geriatric Society et al., 2001). The risk of falling increases linearly with the number of risk factors, from 8.0% with none to 78.0% with four or more risk factors (Tinetti et al., 1988). Furthermore, those who experience falls once have a greater chance of recurrent falls, which may lead to a fear of falling. Some older adults may then begin restricting activities both indoors and outdoors. Not only does this lead to a further lack of physical activity, but research has shown that older persons who restrict activity for fear of falling are more physically frail and have greater burden of chronic conditions and depressive symptoms compared with those who do not restrict activity despite their fear of falls (Murphy et al., 2002).

	Male			Female		
Risk Factor	OR	95%CI	*P*	OR	95%CI	*P*
Age (yr)	1.02	0.95-1.10	NS	1.02	0.99-1.06	NS
Normal walking speed (0.1 m/s)	0.87	0.77-0.97	0.015	0.92	0.88-0.97	0.001
Albumin (g/dl)	1.69	0.45-6.33	NS	1.60	0.88-2.90	NS
25(OH)D (mg/ml)	1	0.95-1.06	NS	0.97	0.94-0.99	0.010

Dependent variable was "fall experience over the previous year" (yes=1; no=0).
NS= not significant

Table 2. Multiple logistic regression model of factors associated with fall experience. (Suzuki, T.; Kwon, J.; Kim, H.; Shimada, H.; Yoshida, Y.; Iwasa, H. & Yoshida, H. (2008). Low serum 25-hydroxyvitamin D levels associated with falls among Japanese community-dwelling elderly. *Journal of Bone and Mineral Research*, Vol.23, No.8, pp. 1309-1317, by permission of the American Society for Bone and Mineral Research.)

2.3 Urinary incontinence

There is general agreement on the multifactorial nature of incontinence. Permanent incontinence also is typically the result of neurological damage or, intrinsic bladder or urethral pathology. However, incontinence is associated with several potentially reversible conditions. Lower urinary tract function, environmental factors, physical and cognitive function, psychological distress, mobility, manual dexterity, medical conditions, and medications may all have an effect on urinary incontinence status in the elderly (Landi et al., 2003). The incidence of urinary incontinence is typically higher in women than men, and those who experience incontinence are usually older with lower functional fitness levels for both sexes. Although there is a large amount of information regarding the mechanisms and treatment options for urinary incontinence, little is known about the potentially reversible causes of this condition in community-dwelling elderly people. Several of the known causes that may be reversible include urinary tract infections, as they can cause the urge to void quite frequently, physical restraints and drastic limitations in mobility, and environmental hazards.

Lifestyle and functional fitness are significantly associated with the onset of urinary incontinence in community-dwelling elderly people (Kim et al., 2004) (Table 3).

3. Treatment for geriatric syndrome

Declines in functional fitness such as walking speed, muscle strength and balance ability in the elderly are strongly associated with the development of geriatric syndromes. Hence, exercise focusing on strength, balance, and mobility improvement, even into advanced age, is usually offered as a strategy for the reduction of frailty, falls, and urinary incontinence in the elderly.

Sex	Variable		OR	95%CI
Male	Age (per 1 yr)		1.23	1.11-1.38
	Plasma albumin (per 0.1 g/dl)		0.70	0.54-0.88
	Smoking status	non-smoker	1.00	
		previous smoker	1.53	0.56-4.59
		current smoker	2.33	0.82-7.61
Female	Grip strength (per 1 kg)		0.92	0.86-0.98
	Social role (per 1 point)		1.81	1.19-2.73
	BMI (per 1 kg/m^2)		1.10	1.01-1.20
	Smoking status	non-smoker	1.00	
		current smoker	7.53	1.36-41.63

Table 3. Multiple logistic regression model of risk factors associated with the onset of urinary incontinence

3.1 Frailty

Aging is characterized by a gradual decrease in muscle mass and muscle strength, which contributes to declines in physical function, increased disability, frailty, and loss of independence. Out of many factors associated with the development of frailty, muscle disuse and nutritional deficiencies are the factors that are potentially reversible or preventable through interventions and a more active lifestyle (Fiatarone et al., 1994).

3.1.1 Nutritional supplementation

Declines in muscle mass are related to declines in muscle protein synthesis rates in older adults. In order to resist and reverse the effects of muscle protein synthesis declines, protein or more specifically, amino-acids, have been the focus of research. Investigators have found that leucine enriched essential amino-acid mixtures are primarily responsible for amino-acid-induced muscle protein anabolism in the elderly. Amino-acid supplementation can increase muscle mass in this population; however, an increase in muscle mass is not always accompanied by an increase in muscle strength (Dillon et al., 2009). Essential amino-acid supplementation alone is probably insufficient in increasing muscle strength. Carbohydrate-rich supplements have also been examined for any effects on muscle strength and muscle mass. However, supplements rich in carbohydrates are inadequate for the purpose of increasing muscle mass and strength (Fiatarone et al., 1994). Vitamin D supplementation, which will be discussed further (see section 3.2.1) has also been shown to increase strength.

3.1.2 Exercise

Exercise in elderly individuals may potentially modify risk factors for age-associated reductions in muscle mass (Liu & Latham, 2009). Research has shown that high intensity resistance training is effective in counteracting muscle weakness and physical frailty in elderly people. More specifically, exercise interventions focused on the major muscle groups that are crucial for performing functional activities, are especially important for the reversal of muscle weakness.

Extensive research has confirmed that doing resistance training two to three times a week can improve physical function and functional limitations, and also reduce disability and muscle weakness in older people. Resistance training in elderly people produces increases in strength from 9 to 15% (Borst, 2004), and about 1.1 kg in lean body mass (Peterson et al., 2011). While more improvements are seen with high intensity and volume resistance training, moderate intensity exercises are also beneficial, and are much safer for aging adults. Exercise prescriptions must be of a safe intensity, duration and frequency to avoid further injury and complications (Taaffe, 2006) (Table 4).

Combinations of both exercise and nutritional supplementation have also been studied by researchers. Amino-acid supplementations alone have beneficial effects such as increasing walking speed, and exercise itself also has beneficial effects of improving physical function. Exercise and amino-acid supplementation together have significant effects in enhancing muscle mass, strength and functional fitness. The combination of high resistance exercise and a high carbohydrate mixture containing small amounts of soy protein is effective in the enhancement of muscle strength. High resistance exercise alone increases both muscle mass and strength, while the carbohydrate supplementation alone does not (Fiatarone et al., 1994). Further research is still needed to investigate which supplementations coupled with exercise, or alone, are most effective.

Resistance training program recommendations	
Exercises	8-10 that target the major muscle groups
Repetitions	8-12 per set. When able to achieve 12 repetitions, increase resistance so that 8 repetitions are possible
Sets	Minimum of 1, preferable 2-3 per exercise with 1-2 minutes rest between sets
Frequency	1-3 days per week with at least 48 hours between sessions
Velocity	2-3 seconds concentric and 2-3 seconds eccentric. Some sets of rapid concentric movements can also be included
Breathing	Normal breathing on each repetition (no breath holding)
Duration	Less than 1 hour

Table 4. Resistance training program recommendations. (Taaffe, DR. (2006). Sarcopenia—exercise as a treatment strategy. *Australian Family Physician*, Vol.35, No.3, pp. 130-134. ©2011 *Australian Family Physician*. Reproduced with permission from The Royal Australian College of General Practitioners. Text and images copyright of *Australian Family Physician*. Permission to reproduce must be sought from the publisher, The Royal Australian College of General Practitioners).

3.2 Falls

The development of effective preventative strategies to reduce the fall rate in community-dwelling elderly people who are at risk of falling require a better understanding of the modifiable risk factors for falling. Among the numerous risk factors for falling, those that are considered modifiable include muscle weakness, impairments in balance and gait, and the use of multiple prescription medications. These risk factors can be modifiable through behavioral strategies such as muscle strengthening exercises, balance and gait training, and education about nonpharmacologic treatments to reduce the number of prescription medications used (Tinetti et al., 1994). Furthermore, the occurrence of falling rises with increasing number of risk factors present; therefore, strategies targeted to reduce these modifiable risk factors may be effective in the prevention of falls.

3.2.1 Vitamin D supplementation

In several trials of older individuals at risk for vitamin D deficiencies, vitamin D supplementation improved strength, function, and balance in a dose-related pattern. A high daily vitamin D supplementation dose (about 700-1000 IU) can reduce the risk of falls by approximately 20%; although small doses (less than 400 or 700 IU) may not be sufficient to reduce falls (Bischoff-Ferrari et al., 2009).

3.2.2 Exercise

Falls in older people are not purely random events but can be predicted by assessing a number of risk factors. Some of these risk factors such as decreased muscle strength, impaired balance, and gait deficit can be modified using exercise, whereas poor vision, and psychoactive medications require different strategies. Exercise can be used as a fall prevention intervention on its own or as a component of a multifaceted program. The pooled estimate of the effects of exercise was that it reduced the rate of falling by 17.0% (Sherrington et al., 2008). Home-based and tailored group exercise classes seem to be effective in reducing falls by improving balance and muscular strength. Also, while home hazard management (e.g. removing tripping hazards) and vision screening are not markedly effective in reducing falls when used alone, they add value when combined with an exercise program (Day et al., 2002).

3.2.3 An exercise-based falls prevention program

Exercise programs designed for fall prevention in elderly people should address three major areas - strength, balance and gait. People at high risk of falling due to muscle weakness, balance impairment, and gait deficit should be instructed to perform low or moderate intensity exercise containing safe and simple movements at entry level.

Strength training

A moderate-intensity strength training program aimed to reduce falls should target the major muscles such as the tibialis anterior, soleus, quadriceps femoris, iliopsoas, tensor fasciae latae, and sartorius (Fig. 3). Tripping is a leading cause of falls in community-dwelling elderly people, responsible for up to 53% of falls in this population (Blake et al., 1988). Trips may be associated with weakness of the tibialis anterior muscle, which would cause low toe-clearance or walking in a "shuffling" manner where the toes do not lift off the ground sufficiently to avoid small obstacles that may cause trips.

Target Muscle		Exercise		Exercise Description
Tibialis Anterior	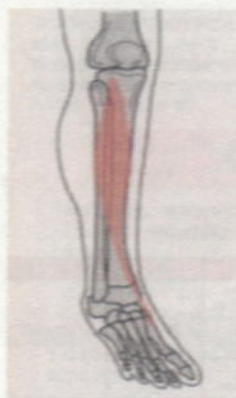	Seated Toe Raises	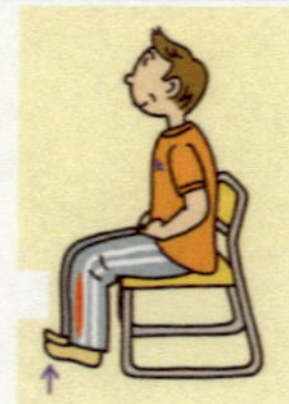	Place hands in comfortable position while seated. Lift toes of both feet as high as possible with the heels still on the floor. Hold for 3-5 seconds, breath normally, and slowly lower toes to the floor. Perform 8-10 repetitions. Remind participants to not rock the body back when raising toes.
Quadriceps	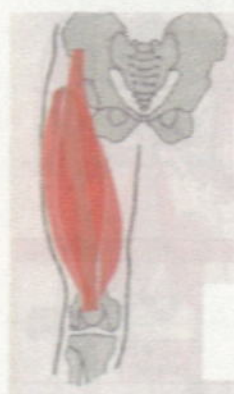	Seated Knee Extension	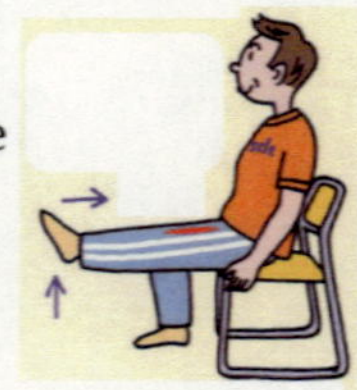	Lift one leg still bent at the knee while inhaling, and extend the leg without "locking" the knee (keep knee slightly bent) while exhaling. Bend the knee again, with the hip still flexed, and place the foot on the floor. Perform 8-12 repetitions, and repeat on the other side. Remind participants to not lean back while lifting the leg, or extending the knee.
Soleus and Gastrocnemius	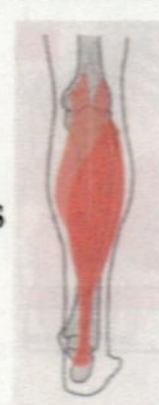	Heel Raises	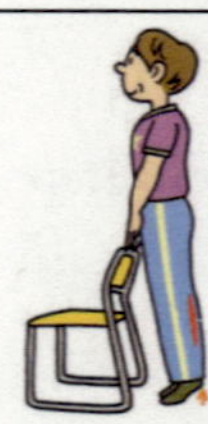	Stand tall with feet flat, shoulder-width apart. Hold on to back of a chair for support. Slowly lift both heels off the floor while exhaling. Hold for 5-10 seconds, breath normally, and slowly lower the heels to the floor. Repeat 10 times.

Fig. 3. Examples of lower extremity strength training exercises.

Balance and gait training

Training is crucial for the improvement of balance in the elderly, and static as well as dynamic and lateral balance exercise have been recommended for reducing falls. Balance exercises progress from holding on to a stable supporting structure such as a chair, to performing the exercises independent of support. Not all elderly people will necessarily start at the first level of each exercise or be prescribed all the balance exercise such as one-leg standing, tandem stance, tandem walking, and side step (Fig. 4).

The results of a large scale study, known as the Frailty and Injuries: Cooperative Studies of Intervention Techniques (FICSIT) trials, suggest that exercise interventions (flexibility, resistance, balance) and Tai Chi for elderly people reduce the risk of falls (Province et al., 1995). To evaluate the effect of Tai Chi on functional fitness and falls, it is necessary to analyze the characteristic movements of Tai Chi. Tai Chi consists of a series of smooth movements linked together in a continuous sequence of whole body weight-shifting, with a low center of gravity. Also, Tai Chi movements involves shifting the weight forward and standing on one foot while lifting the other foot an inch off the floor, which contributes to the improvement of static balance. Moreover, the safe completion of the steps requires an adequate amount of dynamic balance, postural strength, and lateral stability (Li et al., 2004). Participants in the FICSIT trial were instructed on correct foot placement and posture, standing in a semi-squat position, which requires substantial lower extremity strength. These movements are directly or indirectly related to improvement of functional fitness.

Target Balance Type	Exercise		Exercise Description
Static Balance	One-Leg Stand	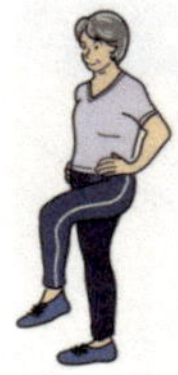	Stand tall with feet flat, shoulder-width apart. Lightly hold on to back of a chair for support or place hands on the hips. Slowly lift one foot off the floor while exhaling. Hold position for 10 seconds, breath normally, and slowly lower the foot to the floor. Repeat by lifting the other leg. Perform 2-3 sets per day.
Dynamic Balance	Tandem Walk	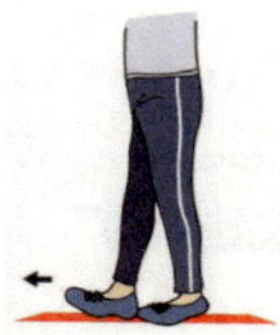	Stand tall with feet flat on the floor, near a wall or railing for safety. Place one foot directly in front of the other foot, allowing the heel of the front foot to touch the toes of the back foot. Repeat with the other foot. Continue for 10 steps.
Lateral Balance	Cross Step	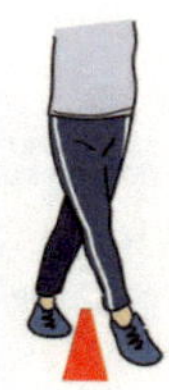	Place a piece of tape or draw a line (refrain from anything that may cause trips) on the floor. Begin by standing with both feet together on one side of the tape. Lift the foot farther from the tape, and place it forward (diagonal) on the other side of the tape in a cross-fashion. Shift weight to the front foot, cross the other foot and place on the other side of tape. Note: Both feet do not come together. Continue for 10 steps.

Fig. 4. Examples of balance and gait exercises.

3.3 Urinary incontinence

The common treatments for urinary incontinence include surgery, drug therapies, and behavioral treatments. Behavioral treatments such as pelvic floor muscle (PFM) exercises and bladder training are recommended as a first line of treatment in the management of urinary incontinence, because of the potential benefits with few risks and no side effects. Urinary incontinence is usually classified into three different types: stress, urge, and mixed. Stress incontinence is urine leakage associated with increased abdominal pressure such as coughing, sneezing, laughing, heavy lifting, standing, running, or other types of physical activity. Urge incontinence is leakage associated with running water, or an urge to void and not being able to reach the toilet in time. Mixed urinary incontinence is when characteristics of both stress and urge incontinence types are present.

3.3.1 Pelvic floor muscle exercise

PFM exercises (Fig. 5), initiated by Kegal in 1948, is hypothesized to enhance urethral resistance by increasing the strength and endurance of the periurethral and perivaginal muscles and by improving the anatomic support to the bladder neck and proximal urethra (Kegel, 1948). These exercises are the preferred treatment for stress incontinence but have recently been recommended for urge or mixed incontinence because of reflex bladder inhibition associated with pelvic floor muscle contraction. The efficacy of PFM exercises in improving urine leakage has been validated by many investigators, and the improvement rate has been reported to range widely from 17 to 84% (Bo, 1995).

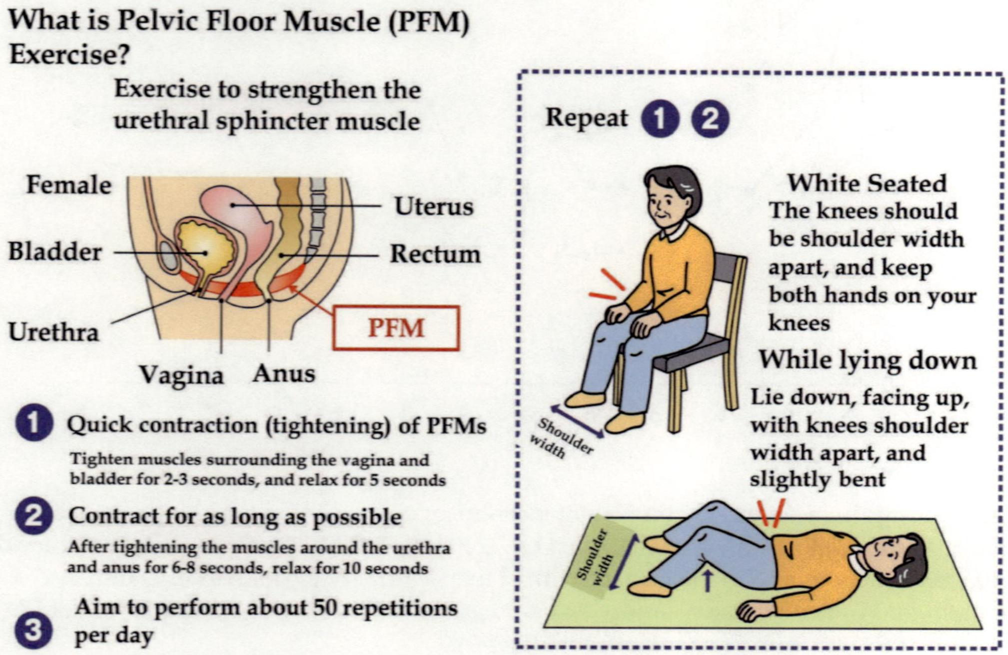

Fig. 5. Pelvic floor muscle exercise for the prevention of urinary incontinence.

At the beginning of PFM training, it is important to teach the elderly people participating in a training program, the structure of the PFM in order to gain awareness of these muscles. The participants should be taught that straining the abdomen would increase the abdominal pressure and would exert load on the PFM. Training should focus on how to exert force on the PFM without excessively straining the abdomen. Most exercise regimens are designed to strengthen the fast and slow-twitch fibers located at the pelvic floor. PFM exercise programs often incorporate alternations of fast contractions, usually held only for about three seconds, sustained contractions, where the participants would hold the contraction for about six to eight seconds, and ten-second relaxation periods between the contractions. The PFM exercises are usually performed in the seated, lying, and standing positions with the legs apart, and the emphasis placed on training of the PFM and relaxing of the other muscles.

The durations of the exercise training periods vary between 3 weeks and 6 months. Bladder training appears to have its greatest efficacy at 6 weeks; PFM exercise appears to be best between 11 to 12 weeks; and combined bladder training and PFM exercise seems to be most effective between 8 to 12 weeks of training (Wyman et al., 1998) (Fig. 6).

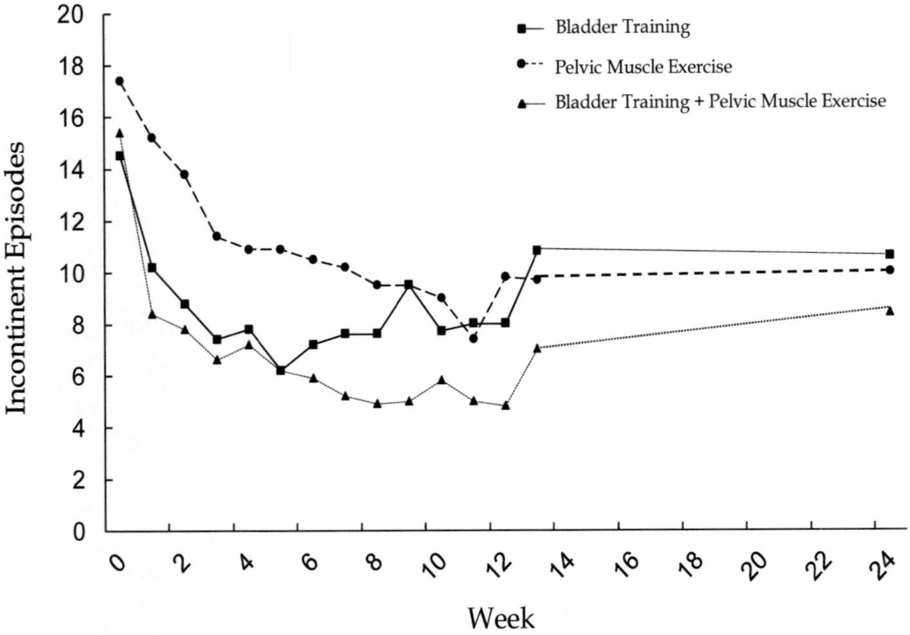

Fig. 6. Change in mean weekly number of incontinent episodes over time by treatment group. (Wyman, J.F.; Fantl, J.A.; McClish, D.K. & Bump, R.C. (1998). Comparative efficacy of behavioral interventions in the management of female urinary incontinence. Continence Program for Women Research Group. *American Journal of Obstetrics and Gynecology*, Vol.179, No.4, pp. 999-1007, with permission from Elsevier).

3.3.2 Fitness exercise

Several studies have reported that obesity and high body mass index (BMI) are associated with urinary incontinence. Presumably, increases in body weight causes increases in abdominal-wall weight, hence increasing intra-abdominal pressure and intra-vesicular pressure (Bo, 2004). Therefore, reductions in abdominal fat from exercise may contribute to decreasing intra-abdominal pressure, causes improvements in urethral sphincter contraction, and therefore decreased risk of urinary incontinence (Fig. 7; Fig. 8). Weight reduction is desirable for women complaining of urinary incontinence (Subak et al., 2009). Bump et al. (1992) found that surgically induced weight loss in obese women significantly reduces weekly incontinence episodes.

Although a direct cause-effect relationship between obesity and incontinence has not yet been established, there is evidence that weight reduction or decrease in BMI may be beneficial for treatment of incontinence. Kim et al. (2007) investigated the distribution of subjects cured from urinary incontinence according to tertiles of BMI, maximum walking speed, and adductor muscle strength, found that a significantly higher proportion among those who were cured of incontinence episodes, demonstrated improvements in BMI and walking speeds (Kim et al., 2007). Therefore, weight reduction, decrease in BMI, and increase in walking ability are desirable qualities for the treatment of urinary incontinence (Table 5).

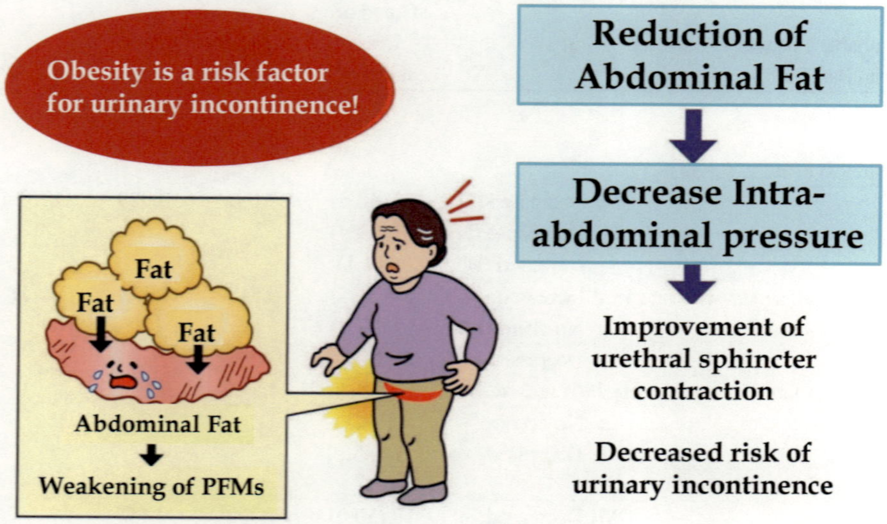

Fig. 7. Strengthening exercises to reduce abdominal fat prevents urinary incontinence

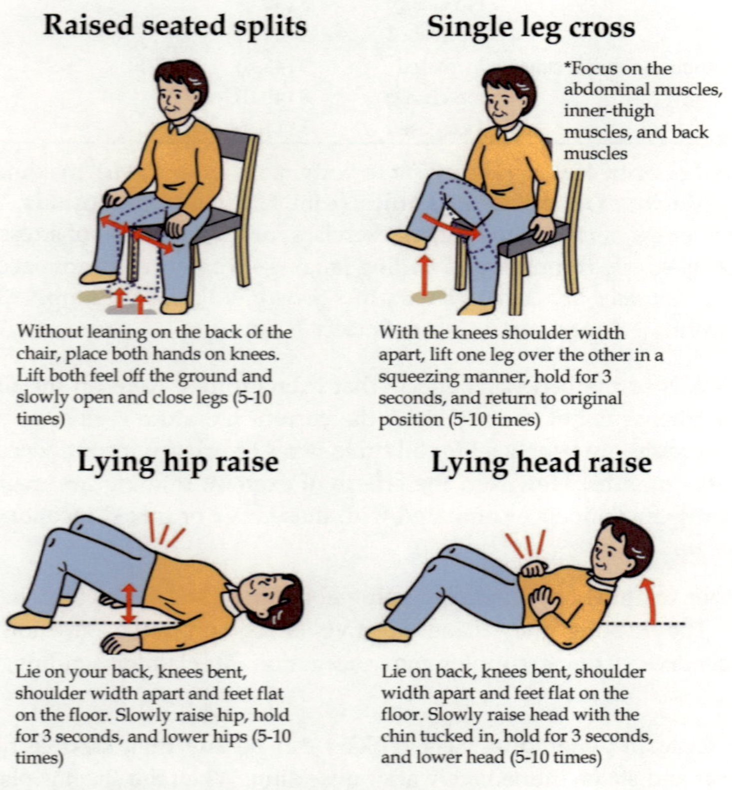

Fig. 8. Examples of exercises aimed to reduce abdominal fat.

Variable Changes Compared with Baseline		Cured of Urine Leakage n(%)	Cochran's Q value	p- value	Post-hoc †
3-month exercise (n=33)					
BMI	Decreased (D)	16 (48.5)	7.091	0.029	D,N>I
	No change (N)	13 (39.4)			
	Increased (I)	4 (12.1)			
Maximum walking speed	Increased	17 (51.5)	6.545	0.038	I>D
	No change	11 (33.3)			
	Decreased	5 (15.2)			
Adductor muscle strength	Increased	11 (33.3)	4.545	0.103	
	No change	6 (18.2)			
	Decreased	16 (48.5)			
1-Year Follow-up (n=20)					
BMI	Decreased	10 (50.0)	3.700	0.157	
	No change	3 (15.0)			
	Increased	7 (35.0)			
Maximumn walking speed	Increased	10 (50.0)	6.100	0.047	I>D
	No change	8 (40.0)			
	Decreased	2 (10.0)			
Adductor muscle strength	Increased	9 (45.0)	3.100	0.212	
	No change	8 (40.0)			
	Decreased	3 (15.0)			

Table 5. Cured of urine leakage according to body mass index (BMI), maximum walking speed, and adductor muscle strength tertiles. (Kim, H.; Suzuki, T.; Yoshida, Y. & Yoshida, H. (2007). Effectiveness of multidimensional exercises for the treatment of stress urinary incontinence in elderly community-dwelling Japanese women: a randomized, controlled, crossover trial. *Journal of the American Geriatrics Society*, Vol.55, No.12, pp. 1932-1939, with permission from the American Geriatrics Society.)

While the details of the beneficial effects that exercise may have on the different types of urinary incontinence is not entirely clear, the current literature seems to suggest that PFM and fitness exercises are beneficial for all three types of urinary incontinence after a training period of three months. However, the effects of exercise training are maintained more in those with stress incontinence compared with those urge or mixed incontinence (Kim et al., 2011a) (Table 6).

Recently, other treatment methods including abdominal and lower back heating have been introduced. The heating may have positive effects on renal function such as renal sympathetic nerve activity suppression, promotion of bladder voiding, and increasing frequency of urination.

The heat and steam generating sheet (HSGS) can be any thin, flexible filmed sheet that generates heat and steam immediately after unsealing. When the sheet is placed on the body, the temperature of the skin surface rises to 38 to 40℃and it continues to generate heat

Variables[a]	G[b]	Baseline	3-month exercise	7-month follow-up	ANOVA[c] G×T	p Value
Body Weight (kg)	I	52.0 ± 8.9	51.9 ± 8.8	50.9 ± 8.9	F=5.78	0.018
	C	53.9 ± 8.2	53.9 ± 8.2	53.9 ± 8.1		
BMI (kg/m^2)	I	23.7 ± 3.4	23.5 ± 3.0	23.2 ± 3.1	F=11.49	0.001
	C	24.1 ± 2.9	24.0 ± 2.7	24.4 ± 3.4		
WC (cm)	I	78.8 ± 10.3	77.8 ± 9.7	77.7 ± 9.9	F=4.06	0.041
	C	79.3 ± 10.4	79.2 ± 10.5	78.9 ± 9.6		
UWS (m/sec)	I	1.2 ± 0.2	1.2 ± 0.2	1.2 ± 0.2	F=2.79	0.099
	C	1.1 ± 0.3	1.1 ± 0.3	1.1 ± 0.2		
MWS(m/sec)	I	1.7 ± 0.4	1.8 ± 0.4	1.8 ± 0.4	F=5.10	0.027
	C	1.7 ± 0.4	1.6 ± 0.3	1.6 ± 0.4		
GS (kg)	I	19.0 ± 4.7	20.7 ± 5.0	19.8 ± 5.7	F=0.37	0.547
	C	19.0 ± 4.2	20.2 ± 3.5	19.5 ± 3.8		
AMS (kg)	I	20.5 ± 7.1	24.1 ± 7.7	24.3 ± 7.9	F=11.00	0.001
	C	21.2 ± 4.8	22.1 ± 4.8	21.8 ± 4.9		
ULS (point)	I	5.0 ± 1.0	3.0 ± 2.0	3.6 ± 2.2	F=7.64	0.007
	C	5.1 ± 1.0	4.4 ± 1.6	4.8 ± 1.6		
Cure of urine leakage	I	0.0	44.1	39.3	21.96	<0.001
	C	0.0	1.6	1.6		
Cure of urine leakage in intervention group	Stress	0.0	63.2[d]	66.7[e]	15.77	<0.001
	Urge	0.0	35.0[d]	26.1[e]	7.49	0.032
	Mixed	0.0	40.0[d]	30.0[e]	9.56	0.016

[a] Data are presented as mean and standard deviation.
WC=waist circumference; UWS=usual walking speed; MWS=maximum walking speed; GS=Grip strength; Ams=adductor muscle strenght; ILS=urine leaking score.
[b] G=group, I=intervention group, C=control group
[c] ANOVA=analysis of variance, T=time.
Chi-square and p values are from generalized estimating wquation.
Cochran's Q-value.
[d] Kruskal-Wallis test : chi-square=1.99, p=0.391
[e] Kruskal-Wallis test : chi-square=10.28, p=0.008
(Scheffe's *post-hoc*=stress >urge, mixed urinary incontinence)

Table 6. Cured of urine leakage after the 3-month exercise between the intervention and control groups. (Kim, H.; Yoshida, H. & Suzuki, T. (2011a). The effects of multidimensional exercise treatment on community-dwelling elderly Japanese women with stress, urge, and mixed urinary incontinence: A randomized controlled trial. *International Journal of Nursing Studies*, doi:10.1016/j.ijnurstu.2011.02.016, with permission from Elsevier.)

and steam for over 5 hours. Research has suggested that the HSGS in combination with exercise yields the highest cure rates of urinary incontinence compared with exercise or the HSGS alone. The HSGS also has beneficial effects for the different urinary incontinence types. Research reveals higher cure rates in those with stress urinary incontinence with the combination of both exercise and heat; however, there is strong evidence that the HSGS can be used as a supplementary treatment method in order to enhance the effects of exercise on those with urge, mixed, and stress urinary incontinence (Kim et al., 2011b) (Table 7).

Type of UI	Ex+HSGS n=37	Ex n=35	HSGS n=37	GE n=34	χ^2 value	*P*-value*
Stress UI, %(n)	61.5(8)	53.8(7)	25.0(3)	9.1(1)	8.94	0.030
Urge UI, %(n)	50.0(7)	16.7(2)	13.3(2)	0.0(0)	12.88	0.005
Mixed UI, %(n)	40.0(4)	30.0(3)	30.0(3)	0.0(0)	3.02	0.389
Total cure rate	51.4(19)	34.3(12)	21.6(1)	2.9(1)	21.89	<0.001

UI=urinary incontinence; Ex=exercise group; HSGS=heat and steam generating sheet group; GE=general education group.
*Kruskal-Wallis test.

Table 7. Cure rate of urinary incontinence according to urinary incontinence type and intervention group. (Kim, H.; Yoshida, H. & Suzuki, T. (2011b). Effects of exercise treatment with or without heat and steam generating sheet on urine loss in community-dwelling Japanese elderly women with urinary incontinence. *Geriatrics and Gerontology International*, doi: 10.1111/j.1447-0594.2011.00705.x, with permission from the Japan Geriatrics Society.)

	After 3-month exercise			After 7-month follow-up		
Variable	Adjusted OR *	95%CI	*p* Value	Adjusted OR *	95%CI	*p* Value
Amount of urine leakage	0.69	0.39-0.98	0.049	0.78	0.26-1.88	0.600
Frequency of urine leakage	1.16	0.24-5.79	0.856	1.63	0.73-4.01	0.248
Compliance to exercise	1.03	1.01-1.16	0.048	1.13	1.02-1.29	0.031
Decreased of BMI	0.67	0.48-0.89	0.011	0.78	0.60-0.96	0.028
Increased of walking speed	0.97	0.91-1.04	0.414	0.99	0.94-1.06	0.913
Period of urine leakage	1.01	0.91-1.13	0.919	1.01	0.91-1.14	0.913

Table 8. Adjusted odds ratios for cure of urine leakage after intervention and the 7-month follow-up. (Kim, H.; Yoshida, H. & Suzuki, T. (2011a). The effects of multidimensional exercise treatment on community-dwelling elderly Japanese women with stress, urge, and mixed urinary incontinence: A randomized controlled trial. *International Journal of Nursing Studies*, doi:10.1016/j.ijnurstu.2011.02.016, with permission from Elsevier.)

3.3.3 Predictor variables

Multiple characteristics that may influence the treatment outcome such as age, gender, urine loss frequency and amount, incontinence type, duration of urinary incontinence, chronic conditions, medications, and functional fitness as well as adherence to the prescribed exercise regimen have been examined. Many previous studies have emphasized that compliance to exercise is the key factor to long-term success (Lagro-Janssen & van Weel., 1998; McDowell et al., 1999), and confirmed that BMI reduction have positive influences on urge, mixed and stress UI treatment (Kim et al., 2011a) (Table 8).

4. Conclusion

Geriatric syndromes are highly prevalent and associated with substantial morbidity and poor outcomes. Various factors cause frailty, falls, and urinary incontinence in elderly people including chronic disease, lack of physical activity, malnutrition, and aging itself, some of which are unpreventable. Exercise and nutritional supplementation are among the beneficial treatments promoting healthy and independent lifestyles in the elderly.

Evidence reveals that exercise targeted at reducing risk factors is an effective strategy for treating geriatric syndromes in elderly people. Progressive and moderate-intensity exercise should be encouraged among elderly people to minimize the degenerative physical and mental function that occurs with aging.

5. References

American Geriatrics Society, British Geriatrics Society, & American Academy of Orthopaedic Surgeons Panel on Falls Prevention. (2001). Guideline for the prevention of falls in older persons. *Journal of the American Geriatrics Society*, Vol.49, No.5, pp. 664-672.

Bischoff-Ferrari, H.A.; Dawson-Hughes, B.; Staehelin, H.B.; Orav, J.E.; Stuck, A.E.; Theiler, R.; Wong, J.B.; Egli, A.; Kiel, D.P. & Henschkowski, J. (2009). Fall prevention with supplemental and active forms of vitamin D: a meta-analysis of randomized controlled trials. *British Medical Journal*, Vol.399, pp. 843-846.

Blake A.J.; Morgan, K.; Bendall, M.J.; Dallosso, H.; Ebrahim, S.B.J.; Arie, T.H.D.; Fentem, P.H. & Bassey, E.J. (1988). Falls by elderly people at home: prevalence and associated factors. *Age and Ageing*, Vol.17, No.6, pp. 365-372.

Bo, K. (1995). Pelvic floor muscle exercise for the treatment of stress urinary incontinence: an exercise physiology perspective. *International Urogynecology Journal*, Vol.6, pp. 282-291.

Bo, K. (2004). Pelvic floor muscle training is effective in treatment of female stress urinary incontinence, but how does it work? *International Urogynecology Journal*, Vol.15, pp. 76-84.

Borst, S.E. (2004). Interventions for sarcopenia and muscle weakness in older people. *Age and Ageing*, Vol.33, No.6, pp. 548-555.

Bump, R.C.; Sugerman, H.J.; Fantl, JA. & McClish, D.K. (1992). Obesity and lower urinary tract function in women: effect of surgically induced weight loss. *American Journal of Obstetrics and Gynecology*, Vol.167, No.2, pp. 392-397.

Day, L.; Fildes, B.; Gordon, I.; Fitzharris, M.; Flamer, H. & Lord, S. (2002). Randomised factorial trial of falls prevention among older people living in their own homes. *British Medical Journal*, Vol.325, No.7356, pp. 128-134.

Dillon, E.L.; Sheffield-Moore, M.; Paddon-Jones, D.; Gilkison, C.; Sanford, A.P.; Casperson, S.L.; Jiang, J.; Chinkes, D.L. & Urban, R.J. (2009). Amino acid supplementation increase lean body mass, basal muscle protein synthesis, and insulin-like growth factor-1 expression in older women. *The Journal of Clinical Endocrinology and Metabolism*, Vol.94, No.5, pp. 1630-16347.

Fiatarone, M.A.; O'Neill, E.F.; Ryan, N.D.; Clements, K.M.; Solares, G.R.; Nelson, M.E.; Roberts, S.B.; Kehayias, J.J.; Lipsitz, L.A. & Evans, W.J. (1994). Exercise training and nutritional supplementation for physical frailty in very elderly people. *The New England Journal of Medicine*, Vol.330, No.25, pp. 1769-1775.

Fried, L.P.; Tangen, C.M.; Walston, J.; Newman, A.B.; Hirsch, C.; Gottdiener, J.; Seeman, T.; Tracy, R.; Kop, W.J.; Burke, G. & McBurnie, M.A. (2001). Frailty in older adults: evidence for a phenotype. *The Journals of Gerontology. Series A, Biological Sciences and Medical Sciences*, Vol.56, No.3, pp. M146-456.

Fried, L.P.; Ferrucci, L.; Darer, J.; Williamson, J.D. & Anderson, G. (2004). Untangling the concepts of disability, frailty, and comorbidity: implications for improved targeting and care. *The Journals of Gerontology. Series A, Biological Sciences and Medical Sciences*, Vol.59, No.3, pp. 255-263.

Inouye, S.K.; Studenski, S.; Tinetti, M.E. & Kuchel, G.A. (2007). Geriatric syndromes: clinical, research, and policy implications of a core geriatric concept. *Journal of the American Geriatrics Society*, Vol.55, No.5, pp. 780-791.

Kegel, A.H. (1948). Progressive resistance exercise in the functional restoration of the perineal muscles. *American Journal of Obstetrics and Gynecology*, Vol.56, No.2, pp. 238-248.

Kim, H.; Yoshida, H.; Hu, X.; Yukawa, H.; Shinkai, S.; Kumagai, S.; Fujiwara, Y.; Yoshida, Y.; Furuna, T.; Sugiura, M.; Ishizaki, T. & Suzuki, T. (2004). Risk factors associated with onset of urinary incontinence in community-dwelling elderly population: a 4-year follow-up study. *Nihon Koshu Eisei Zasshi*, Vol.51, No.8, pp. 612-622 [Article in Japanese].

Kim, H.; Suzuki, T.; Yoshida, Y. & Yoshida, H. (2007). Effectiveness of multidimensional exercises for the treatment of stress urinary incontinence in elderly community-dwelling Japanese women: a randomized, controlled, crossover trial. *Journal of the American Geriatrics Society*, Vol.55, No.12, pp. 1932-1939.

Kim, H.; Yoshida, H. & Suzuki, T. (2011a). The effects of multidimensional exercise treatment on community-dwelling elderly Japanese women with stress, urge, and mixed urinary incontinence: A randomized controlled trial. *International Journal of Nursing Studies*, Vol.48, pp.1165-1172.

Kim, H.; Yoshida, H. & Suzuki, T. (2011b). Effects of exercise treatment with or without heat and steam generating sheet on urine loss in community-dwelling Japanese elderly women with urinary incontinence. *Geriatrics and Gerontology International*, Vol.11, pp.452-459.

Lagro-Janssen, T. & van Weel, C. (1998). Long-term effect of treatment of female incontinence in general practice. *British Journal of General Practice*, Vol.48, pp. 1735-1738.

Landi, F.; Cesari, M.; Russo, A.; Onder, G.; Lattanzio, F. & Bernabei, R. (2003). Potentially reversible risk factors and urinary incontinence in frail older people living in community. *Age and Ageing*, Vol.32, No.2, pp. 194-199.

Li, F.; Fisher, K.J.; Harmer, P.; Irbe, D.; Tearse, R.G. & Weimer, C. (2004). Tai chi and self-rated quality of sleep and daytime sleepiness in older adults: A randomized controlled trial. *Journal of the American Geriatrics Society*, Vol.52, pp. 892-900.

Liu, C.J. & Latham, N.K. (2009). Progressive resistance strength training for improving physical function in older adults. *Cochrane Database of Systematic Reviews*, Vol.8, No.3, CD002759.

Magaziner, J.; Simonsick, E.M.; Kashner, T.M.; Hebel, J.R. & Kenzora, J.E. (1989). Survival experience of aged hip fracture in patients. *American Journal of Public Health*, Vol.79, No.3, pp. 274-278.

McDowell, B.J.; Engberg, S.; Sereika, S.; Donovan, N.; Jubeck, M.E.; Weber, E. & Engberg, R. (1999). Effectiveness of behavioral therapy to treat incontinence in homebound older adults. *Journal of the American Geriatrics Society*, Vol.47, pp. 309-318.

Murphy, S.L.; Williams, C.S. & Gill, T.M. (2002). Characteristics associated with fear of falling and activity restriction in community-living older persons. *Journal of the American Geriatrics Society*, Vol.50, pp. 516-520.

Peterson, M.D.; Sen, A. & Gordon, P.M. (2011). Influence of resistance exercise on lead body mass in aging adults: A meta-analysis. *Medicine and Science in Sports and Exercise*, Vol.43, No.2, pp. 249-258.

Province, M.A.; Hadley, E.C.; Hornbrook, M.C.; Lipsitz, L.A.; Miller, J.P.; Mulrow, C.D.; Ory, M.G.; Sattin, R.W.; Tinetti, M.E. & Wolf, S.L. (1995) The effects of exercise on falls in elderly patients. A preplanned meta-analysis of the FICSIT Trials. Frailty and Injuries: Cooperative Studies of Intervention Techniques. *The Journal of the American Medical Association*, Vol.273, No.17, pp. 1341-1347.

Sherrington, C.; Whitney, J.C.; Lord, S.R.; Herbert, R.D; Cumming, R.G & Close, J.C.T. (2008). *Journal of the American Geriatrics Society*, Vol.56, pp. 2234-2243.

Subak, L.L.; Wing, R.; West, D.S.; Franklin, F.; Vittinghoff, E.; Creasman, J.M.; Richter, H.E.; Myers, D.; Burgio, K.L.; Gorin, A.A.; Macer, J.; Kusek, J.W. & Grady, D. (2009). Weight loss to treat urinary incontinence in overweight and obese women. *The New England Journal of Medicine*, Vol.360, No.5, pp. 481-490.

Suzuki, T.; Kwon, J.; Kim, H.; Shimada, H.; Yoshida, Y.; Iwasa, H. & Yoshida, H. (2008). Low serum 25-hydroxyvitamin D levels associated with falls among Japanese community-dwelling elderly. *Journal of Bone and Mineral Research*, Vol.23, No.8, pp. 1309-1317.

Taaffe, DR. (2006). Sarcopenia—exercise as a treatment strategy. *Australian Family Physician*, Vol.35, No.3, pp. 130-134.

Tinetti, M.E.; Speechley, M. & Ginter, S.F. (1988). Risk factors for falls among elderly persons living in the community. *The New England Journal of Medicine*, Vol.319, No.26, pp. 1701-1707.

Tinetti, M.E.; Baker, D.I.; McAvay, G.; Claus, E.B.; Garrett, P.; Gottschalk, M.; Koch, M.L.; Trainor, K. & Horwitz, R.I (1994). A multifactorial intervention to reduce the risk of falling among elderly people living in the community. *The New England Journal of Medicine*, Vol.331, No.13, pp. 821-827.

Tinetti, ME.; Inouye, SK.; Gill, TM. & Doucette, JT. (1995). Shared risk factors for falls, incontinence, and functional dependence. *The Journal of the American Medical Association*, Vol.273, No.17, pp. 1348-1353.

Wyman, J.F.; Fantl, J.A.; McClish, D.K. & Bump, R.C. (1998). Comparative efficacy of behavioral interventions in the management of female urinary incontinence. Continence Program for Women Research Group. *American Journal of Obstetrics and Gynecology*, Vol.179, No.4, pp. 999-1007.

Xue, Q.L.; Bandeen-Roche, K.; Varadhan, R.; Zou, J. & Fried, L.P. (2008). Initial manifestations of frailty criteria and the development of frailty phenotype in the Women's Health and Aging Study II. *The Journals of Gerontology. Series A, Biological Sciences and Medical Sciences*, Vol.63, No.9, pp. 984-990.

7

Aging and Exercise Training on the Neuromuscular Functions of Human Movements

Junichiro Yamauchi[1,2]
[1]*Graduate School of Human Health Sciences, Tokyo Metropolitan University;*
[2]*Future Institute for Sport Sciences, Japan*

1. Introduction

The mechanical characteristics of muscles that control the movement are important in determining the human locomotor system and can be modified with aging and exercise training. The function of keeping or improving lower limb muscle is important for elderly individuals because such function is associated with better functional performance such as brisk walking, stair climbing and chair standing. Because many of our daily living activities are multi-joint movements, we have investigated the aging-related changes in muscle functions of the lower limb multi-joint movements over a wide range and large number of people. In this chapter, I address the importance of muscle physiology in human movements with effects of aging and exercise training for elderly individuals.

2. Aging on the neuromuscular system

Aging is associated with impairment of various biological functions, such as decreases in muscle mass, strength, cellular protein synthesis, bone mineral density and hormonal secretion, or an increase in adipose tissue (Goodpaster et al. 2001; Lamberts et al 1997; Snead et al. 1993). The deterioration of skeletal muscle function is one of the primary consequences of aging. Muscular strength or power in humans is usually dependent on the growth process or aging. It is known that the peak of muscular strength is generally achieved between the ages of 20 and 30 years in both men and women, thereafter gradually decreases and begins to accelerate a decline after the ages of 60 to 65 (Hakkinen et al. 1995, 1997; Lindle et al. 1997). Aging can cause to a great decline in the function of neuromuscular system both during dynamic and isometric muscle activities (Bassey & Short, 1990; Hakkinen et al. 1995, 1997). This impairment in muscular force production appears to be dependent on the type of muscular contractions and gender: a decline in concentric strength starts earlier in ages of both men and women than eccentric strength, which also starts to decline earlier in men than in women (Lindle et al. 1997). A decrease in muscle force with aging is also associated with a reduced number of motor units (McComas et al. 1993). Such decrease in neuromuscular function seems to be occurred in selective atrophy of muscle fiber type. With aging process, it is greater loss in fast twitch types than in slow twitch types. Slow-twitch muscle fibers as SO (slow-twitch oxidative) fibers have characteristics in aerobic (oxidative) metabolism, slow contraction speed, and, in return, they are designed to be fatigue resistance. On the contrary, fast-twitch muscle fibers have three times faster intrinsic speeds of contraction and faster time to peak tension, produce higher twitch and tetanic tensions, have higher peak powers and reach peak power at higher speeds of contraction than slow-twitch muscle fibers; in return, they have the smaller number of both capillaries and mitochondria so that they induce fatigue quickly and need the longer recovery time to re-synthesize contractile proteins in accordance with high intensity exercises. Therefore, the aging-related decline in explosive strength can be associated with a decrease in maximum and rapid voluntary motor unit activation as well as atrophy of fast twitch fibers (Hakkinen et al. 1995). The ability of muscle to generate force explosively is especially important to move quickly so as to prevent a fall from a stumble in elderly individuals (Earles et al. 2001). The declines in physical performance or muscle force production of lower limbs among elderly individuals are a serious issue because it can be predictive of subsequent disability, bedridden and eventually early death (Guralnik et al. 1995).

3. Aging related muscle atrophy and changes in contractile properties

The decline in force generating capacity and muscle mass with aging is called sarcopenia. The maximum force production is strongly related to muscle mass or cross sectional area of muscle, so that the decline in maximum force production with aging can be caused by a decrease in muscle mass (Akima et al. 2001). It has been reported that a 31% decrease in the volume of quadriceps femoris is seen in elderly as compared with young individuals (Trappe et al. 2001). Furthermore, the muscle force per cross-sectional fiber area (specific tension) in the quadriceps femoris muscle (Frontera et al. 2000) and vastus lateralis muscle (Trappe et al. 2003) in human does not change with aging, so that an aging-related decrease in muscle mass is one of the key factors for loss of strength in elderly people. On the other hands, other studies have shown the reduction of specific tension in type I and IIa fibers in human vastus lateralis muscle with aging (Frontera et al. 2000; D'Antona et al. 2003; Larsson et al. 1997), implying the impairment of neural factors. In addition, reduction of muscle function and volume with aging is associated with a higher percentage of body fat in elderly individuals, due probably to a decrease in basal metabolism. More interestingly, smaller size of thigh circumference could increase a risk of death in older age (Heitmann & Frederksen, 2009). These suggest that aging-related decline in muscle function and mass have many important aspects of health issues in elderly individuals.

Muscle contractile velocity provides important information about not only mechano-chemical characteristics of the actin-myosin interaction (Huxley and Simmons, 1971) but also the contractile properties of human movements. With aging, no changes in maximum unloaded velocity are reported by the study with single muscle fiber of the vastus lateralis in young and old people (Trappe et al. 2003), although other single fiber studies on human vastus lateralis muscle have reported an inconsistency such that either decreased or unchanged maximum unloaded velocity with aging was observed depending on the type of muscle fibers or genders (D'Antona et al. 2003; Krivickas et al. 2001; Larsson et al. 1997). The animal studies have also shown no consistent results on the changes in maximum unloaded velocity associated with aging, e.g., a decrease in the slow twitch, soleus (Li & Larsson, 1996; Thompson & Brown, 1999) and a decrease in the fast twitch, superficial vastus lateralis muscle fibers (Fitts et al. 1984), while no changes in the slow twitch, soleus muscle fibers (Brooks & Faulkner, 1988; Fitts et al. 1984) and the fast twitch, extensor digitorum longus (Brooks & Faulkner, 1988; Fitts et al. 1984; Li & Larsson, 1996) and flexor digitorum longus muscle fibers (Walters et al. 1990). It seems likely that the reduction of force generation rather than shortening velocity is a major factor for the impairment of physical performance in elderly individuals.

4. Aging on the neuromuscular functions of human movements

Although the contractile properties of isolated muscle have been extensively studied, the influence of aging on contractile properties of muscles that control the multi-joint movements has not been extensively studied. We have developed the dynamometer with a high time-resolution servo system to obtain the isotonic, force-velocity relation of knee-hip extension movements (Yamauchi et al. 2007). By using this method, muscle functions are precisely evaluated with relatively small physical stress; i.e., without generation of large force to accelerate the inertial mass (Yamauchi & Ishii, 2007) and without a large increase in blood pressure (Yamauchi et al. 2008). To understand aging-related differences on the maximum force, unloaded velocity and power of leg multi-joint movements, the dynamometer was used to investigate the isotonic force-velocity and force-power relations of muscles that control leg multi-joint movements, and the maximum isometric force (Fmax), unloaded velocity (Vmax) and power (Pmax) were determined from the force-velocity relation.

We compared muscle functions of bilateral and unilateral knee-hip extension movements between healthy young (age, 19-31yrs) and healthy elderly (age, 60-82yrs) women (Yamauchi et al. 2009a). Figure 1 shows a typical example of force-velocity and force-power relations of knee-hip extension movements in young and elderly individuals. We showed that Fmax and Pmax of bilateral and unilateral knee-hip extension movements were 20-30% lower in elderly than in young women (Figure 2). On the other hand, there was no significant change in Vmax between young and elderly women and between bilateral and unilateral movements. Bilateral deficit was larger as the generation of force was larger in both young and elderly women. Also, bilateral deficit of Fmax and Pmax were not different between young and elderly women. Next, we investigated muscle functions of two hundred eighty-five recreationally active men (n=142) and women (n=143) aged between 18 and 82 year old volunteers for the cross sectional study (Yamauchi et al. 2010). We showed that with increasing age, Fmax/body mass significantly declined in both men ($r=-0.400$, $p<0.001$) and women ($r=-0.587$, $p<0.001$), while Vmax/leg length did not change with age in both men ($r=-0.033$, $p>0.05$) and women ($r=-0.040$, $p>0.05$). Pmax significantly declined with age in both men ($r=-0.370$, $p<0.001$) and women ($r=-0.446$, $p<0.001$). Figure 3 shows that maximum force and maximum power of knee-hip extension movements progressively decrease with increasing age. Both results showed the aging-related decline in maximum force and power output, but no differences in the intrinsic shortening velocity of leg multi-joint movements. This finding suggests that decreases in muscle force generating capacity and power may primarily lead to the loss of mobility and a reduced capability of

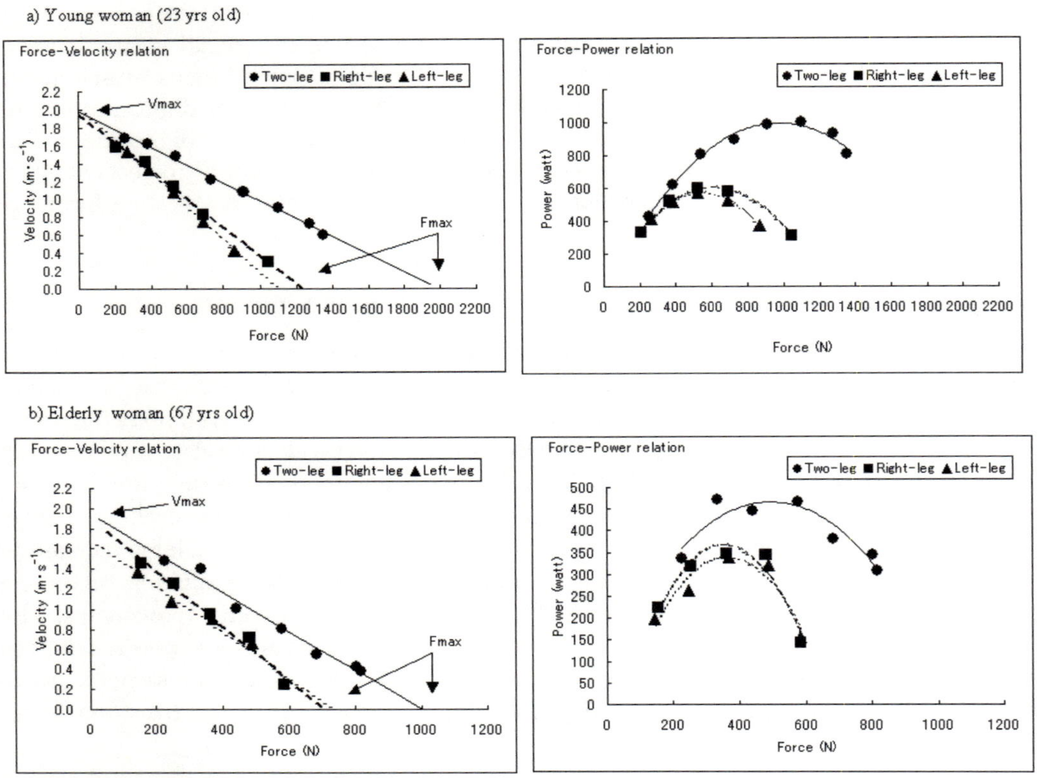

Fig. 1. Representative force-velocity and force-power relationships of bi- and unilateral knee-hip extension movements in young (a) and elderly (b) women (Yamauchi et al. 2009a) Filled circles, bi-lateral contraction (young, r=-0.99; elderly, r=-0.99); filled squares, right unilateral contraction (young, r=-0.99; elderly, r=-0.99); filled triangles, left unilateral contractions (young, r=-0.99; elderly, r=-0.98). Fmax and Vmax were estimated by extrapolations of linear regressions to zero force and velocity, respectively. Pmax was calculated as 0.5Fmax times 0.5Vmax.

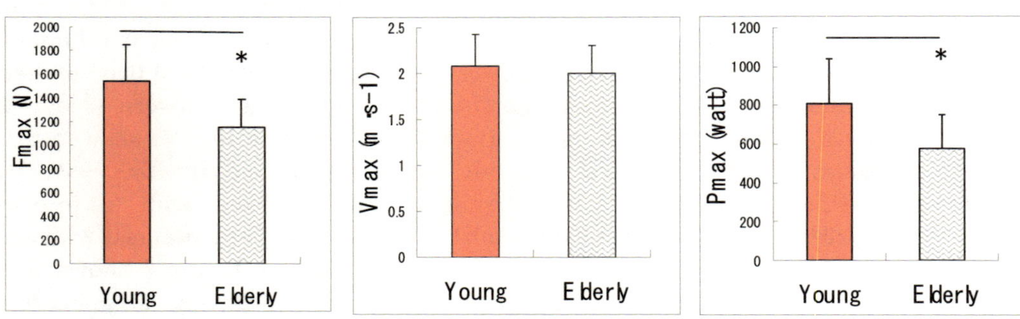

Fig. 2. Maximum isometric force (Fmax), velocity (Vmax) and power (Pmax) of knee-hip extension in young and elderly women (modified from Yamauchi et al. 2009a). Data were expressed as mean and SD. * $p<0.01$ as compared to Y group.

accelerating and decelerating the body mass during the movements. Such decrease in maximum force relative to body mass in elderly individuals indicates an increase in the risk of fall or decrease in quality of active life. This impairment of force generating capacity could be the major cause of aging-associated changes in walking ability, such as decrease in walking distance and speed (Lauretani et al. 2003). Thus, it is important to prevent a loss of force generating capacity of leg multi-joint movements in elderly individuals.

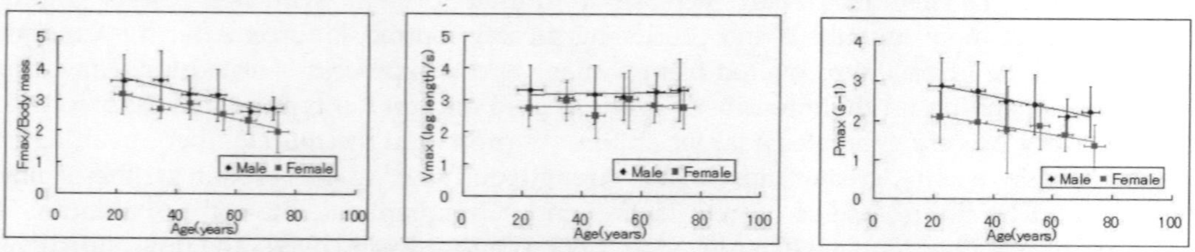

Fig. 3. Aging related changes in muscle functions of lower limb multi-joint movements (modified from Yamauchi et al. 2010)

5. Exercise training adaptation on the neuromuscular system

The exercise training can induce physiological adaptations in the muscle and nervous system (Bosco et al. 1986; Coyle et al. 1981; Hakkinen et al. 1989; McDonagh & Davies, 1984). A greater force production is directly related to the muscular hypertrophy in the long-term adaptation, whereas to the neural adaptation in the short-term adaptation to the exercise training. It is well known that most of untrained individuals can easily increase the voluntary maximum force capacity without muscle hypertrophy in the early phase of strength training. The great increases in force production for untrained individuals during the early phase of training can be explained by neural adaptation in terms of an increase in both muscle activation levels and synchronous activation patterns (Hakkinen, 1989; Kreamer et al. 1996; Ploutz et al. 1994; Staron et al. 1994). As muscle fibers adapt to exercise trainings, adaptation of motoneurons occurred for satisfying a new level of physiological demands; e.g., enlargements of the cell body, nucleus, and nucleolus of the motoneuron are observed after high intensity exercises (Burke, 1975). EMG studies have shown that increases in both recruitment and firing rate as well as various facilatory and inhibitory effects in CNS are recognized during various period of strength training (Sale, 1991). As force increases, both motor unit recruitment and firing rate increase. Such training-induced neural adaptations may lead an increase in the amount of neural input to the trained muscles especially during a short period of time (Hakkinen, 1989), allowing force to develop more rapidly and peak force to be kept for a long period of time (Sale, 1988).

When strength training proceeds to the longer period, more muscular hypertrophy factors, as a result of the synthesis of new protein, will contribute to the improvement of muscle force generating capacity (McDonagh & Davies, 1984). When the effect of muscle fiber hypertrophy increases, the motor unit activation required to produce a given force reduces. An increase in mechanical stress per unit area of activated muscle to lift a given load during exercise training can potentially be a physiological stimulus for strength gain and muscle hypertrophy, thus the strength training must be performed with progressively increases in load and with different types of movement over a exercise period (Kraemer et al. 1996; Ploutz et al. 1994). The muscle hypertrophy effects of exercise training in the human muscle are most prominent in the type II fibers (Komi, 1984; McDonagh & Davies, 1984). Although the cross sectional areas of both slow-twitch and fast-twitch muscle fibers increase after the exercise training (Linossier et al. 1997; MacDougall et al. 1979; Staron et al. 1990, 1991), training-induced hypertrophy appears to be greater in fast-twitch fibers than in slow-twitch fibers. To develop the muscular size, increases in protein synthesis are required as an adaptation to increased mechanical stress (Kraemer et al. 1995; MacDougall et al. 1979; McDonagh & Davies, 1984). An increase in muscle protein synthesis results in the construction of more myofibrils and producing greater contractile force. After the strength training, muscle fibers are recovered from damage and this process is lasted for a day or a few days depending on the intensity of exercise used and on the type of muscle involved. This recovery process generates a larger amount of protein in the muscle fiber, resulting in greater protein density, greater muscle fiber strength and size. Muscle protein synthesis may be increased by the release of growth factors and subsequent satellite cell activation as a result of muscle fiber damage (Chesley et al. 1992; White & Esser, 1989). The time course for changes in muscle protein synthesis after strength training may be related to training variables, such as the intensity and volume of exercise; the muscle or muscle groups involved; the type of muscle contraction performed; the training state of the trainees; and training frequency and subsequent recovery from exercise.

6. Exercise training for elderly individuals

So, how can we prevent a decrease in muscle force and power generating capacities with aging? The maximum force production is related to muscle size and neural factors so that the decline in maximum force production with aging should be caused by a decrease in muscle size and impairment of nervous system. Aging-related loss in muscle mass and rapid voluntary motor unit activation, especially the atrophy of fast twitch muscle fibers, are key factors for loss of muscle force production in lower limb multi-joint movements for elderly people. Scientific research shows that the resistance training is an effective countermeasure against sarcopenia or aging-related loss in muscle mass and functions. Resistance training for elderly individuals has positive effects of insulin action, bone density, energy metabolism and other biological functional status, so as to improve in daily activity. Even in debilitated elderly patients, resistance training for a short period can increase isometric force and physical function (Meuleman et al 2000). Long-term exercise trainings also show the improvement of neurobehavioral functions and the reducing risks of fall in elderly individuals (Fujisawa et al. 2007). Therefore, importance of resistance training for the elderly individuals is increasing in our society.

Most of studies in exercise training are usually using strength training equipment at fitness gym or exercise science laboratory. This may lead to people thinking that it is necessary to go to the fitness gym when they want to strengthen their body. At the fitness gym, fitness trainer can teach you how to train your body more effectively and correctly with using machines. However, once you learned proper exercise with experts, you can do many exercises at home without using machines. This self-managed exercise at home is more important for elderly individuals because older individuals are simply lower in daily activity. For this reason, exercise training at home or a community center without using strength training equipment has become increasingly in demand by elderly individuals. Some home-based exercise programs have shown benefits to functional abilities in daily activities of elderly individuals (King et al. 1991; McMurdo & Johnstone, 1995). It is important to understand how exercise training with using own bodyweight in elderly individuals affects muscle functions that relate to daily activity.

We have shown that exercise training using only body weight for a 10-month period successfully increased maximum force on average 15% and power output 13%, but left unchanged maximum unloaded velocity of leg multi-joint movements (Figure 4). Increased muscle force and power output of the knee–hip extension movement after the exercise training is likely due to an increase in muscle mass and improved muscle activation level. Also, improvement of muscular coordination in lower limbs could give rise to an increase in maximum force and power of knee-hip extension movement. Exercise training with leg multi-joint movements such as squat may largely provide increases in muscle force and power of knee-hip extension movement because specific movements favor to contribute improvement in coordination of agonist-antagonist muscle activity in multi-joint movements.

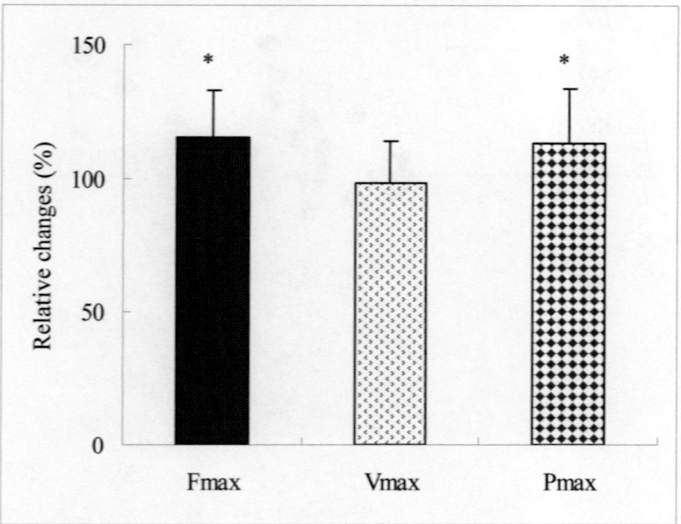

Fig. 4. Relative changes in maximum force (Fmax), velocity (Vmax) and power (Pmax) of lower limb multi-joint movements after the bodyweight based exercise training (modified from Yamauchi et al. 2009b). *Denotes a significant difference from pre-exercise training value ($p<0.001$).

Improvement of lower limb muscle force generating capacity after the exercise training could provide a positive influence on activities of daily living in elderly individuals. Increases in relative force and power reduce a risk of fall and increase quality of active life in elderly individuals (Tinetti et al. 1988). A greater muscle force generation can lead a better capability of accelerating and decelerating bodyweight during the movements and this capability will help elderly individuals to remain independent. The magnitude of increase in maximum force is related to the training intensity in elderly individuals (Figure 5). Individuals with higher exercise intensity gained greater increase in maximum force. This suggests that bodyweight-based resistance exercises could give enough training stimuli for individuals with a lower level of maximum force level, but not for individuals with an already high level. For the bodyweight based exercise training program, body weight relative to maximum force is an important parameter as a training intensity to determine the effects. When exercise trainings with own bodyweight continuously perform for a long term, their effects may dilute as time goes by because of increase in strength or decrease in training intensity. Thus, training intensity should change progressively with external resistance, movement speed, variation of exercise and frequency. It is generally suggested that strength training twice per week or even three times per week is optimal for improvements in strength, power and functional performance in elderly individuals. Further study needs to investigate frequency and other valuables of exercise training with using own bodyweight. Appropriate measurements of muscle function and subsequent exercise prescription in the multi-joint movements of the lower limbs are essential for the aged population.

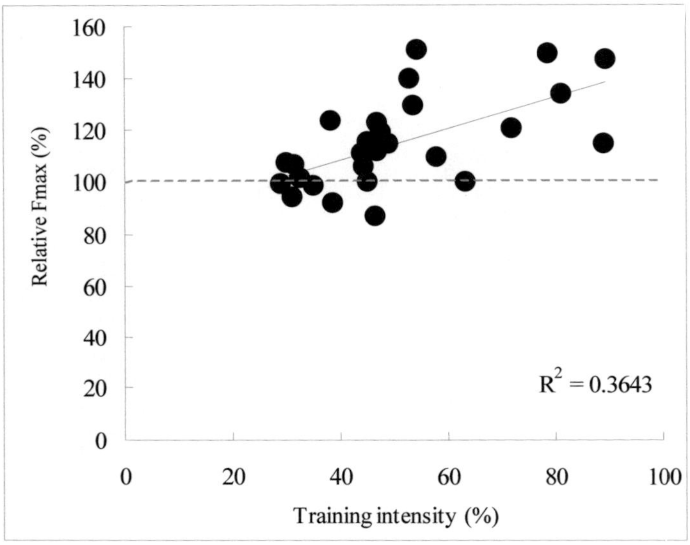

Fig. 5. Relationship between training intensity and % changes in maximum force (Fmax) after the bodyweight based exercise training (Yamauchi et al. 2009b)

7. Conclusion

It is important to understand the aging-related differences in muscle function of lower limb multi-joint movements because they are profoundly related to the movements of daily living. Aging-related decline in muscular power performance of multi-joint movements in the lower limbs has much larger effects on the force generating capacity than on the shortening velocity of muscles, because, with aging process, the maximum force generating capacity declined, whereas the maximum shortening velocity was not affected. This suggests that decreases in muscle force generating capacity and power with aging may primarily cause to the loss of mobility and a reduced capability of accelerating and decelerating body mass during leg multi-joint movements in elderly individuals. On the other hands, the exercise training is considered as important countermeasure against sarcopenia. Exercise training using own bodyweight was effective to increase in muscle force and power of leg multi-joint movements in elderly individuals. An initial training status was important for progressive increases in muscle force of leg multi-joint movements in elderly individuals. Proper assessment of muscle functions prior to exercise training is important for elderly individuals to provide better exercise prescription at home or a community center.

8. References

Akima H, Kano Y, Enomoto Y, Ishizu M, Okada M, Oishi Y, Katsuta S & Kuno S (2001). Muscle function in 164 men and women aged 20--84 yr. Med Sci Sports Exerc 33, 220-226.

Bassey EJ & Short AH (1990). A new method for measuring power output in a single leg extension: feasibility, reliability and validity. Eur J Appl Physiol Occup Physiol 60, 385-390.

Bosco C, Rusko H & Hirvonen J (1986). The effect of extra-load conditioning on muscle performance in athletes. Med Sci Sports Exerc 18, 415-419.

Brooks SV & Faulkner JA (1988). Contractile properties of skeletal muscles from young, adult and aged mice. J Physiol (Lond) 404, 71-82.

Burke RE (1975). Motor unit properties and selective involvement in movement. Exerc Sport Sci Rev 3, 31-81.

Chesley A, MacDougall JD, Tarnopolsky MA, Atkinson SA & Smith K (1992). Changes in human muscle protein synthesis after resistance exercise. J Appl Physiol 73, 1383-1388.

Coyle EF, Feiring DC, Rotkis TC, Cote RW, Roby FB, Lee W & Wilmore JH (1981). Specificity of power improvements through slow and fast isokinetic training. J Appl Physiol 51, 1437-1442.

D'Antona G, Pellegrino MA, Adami R, Rossi R, Carlizzi CN, Canepari M, Saltin B & Bottinelli R (2003). The effect of ageing and immobilization on structure and function of human skeletal muscle fibres. J Physiol (Lond) 552, 499-511.

Earles DR, Judge JO & Gunnarsson OT (2001). Velocity training induces power-specific adaptations in highly functioning older adults. Arch Phys Med Rehabil 82, 872-878.

Fitts RH, Troup JP, Witzmann FA & Holloszy JO (1984). The effect of ageing and exercise on skeletal muscle function. Mech Ageing Dev 27, 161-172.

Frontera WR, Suh D, Krivickas LS, Hughes VA, Goldstein R & Roubenoff R (2000). Skeletal muscle fiber quality in older men and women. Am J Physiol, Cell Physiol 279, C611-C618.

Fujisawa M, Ishine M, Okumiya K, Nishinaga M, Doi Y, Ozawa T & Matsubayashi K (2007). Effects of long-term exercise class on prevention of falls in community-dwelling elderly: Kahoku longitudinal aging study. Geriatr Gerontol Int 7: 357-362.

Goodpaster BH, Carlson CL, Visser M, Kelley DE, Scherzinger A, Harris TB, Stamm E & Newman AB (2001). Attenuation of skeletal muscle and strength in the elderly: The Health ABC Study. J Appl Physiol 90, 2157-2165.

Guralnik JM, Ferrucci L, Simonsick EM, Salive ME & Wallace RB (1995). Lower-extremity function in persons over the age of 70 years as a predictor of subsequent disability. N Engl J Med 332, 556-561.

Häkkinen K (1989). Neuromuscular and hormonal adaptations during strength and power training. A review. J Sports Med Phys Fitness 29, 9-26.

Häkkinen K, Kraemer WJ & Newton RU (1997). Muscle activation and force production during bilateral and unilateral concentric and isometric contractions of the knee extensors in men and women at different ages. Electromyogr Clin Neurophysiol 37, 131-142.

Häkkinen K, Pastinen UM, Karsikas R & Linnamo V (1995). Neuromuscular performance in voluntary bilateral and unilateral contraction and during electrical stimulation in men at different ages. Eur J Appl Physiol Occup Physiol 70, 518-527.

Häkkinen K, Mero A & Kauhanen H (1989). Specificity of endurance, sprint and strength training on physical performance capacity in young athletes. J Sports Med Phys Fitness 29, 27-35.

Heitmann & Frederksen (2009). Thigh circumference and risk of heart disease and premature death: prospective cohort study. BMJ. 339:b3292.

Huxley & Simmons (1971). Proposed mechanism of force generation in striated muscle. Nature 233, 533-538.

King AC, Haskell WL, Taylor CB, Kraemer HC & DeBusk RF (1991). Group- vs home-based exercise training in healthy older men and women. A community-based clinical trial. JAMA 266: 1535-42.

Komi PV (1984). Biomechanics and neuromuscular performance. Med Sci Sports Exerc 16, 26-28.

Kraemer WJ, Fleck SJ & Evans WJ (1996). Strength and power training: physiological mechanisms of adaptation. Exerc Sport Sci Rev 24, 363-397.

Kraemer WJ, Patton JF, Gordon SE, Harman EA, Deschenes MR, Reynolds K, Newton RU, Triplett NT & Dziados JE (1995). Compatibility of high-intensity strength and endurance training on hormonal and skeletal muscle adaptations. J Appl Physiol 78, 976-989.

Krivickas LS, Suh D, Wilkins J, Hughes VA, Roubenoff R & Frontera WR (2001). Age- and gender-related differences in maximum shortening velocity of skeletal muscle fibers. Am J Phys Med Rehabil 80, 447-455 quiz 456-7.

Lamberts SW, van den Beld AW & van der Lely AJ (1997). The endocrinology of aging. Science 278, 419-424.

Larsson L, Li X & Frontera WR (1997). Effects of aging on shortening velocity and myosin isoform composition in single human skeletal muscle cells. Am J Physiol 272, C638-C649.

Lauretani F, Russo CR, Bandinelli S, Bartali B, Cavazzini C, Di Iorio A, Corsi AM, Rantanen T, Guralnik JM & Ferrucci L (2003). Age-associated changes in skeletal muscles and their effect on mobility: an operational diagnosis of sarcopenia. J Appl Physiol 95:1851-60.

Li X & Larsson L (1996). Maximum shortening velocity and myosin isoforms in single muscle fibers from young and old rats. Am J Physiol 270, C352-C360.

Lindle RS, Metter EJ, Lynch NA, Fleg JL, Fozard JL, Tobin J, Roy TA & Hurley BF (1997). Age and gender comparisons of muscle strength in 654 women and men aged 20-93 yr. J Appl Physiol 83, 1581-1587.

Linossier MT, Dormois D, Geyssant A & Denis C (1997). Performance and fibre characteristics of human skeletal muscle during short sprint training and detraining on a cycle ergometer. Eur J Appl Physiol Occup Physiol 75, 491-498

MacDougall JD, Sale DG, Moroz JR, Elder GC, Sutton JR & Howald H (1979). Mitochondrial volume density in human skeletal muscle following heavy resistance training. Med Sci Sports 11, 164-166.

McComas AJ, Galea V & de Bruin H (1993). Motor unit populations in healthy and diseased muscles. Phys Ther 73, 868-877.

McDonagh MJ & Davies CT (1984). Adaptive response of mammalian skeletal muscle to exercise with high loads. Eur J Appl Physiol Occup Physiol 52, 139-155.

McMurdo ME & Johnstone R (1995). A randomized controlled trial of a home exercise programme for elderly people with poor mobility. Age Ageing 24: 425-8.

Meuleman JR, Brechue WF, Kubilis PS & Lowenthal DT (2000). Exercise training in the debilitated aged: strength and functional outcomes. Arch Phys Med Rehabil 81: 312-318.

Ploutz LL, Tesch PA, Biro RL & Dudley GA (1994). Effect of resistance training on muscle use during exercise. J Appl Physiol 76, 1675-1681.

Sale DG (1988). Neural adaptation to resistance training. Med Sci Sports Exerc 20, S135-S145.

Sale DG (1991). Neural Adaptation to Strength Training. In Strength and Power in Sport, ed. Komi PV, pp. 249-265. Blackwell Science, Oxford.

Snead DB, Birge SJ & Kohrt WM (1993). Age-related differences in body composition by hydrodensitometry and dual-energy X-ray absorptiometry. J Appl Physiol 74, 770-775.

Staron RS, Karapondo DL, Kraemer WJ, Fry AC, Gordon SE, Falkel JE, Hagerman FC & Hikida RS (1994). Skeletal muscle adaptations during early phase of heavy-resistance training in men and women. J Appl Physiol 76, 1247-1255.

Staron RS, Leonardi MJ, Karapondo DL, Malicky ES, Falkel JE, Hagerman FC & Hikida RS (1991). Strength and skeletal muscle adaptations in heavy-resistance-trained women after detraining and retraining. J Appl Physiol 70, 631-640.

Staron RS, Malicky ES, Leonardi MJ, Falkel JE, Hagerman FC & Dudley GA (1990). Muscle hypertrophy and fast fiber type conversions in heavy resistance-trained women. Eur J Appl Physiol Occup Physiol 60, 71-79.

Thompson LV & Brown M (1999). Age-related changes in contractile properties of single skeletal fibers from the soleus muscle. J Appl Physiol 86, 881-886.

Tinetti ME, Speechley M & Ginter SF (1988). Risk factors for falls among elderly persons living in the community. N Engl J Med 319: 1701-1707.

Trappe S, Gallagher P, Harber M, Carrithers J, Fluckey J & Trappe T (2003). Single muscle fibre contractile properties in young and old men and women. J Physiol (Lond) 552, 47-58.

Trappe TA, Lindquist DM & Carrithers JA (2001). Muscle-specific atrophy of the quadriceps femoris with aging. J Appl Physiol 90, 2070-2074.

Walters TJ, Sweeney HL & Farrar RP (1990). Aging does not affect contractile properties of type IIb FDL muscle in Fischer 344 rats. Am J Physiol 258, C1031-C1035.

White TP & Esser KA (1989). Satellite cell and growth factor involvement in skeletal muscle growth. Med Sci Sports Exerc 21, S158-S163.

Yamauchi J & Ishii N (2007). Relations between force-velocity characteristics of the knee-hip extension movement and vertical jump performance. Journal of Strength and Conditioning Research 21: 703-709.

Yamauchi J, Mishima C, Fujiwara M, Nakayama S & Ishii N (2007). Steady-state force-velocity relation in human multi-joint movement determined with force clamp analysis. J Biomech 40: 1433-42.

Yamauchi J, Mishima C, Nakayama S & Ishii N (2010). Ageing related differences in maximum force, unloaded velocity and power of human leg multi-joint movement. Gerontology 56: 167-174.

Yamauchi J, Mishima C, Nakayama S & Ishii N (2009a). Force-velocity, force-power relationships of bilateral and unilateral leg multi-joint movements in young and elderly women. Journal of Biomechanics 42: 2151-2157.

Yamauchi J, Nakayama S & Ishii N (2008). Blood pressure response to force-velocity properties of the knee-hip extension movement. Eur J Appl Physiol 102: 569-575.

Yamauchi J, Nakayama S & Ishii N (2009b). Effects of bodyweight-based exercise training on muscle functions of leg multi-joint movement in elderly individuals. Geriatrics & Gerontology International 9: 262-269.

8

Tailor-Made Programs for Preventive Falls that Match the Level of Physical Well-Being in Community-Dwelling Older Adults

Minoru Yamada, Tomoki Aoyama and Hidenori Arai
Kyoto University,
Japan

1. Introduction

Falls are relatively common in the elderly, with approximately 30% of individuals aged 65 and older falling at least once a year and approximately half of them experiencing repeated falls (Tinetti et al., 1988). Falls and fractures have a major impact on elderly individuals, their caregivers, health service providers, and the community. Sherrington et al. reported that up to 42% of falls can be prevented by well-designed exercise programs that target balance and involve a good amount of exercise (Sherrington et al., 2008).

In daily life, locomotion occurs under complicated circumstances, with cognitive attention focused on a particular task, such as watching the traffic or reading street signs, rather than on performing a simple motor task such as walking. A seminal study demonstrating that the characteristic "stops walking when talking" could serve as a predictor of falls introduced a novel method for predicting falls based on dual-task (DT) performance (Lundin-Olsson et al., 1997). Our recent study indicated that different factors may be related to fall incidents depending on the level of frailty of the community-dwelling elderly adults (Yamada et al., 2011a). These findings suggest that fall prevention programs should be tailored to the elderly adult's level of physical well-being. The purpose of this review is to review approaches to fall prevention tailored to an individual's level of physical well-being.

2. What is "Dual-task"?

Recently, several investigators have reported that DT gait is associated with fall incidents in elderly adults. A summary of these DT studies is shown in Table 1.

3. How can we use DT to assess fall risk in the elderly?

3.1 Game-based fall risk assessment

DT performance may be a reliable predictor of falls in elderly adults. The Nintendo Wii Fit program requires the distribution of attention to the motor task and the monitor (cognitive task). Thus, it is assumed that this program includes a constituent of DT. We examined whether the Wii Fit program's Basic Step can be used for fall risk assessment in healthy,

	Primary task	Secondary task	Fall related
Beauchet et al., 2008	Walk	Cognitive task	○
Beauchet et al., 2008	Walk	Cognitive task	○
Kressing RW et al, 2008	Walk	Cognitive task	○
Beauchet et al., 2007	Walk	Cognitive task	○
Faulkner KA et al, 2007	Walk	Cognitive task	○
Toulotte C et al, 2006	Walk	Manual task	○
Springer S et al, 2006	Walk	Cognitive task	×
Bootsma-vander Wiel A et al, 2003	Walk	Cognitive task	×
Verghese et al., 2002	Walk	Cognitive task	○
Stalenhoef PA et al, 2002	Walk	Cognitive task	×
Lundin-Olsson L et al, 1997	Walk	Cognitive task	○

○, related to falls; x, non-related to falls

Table 1. Effect of dual tasking on falls.

community-dwelling elderly adults (Yamada et al., 2011b). The results suggested that game-based fall risk assessment has a high generality and is very useful for assessing community-dwelling elderly adults (Fig. 1).

This study included a Wii Fit Balance Board, which was placed under the participants' feet. A score of 111 points on Basic Step was used to classify 88.6% of the cases correctly ($p < 0.001$). The horizontal demonstrates the cutoff point.

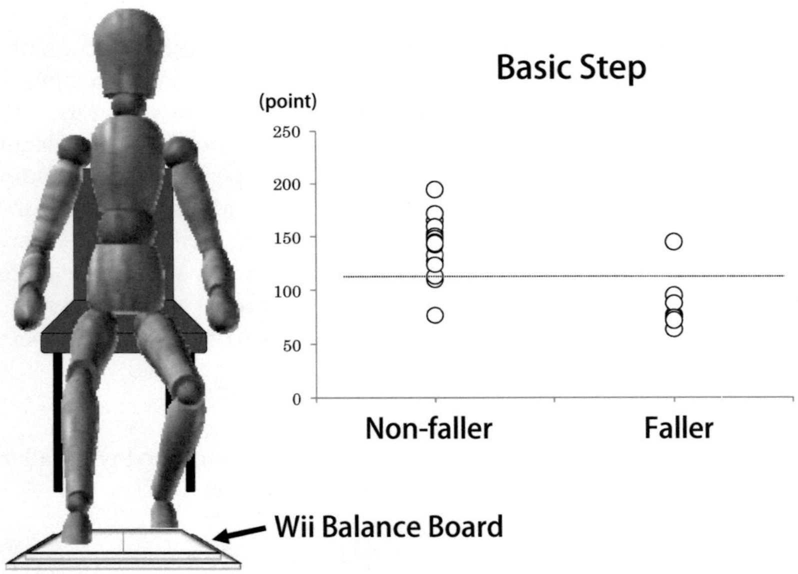

Fig. 1. Schematic diagram of Basic Step as played in a sitting position and scatter chart.

3.2 Smartphone-based fall risk assessment

The Android-based Smartphone can be used to develop applications freely. These applications can then be disseminated across the world via the internet. The use of Android-based applications is advantageous because they are free to develop, offer flexible design options, and can be easily and rapidly distributed over the internet. We developed an Android application (RollingBall) for the assessment of fall risk (available for download at http://www.kuhp.kyoto-u.ac.jp/~kazuya/RollingBall.apk) in which a small blue ball (1.5 cm in diameter) is moved on a large white circle (4 cm in diameter) by tilting the phone. The angle of the phone is determined by triaxial accelerometers (Fig. 2). The Android application also calculates a score on the basis of the coordinate data of the ball on the circle; higher scores indicate that the blue ball is closer to the center of the circle. The application was based on the "walking while carrying a ball on a tray" task. We previously examined whether the score determined by the Android application for DT-based fall risk assessment was related to falls in a population of community-dwelling elderly people (Yamada et al., 2011c). The results suggested that the Android application is very useful for fall risk assessment in elderly adults (Fig. 2).

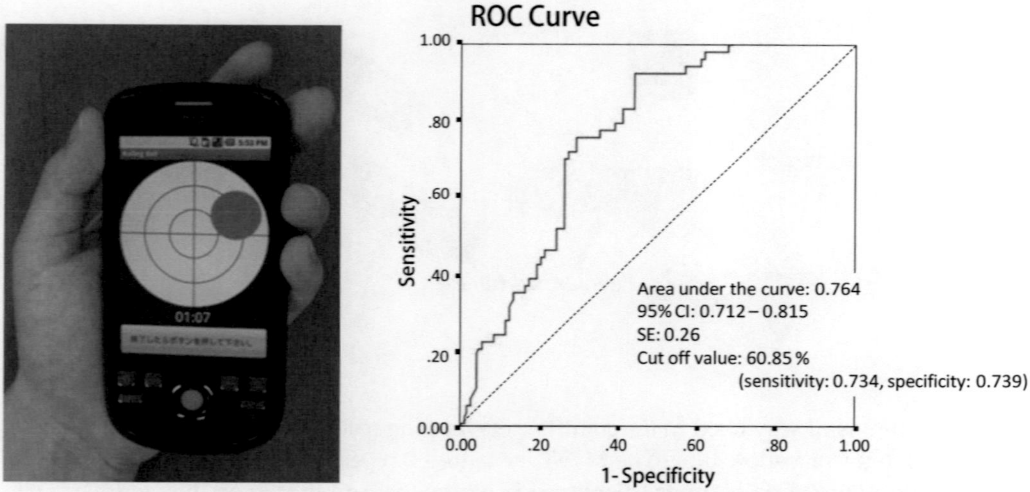

Fig. 2. An Android application allows users to control the position of a small blue circle (1.5 cm in diameter) on a large white circle (4 cm in diameter). Scores are automatically calculated on the basis of coordinate tracking data for the blue circle.

ROC (receiver operating characteristic) curve of the dual tasking (DT) total cost for the classification of fall risk. The area under the curve was 0.764. For the DT total cost, the cut-off value was 60.85% (sensitivity = 73.4%, specificity = 73.9%). CI, confidence interval

3.3 Multitarget Stepping Test (MTST)

We developed a walking test, the multitarget stepping test (MTST) (Yamada et al., 2011d). During the test, stepping and avoidance failures were measured while participants walked along a 10-m walkway and stepped on multiple targets. The MTST was performed on a black elastic mat (10 m long × 1 m wide). Forty-five 10 cm × 10 cm squares were on the mat (see Fig. 3). These squares were arranged into 3 rows (15 cm between each row) and 15 lines (61 cm between each line). Each square was marked with red, blue, or yellow tape. Each line had one of the 3 colored squares in a random order. One square (blue or yellow) was the footfall target, whereas the others were distracters. The color of the footfall target was counterbalanced among the participants and announced to each participant before he or she began walking.

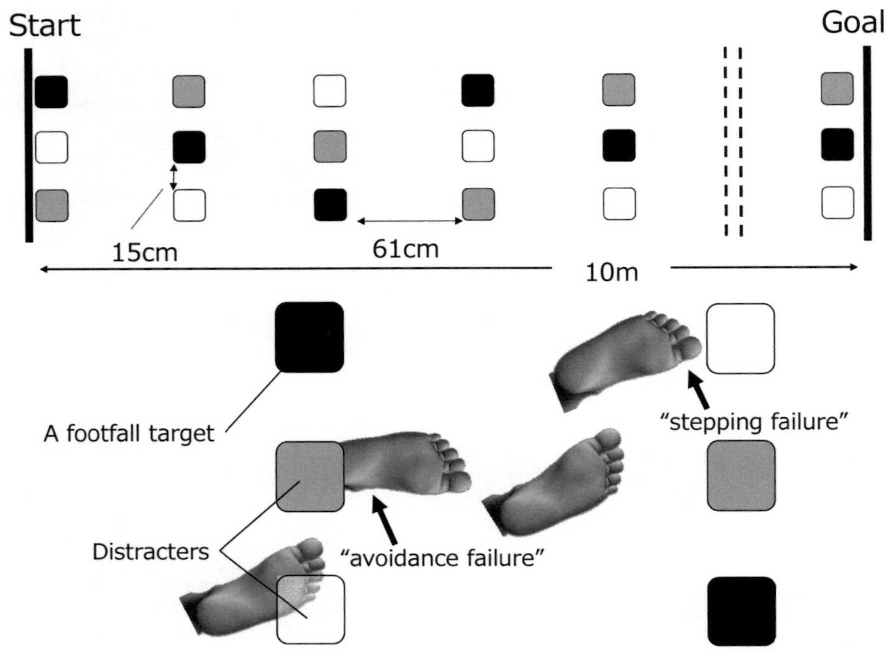

Fig. 3. The 10-m walkway used in the multitarget stepping test (MTST): Each square was made of red, blue, or yellow tape. The MTST measured 2 types of failure. A participant intended to step on footfall targets (displayed in white). Failure to step on the footfall target was regarded as a stepping error. Failure to avoid a distracter was regarded as an avoidance failure. As shown in this figure, avoidance failure was always the result of an accidental step as the participant walked from target to target; it did not occur because of selecting the wrong target out of the 3 squares on the line on which the participant intended to step.

The participants walked on the mat at a self-selected pace while stepping on the target square placed on each line. The participants were instructed (a) to step on a footfall target with either side of the foot and any part of the sole, (b) to take as many steps as necessary while walking between the lines to comfortably walk toward the next footfall target, and (c) to not step on the distracters. The main dependent measures were 2 types of failure indicating less accurate stepping performance: a stepping failure (i.e., failure to step on the footfall target) and an avoidance failure (i.e., failure to avoid distracters).

The results demonstrated that the stepping failure was independently associated with falling (odds ratio [OR] = 19.365, 95% confidence interval [CI] = 3.28–113.95; $p < 0.001$). Hence, measurements of stepping accuracy while performing the MTST, particularly precise stepping failure, could help identify elderly individuals at high risk for a fall.

3.4 Questionnaire-based fall risk assessment

As discussed, DT walking, game-based assessment, Smartphone assessment, and/or MTST can be used to identify elderly adults at high risk of falling. However, more simple and reliable assessment methods are necessary for community-dwelling elderly people. We previously examined whether a newly developed index we had designed to assess complex-task locomotion was related to falls in a robust elderly population (Yamada et al., in press a). The results suggested that a score of more than 1 point on the new index can predict falls in elderly adults (Table 2, Fig. 4).

	Item	0	1
1)	Can you stand up without a support?	Yes	No
2)	Can you turn in the opposite way, while holding an empty glass?	Yes	No
3)	Can you walk without dropping a glass of water?	Yes	No
4)	Have you ever tripped over an obstacle while going to the bathroom or picking up the telephone?	No	Yes

Table 2. Newly developed index

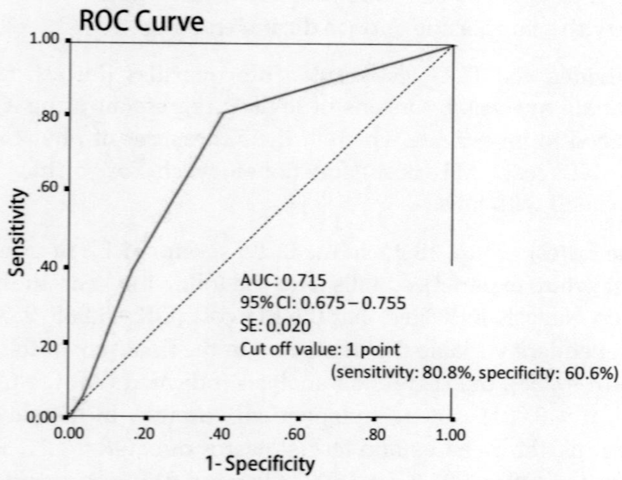

Fig. 4. The ROC (receiver operating characteristic) curve for the total points used for the classification of fall risk: The area under the curve (AUC) was 0.715. Concerning the total points, the cut-off value was determined at 1 point (sensitivity, 80.8%; specificity, 60.6%). CI, confidence interval

4. Different factors related to fall incidents

Our research has indicated that different factors may be related to fall incidents depending on the level of frailty in community-dwelling elderly adults.

One study population consisted of 1038 elderly Japanese subjects aged 65 years or older living in a community (401 men, 637 women; mean age, 77 ± 8 years). We assessed 6 items of physical functioning: timed up and go (TUG), functional reach, 5-chair stand, single-task (ST) 10-m walking time, and DT (CT [cognitive task], MT [manual task]) 10-m walking time.

In the TUG test, participants were asked to stand up from a standard chair with a seat height of 40 cm, walk a distance of 3 m at a maximum pace, turn, walk back to the chair, and sit down (Podsiadlo et al., 1991). Functional reach was measured using a simple clinical apparatus consisting of a yardstick secured to the wall at right acromion height as previously described (Duncan et al., 1990). In the 5-chair stand, participants were asked to stand up and sit down 5 times as quickly as possible and were timed from the initial sitting position to the final standing position at the end of the fifth stand (Guralnik et al., 1994). In ST walking, the participants were asked to walk as fast as possible along a 10-m straight line, with a 1-m approach at both ends, for a total length of 12 m. The time required was measured. In CT walking, participants walked 15 m at the most comfortable speed while counting numbers aloud in reverse order starting at 100. In MT walking, participants walked 15 m at the most comfortable speed while carrying a ball (7 cm in diameter, 150 g in weight) on a tray (17 cm in diameter, 50 g in weight). The DT cost (CT and MT) was then calculated as follows: DT cost [%] = 100 × (DT walking time - ST walking time)/([ST walking time + DT walking time]/2).

Information on fall incidents over the following year was collected from participants via a monthly telephone interview. A fall was defined as any event that led to unplanned, unexpected contact with a supporting surface during walking.

For analysis, we divided the TUG test results into quartiles (fastest, faster, slower, and slowest). A multivariate analysis by means of logistic regression using a stepwise-forward method was performed to investigate which of the 5 measures of physical functioning (i.e., ST walking time, CT cost, MT cost, functional reach, or 5-chair stand test) was independently associated with falls.

A total of 20% in the fastest group, 18.2% in the faster group, 34.1% in the slower group, and 44.1% in the slowest group experienced falls over the following year. In the fastest group (n = 230), the regression analysis indicated that the MT cost (OR = 1.068, 95% CI = 1.04–1.10; $p < 0.001$) was an independent variable that remained in the final step of the regression model. In the faster group (n = 258), the regression analysis indicated that the CT cost (OR = 1.03, 95% CI = 1.01–1.04; $p < 0.001$) was an independent variable. In the slower (n = 264) and slowest (n = 286) groups, the 5-chair stand test (slower group: OR = 1.11, 95% CI = 1.03–1.19; $p < 0.001$; slowest group: OR = 1.05, CI = 1.01–1.09; $p < 0.045$) was found to be a significant and independent variable of falls. A summary of these results is shown in Fig. 5.

5. Fall prevention programs tailored to levels of physical well-being

Fig. 5 shows that different factors may be related to fall incidents depending on one's level of physical well-being. DT walking is associated with falls in the robust elderly population, and thus this population should be given the rhythmic stepping exercise (Yamada et al., 2011e). DT walking and muscle strength are associated with falls in the intermediate elderly population, and thus this population should be given the seated stepping exercise (Yamada et al., 2010a). Muscle strength and DT walking are associated with falls in the pre-frail elderly population (Yamada et al., 2010b) and thus this population should be given the trail walking exercise. Finally, muscle strength is associated with falls in the frail elderly population, and thus this population should be given resistance exercise (Yamada et al., 2011f).

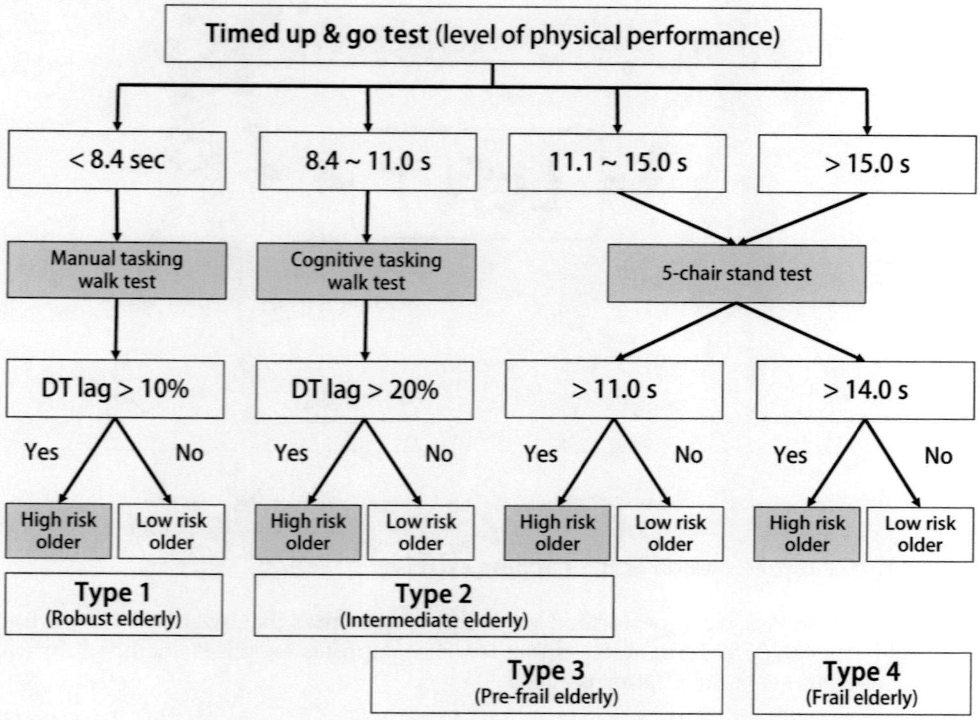

Fig. 5. Flow chart showing that the different factors may be related to fall incidents depending on an individual's level of physical well-being; DT, dual tasking

5.1 Rhythmic stepping exercise

Rhythmic stepping exercises were performed on a thin elastic mat (150 × 150 cm) that was partitioned into 5 squares (50 cm each) to form a cross (Fig. 6). The stepping exercises included forward, backward, and sideways step patterns. The participants were required to step at a tempo of 60–120 beats/min along with the accompanying rhythm sound and to step into the square indicated verbally by the supervisor (e.g., "right," "forward," "back"). Cognitive functioning (reaction, short-term memory, etc.) and motor functioning (stepping in multiple directions) were simultaneously required of the participants. In order to change the level of difficulty, the instruction method transposed not only direction but also color (e.g., "red," "blue") or number (e.g., "3," "7"). The participants completed 5 sets of 1 min per set of stepping exercises between weeks 1 and 8, which was then increased to 3 sets of 3 min per set between weeks 9 and 16 and 3 sets of 5 min per set between weeks 17 and 24. The instructions given at the beginning of each class were as follows: "Please step as correctly as possible, and avoid making mistakes as much as you can."

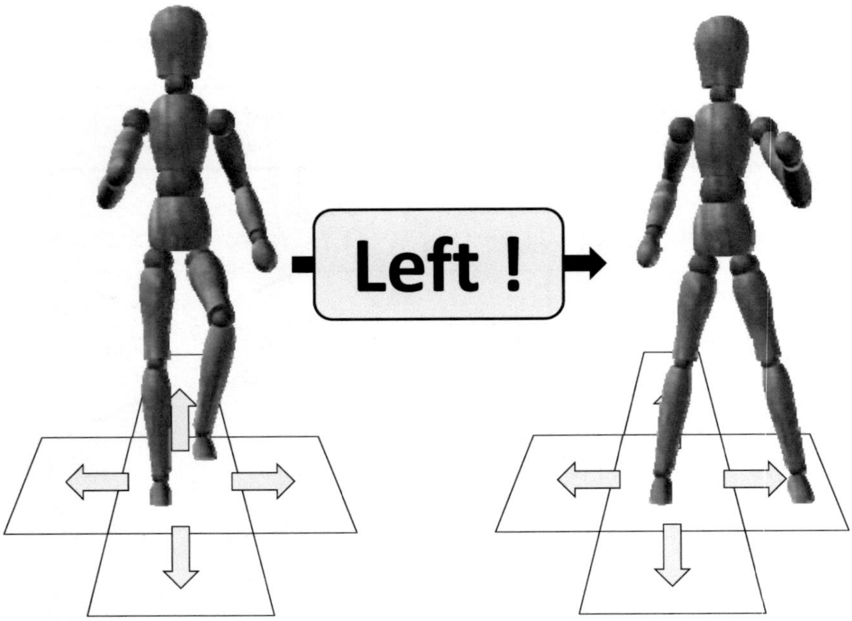

Fig. 6. Schematic representation of the stepping exercises.

The stepping exercises were performed on a thin elastic mat that was partitioned into 5 squares (50 cm each) to form a cross shape. The stepping exercises included forward, backward, and sideways step patterns.

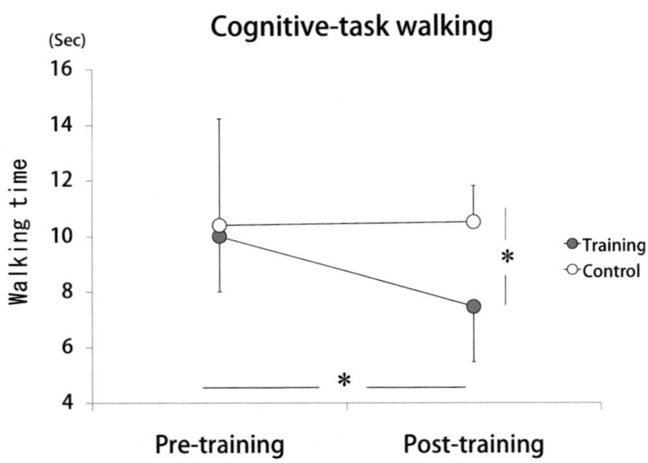

Fig. 7. Cognitive task walk time in training (rhythmic stepping exercise) and control groups during pre- and post-training. Significant differences were observed between the 2 groups ($p < 0.05$).

We evaluated whether a 24-week rhythmic stepping exercise program would effectively improve physical functioning and reduce fear of falling in community-dwelling elderly adults. The results of this study suggested that the rhythmic stepping exercise program was indeed effective at improving DT walking ability and fear of falling (Yamada et al., 2011e).

5.2 Seated stepping exercise

The participants were instructed on how to perform the seated stepping exercises by using a standard dining room chair (Fig. 8). The participants stepped up and down alternating between left and right legs as quickly as possible while returning the legs to the initial starting position. The minimum lifting height for stepping was the lifting of the plantar surface above the ground. The intensity of the exercise was increased over the 12-week period by increasing the total stepping time. The participants completed 10 sets of 5 s per set in weeks 1–12, increasing to 10 sets of 10 s per set in weeks 13–24. The participants were asked to perform a verbal fluency task during stepping (DT condition). This task consisted of listing words within a category (e.g., animals, vegetables, fruits, fish) or by letter (e.g., a word that begins with "A") at a self-selected speed. This task was self-generated; the participants did not read from a list but had to conceptualize and vocalize each word. The verbal fluency task was changed for each exercise session. The participants were not specifically instructed to prioritize either task but were asked to combine both tasks as much as they could. The instructions were as follows: "Please step as quickly as possible, and avoid making mistakes as much as you can."

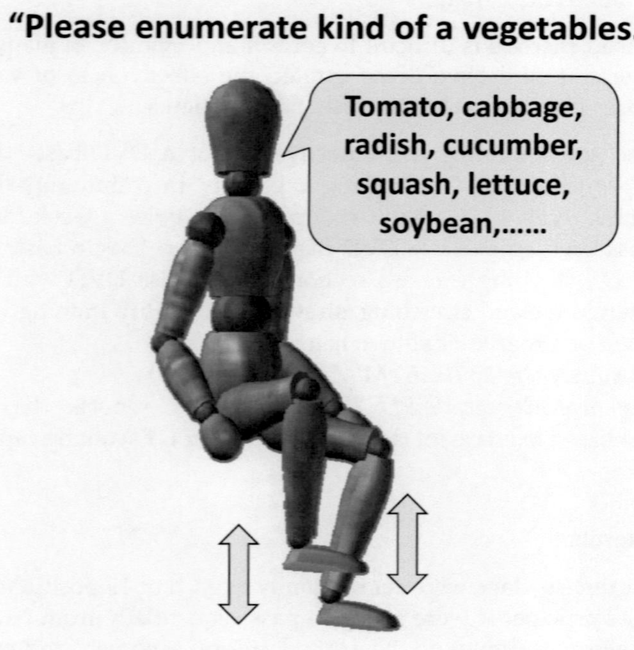

Fig. 8. Schematic representation of the seated stepping exercise

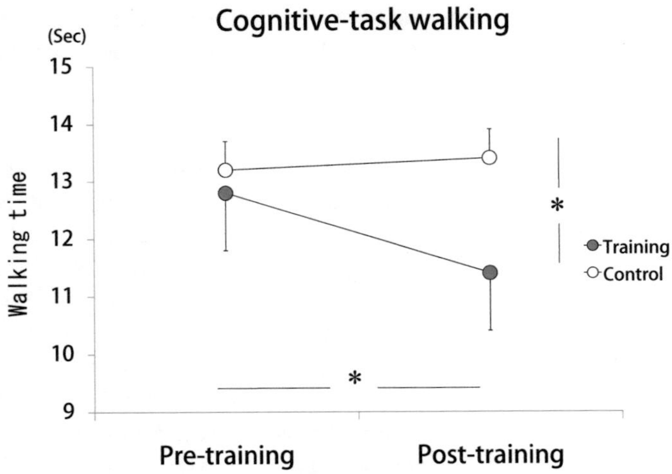

Fig. 9. Cognitive task walk time in training (seated stepping exercise) and control groups during pre- and post-training. Significant differences were observed between the 2 groups ($p < 0.05$).

We evaluated whether a 24-week seated stepping exercise program would effectively improve physical functioning in community-dwelling elderly adults. The results of this trial suggested that the seated stepping exercise program was indeed effective at improving DT walking ability (Yamada et al., 2010a).

However, unsupervised exercise is difficult to control and monitor in many elderly adults. In recent years, several studies have demonstrated the effectiveness of various video- or internet-based exercises in elderly adults or orthopedic patients.

We also investigated the feasibility and effectiveness of a DVD-based seated stepping exercise for the improvement of DT walking capability in community-dwelling elderly adults. The participants received 20 min of group training twice a week for 24 weeks (Fig. 10). The exercise class used an exercise DVD that included a 15-min basic exercise section and a 5-min seated DT stepping exercise section. An exercise DVD with 4 volumes was used. The basic training involved stretching, strength, and agility training while seated. An example from the exercise program is shown below: *http://www.youtube.com/watch?v=1391kzEYMJM* and *http://www.youtube.com/watch?v=mcaWhPLN7Es*. This study reports the feasibility and effectiveness of DVD-based exercise for the improvement of DT walking capability (Yamada et al., in press b).

5.3 Trail walking exercise

In the trail walking exercise, flags were set randomly at each of 15 positions in a 25-m^2 area (5 m × 5 m; Fig. 12). Participants were asked to pass sequentially from No. 1 to No. 15. A circle 30 cm in diameter was drawn on the ground around each flag, and participants were required to step in the circle to pass the flag. The height of the flag was 30 cm. The tester gave the following instructions to the participants: "Please move to No. 15 as quickly and correctly as possible." The 24-week program included a progressive aspect in which the

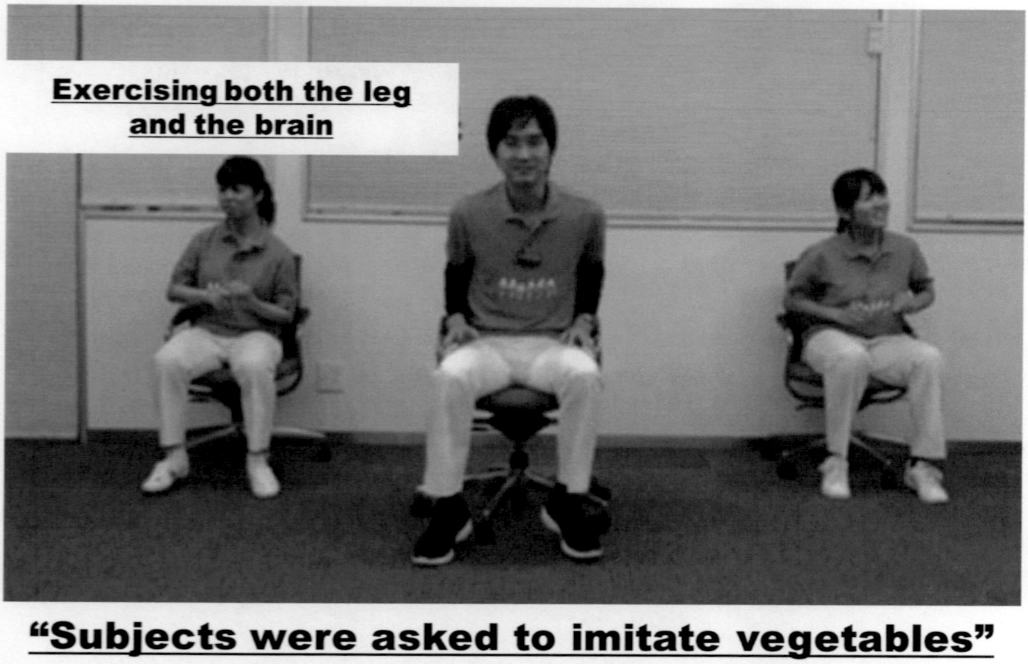

Fig. 10. Schematic representation of the DVD-based seated stepping exercise.

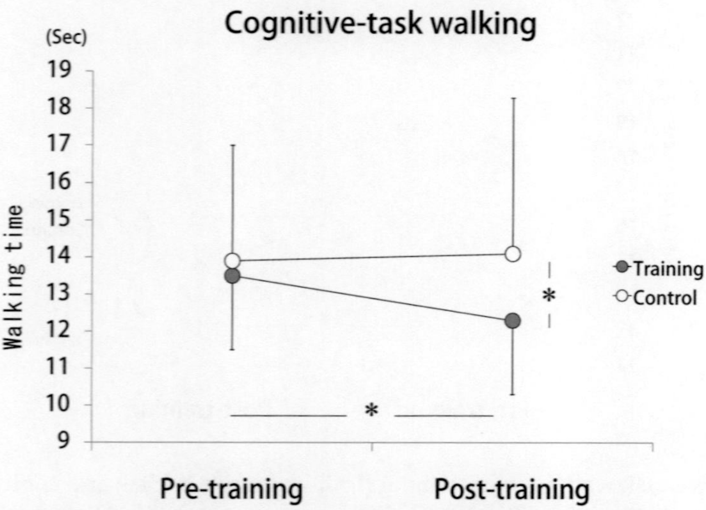

Fig. 11. Cognitive task walk time in training (DVD-based seated stepping exercise) and control groups during pre- and post-training. Significant differences were observed between the 2 groups ($p < 0.05$).

participants were asked to pass sequentially from No. 1 to No. 15 during weeks 1 to 12 but were asked to pass sequentially from No. 15 to No. 1 during weeks 13 to 24. The flag positions were changed for each day of training.

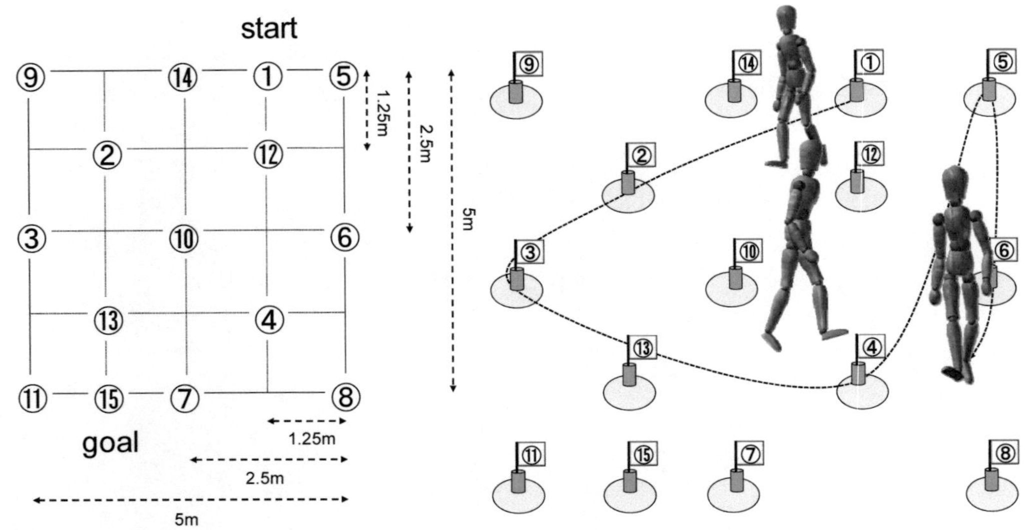

Fig. 12. Schematic representation of the trail walking exercise

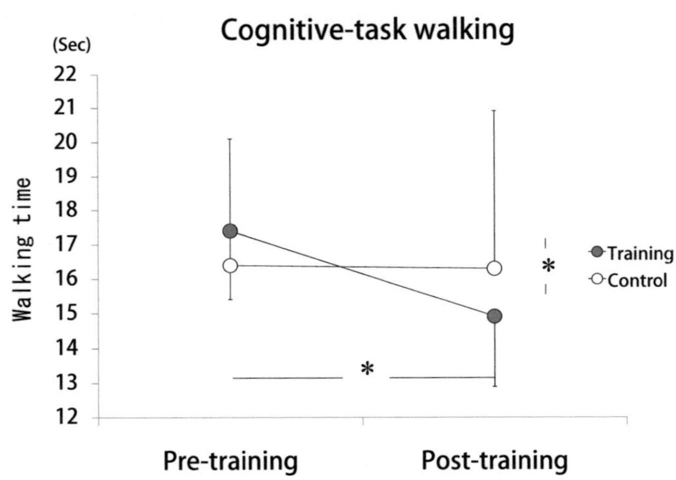

Fig. 13. Cognitive task walk time in training (trail-walking exercise) and control groups during pre- and post-training. Significant differences were observed between the 2 groups ($p < 0.05$).

We evaluated whether a 16-week trail walking exercise program would effectively improve physical functioning and reduce fall incidents in community-dwelling elderly adults. The results of this trial suggested that the trail walking exercise program was indeed effective at improving DT walking ability and decreasing the incident rate of falls 6 months after trial completion (Yamada et al., 2010b).

5.4 Resistance exercise for frail elderly adults

The participants underwent resistance training sessions twice a week for 24 weeks. All participants performed seated row, leg press, leg curl, and leg extension exercises on resistance training machines. Training loads were chosen using the 10-repetition maximum (10-RM; the maximum weight that can be lifted 10 times). The participants used the 10-RM for 3 sets of 10 repetitions for each machine exercise. The participants were required to adjust the training weight to ensure failure at the 10-RM. It took approximately 1 h to finish all sessions, with a 15-min warm-up at the beginning and a 10-min cool-down stretch at the end.

We compared the effects of resistance training on skeletal muscle mass, physical performance, and fear of falling in pre-frail and frail elderly adults. The results of this trial suggested that the skeletal muscle mass was increased by the resistance training program in both groups. However, improvements in the fear of falling and physical functioning were limited to the frail elderly adults (Yamada et al., 2011f).

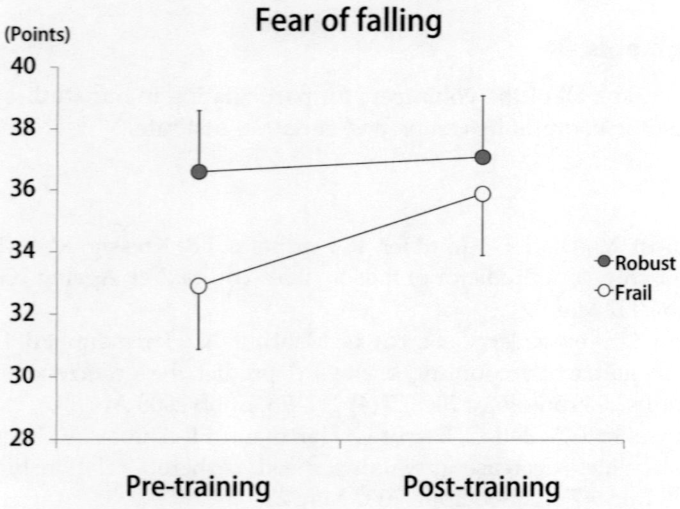

Fig. 14. Fear of falling in robust and frail groups during pre- and post-resistance training. Significant differences were observed between the 2 groups ($p < 0.05$).

6. Conclusions

The findings of this review suggest that fall prevention programs should be tailored to an individual's level of physical well-being; robust elderly adults should be given the rhythmic stepping exercise; intermediate elderly adults, the trail walking exercise; pre-frail elderly adults, the seated stepping exercise; and frail elderly adults, resistance exercises. A summary of interventions tailored to the individuals' levels of physical well-being is shown in Fig. 15.

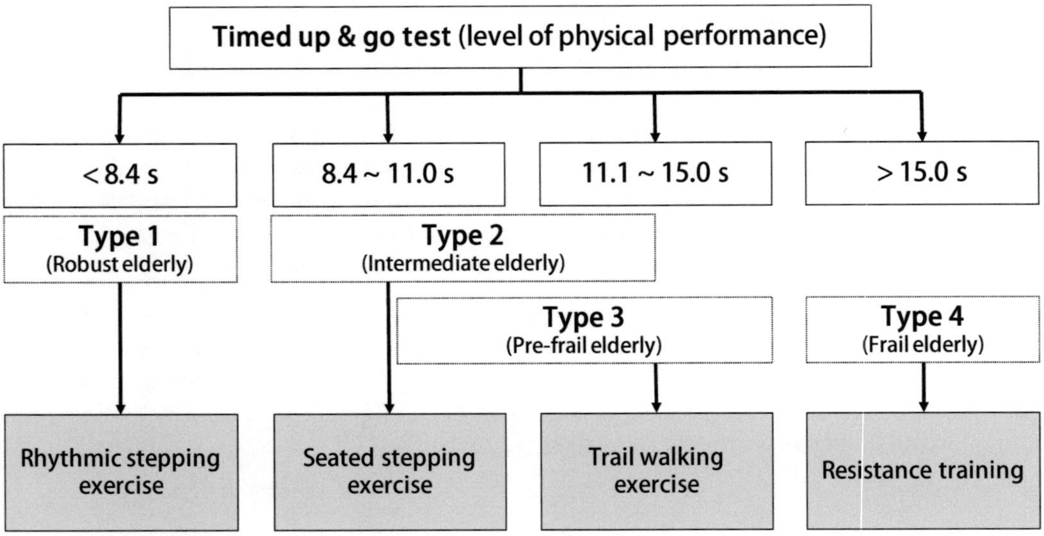

Fig. 15. Flow chart showing interventions tailored to levels of physical well-being.

7. Acknowledgments

We would like to thank all of the volunteers for participating in our studies and the staff of the day-service center, community center, and geriatrics institute.

8. References

Beauchet O, Dubost V, Allali G, Gonthier R, Hermann FR, Kressig RW. 'Faster counting while walking' as a predictor of falls in older adults. Age Ageing 2007 Jul;36(4):418–23. Epub 2007 Mar 9.

Beauchet O, Allali G, Annweiler C, Berrut G, Maarouf N, Herrmann FR, Dubost V. Does change in gait while counting backward predict the occurrence of a first fall in older adults? Gerontology 2008;54(4):217–23. Epub 2008 Apr 14.

Beauchet O, Annweiler C, Allali G, Berrut G, Herrmann FR, Dubost V. Recurrent falls and dual task-related decrease in walking speed: is there a relationship? J Am Geriatr Soc. 2008 Jul;56(7):1265-9. Epub 2008 May 26.

Bootsma-van der Wiel A, Gussekloo J, de Craen AJ, van Exel E, Bloem BR, Westendorp RG.: Walking and talking as predictors of falls in the general population: the Leiden 85-Plus Study. J Am Geriatr Soc 51: 1466-71, 2003

Duncan PW, Weiner DK, Chandler J, Studenski S. Functional reach: a new clinical measure of balance. J Gerontol 1990;45:M192–M197.

Faulkner KA, Redfern MS, Cauley JA, Landsittel DP, Studenski SA, Rosano C, Simonsick EM, Harris TB, Shorr RI, Ayonayon HN, Newman AB; Health, Aging, and Body Composition Study.: Multitasking: association between poorer performance and a history of recurrent falls. J Am Geriatr Soc 55: 570-6, 2007

Guralnik JM, Simonsick EM, Ferrucci L, Glynn RJ, Berkman LF, Blazer DG, et al. A short physical performance battery assessing lower extremity function: association with self-reported disability and prediction of mortality and nursing home admission. J Gerontol 1994; 49: M85–M94.

Kressing RW, Herrmann FR, Grandjean R, Michel JP, Beauchet O.: Gait variability while dual-tasking: fall predictor in older inpatients?. Aging Clin Exp Res 20: 123-130, 2008

Lundin-Olsson L, Nyberg L, Gustafson Y. "Stops walking when talking" as a predictor of falls in elderly people. Lancet 1997; 349: 617.

Podsiadlo D, Richardson S. The timed "Up & Go": a test of basic functional mobility for frail elderly persons. J Am Geriatr Soc 1991; 39: 142–8.

Sherrington C, Whitney JC, Lord SR, Herbert RD, Cumming RG, Close JC. Effective exercise for the prevention of falls: a systematic review and meta-analysis. J Am Geriatr Soc 2008 Dec;56(12):2234–43.

Springer S, Giladi N, Peretz C, Yogev G, Simon ES, Hausdorff JM.: Dual-tasking effects on gait variability: the role of aging, falls, and executive function. Mov Disord 21:950-7, 2006

Stalenhoef PA, Diederiks JP, Knottnerus JA, Kester AD, Crebolder HF. A risk model for the prediction of recurrent falls in community-dwelling elderly: a prospective cohort study. J Clin Epidemiol. 2002 Nov;55(11):1088–94.

Tinetti ME, Speechley M, Ginter SF. Risk factors for falls among elderly persons living in the community. N Engl J Med 1988; 319:1701–7.

Toulotte C, Thevenon A, Watelain E, Fabre C.: Identification of healthy elderly fallers and non-fallers by gait analysis under dual-task conditions. Clin Rehabil 20: 269-76, 2006

Verghese J, Buschke H, Viola L, Katz M, Hall C, Kuslansky G, Lipton R. Validity of divided attention tasks in predicting falls in older individuals: a preliminary study. J Am Geriatr Soc 2002 Sep;50(9):1572–6.

Yamada M, Arai H, Nagai K, Tanaka B, Uehara T, Aoyama T. Development of a new index for fall risk assessment in older adults. Int J Gerontol (in press a)

Yamada M, Aoyama T, Hikida Y, Takamura M, Tanaka Y, Kajiwara Y, Nagai K, Uemura K, Mori S, Tanaka B. Effects of a DVD-based seated dual-task stepping exercise on the fall risk factors among community-dwelling elderly adults: A pilot feasibility study. Telemed J E-Health (in press b)

Yamada M, Aoyama T, Arai H, Nagai K, Tanaka B, Uemura K, Mori S, Ichihashi N. Dual-task walk is a reliable predictor of falls in robust elderly adults. J Am Geriatr Soc 2011a; 59: 163–4.

Yamada M, Aoyama T, Nakamura M, Tanaka B, Nagai K, Tatematsu N, Uemura K, Nakamura T, Tsuboyama T, Ichihashi N. The reliability and preliminary validity of game-based fall risk assessment in community-dwelling older adults. Geriatr Nurs 2011b: 32(3):188–94.

Yamada M, Aoyama T, Okamoto K, Nagai K, Tanaka B, Takemura T. Using a Smartphone while walking: a measure of dual-tasking ability as a falls risk assessment tool. Age Ageing 2011c;40(4):516–9.

Yamada M, Higuchi T, Tanaka B, Nagai K, Uemura K, Aoyama T, Ichihashi N. Measurements of stepping accuracy in a multitarget stepping task as a potential indicator of fall risk in elderly individuals. J Gerontol A Biol Sci Med Sci 2011d Jul 11. [Epub ahead of print]

Yamada M, Tanaka B, Nagai K, Aoyama T, Ichihashi N. Rhythmic stepping exercise under cognitive condition improves fall risk factors in community-dwelling older adults: preliminary results of cluster-randomized controlled trial. Aging Ment Health 2011e: 15; 647–53.

Yamada M, Arai H, Uemura K, Mori S, Nagai K, Tanaka B, Terasaki Y, Iguchi M, Aoyama T. Effect of resistance training on physical performance and fear of falling in elderly with different levels of physical well-being. Age Ageing 2011f. [Epub ahead of print]

Yamada M, Aoyama T, Tanaka B, Nagai K, Ichihashi N. Seated stepping exercise under a dual-task condition improves ambulatory function with a secondary task: a randomized controlled trial. Aging Clin Exp Res 2010a [Epub ahead of print]

Yamada M, Tanaka B, Nagai K, Aoyama T, Ichihashi N. Trail-walking exercise and fall risk factors in community-dwelling older adults: preliminary results of a randomized controlled trial. J Am Geriatr Soc 2010b: 58(10):1946–51.

9

Vaccine-Preventable Infectious Respiratory Diseases in the Elderly

Noriko Kojimahara
Tokyo Women's Medical University,
Japan

1. Introduction

Many infections occur more frequently in the elderly and are often associated with morbidity and mortality. Pneumonia, particularly due to *Streptococcus pnuemoniae,* is the most frequent cause of death in geriatric patients. After suffering influenza, there is a problem in that the elderly tend to get pneumonia as an influenza-related disease. Therefore, annual immunization against influenza and pneumococcal vaccines at the age of 65 years are recommended for all adults who are 65 years old and older (1). In this review, we address whether the protective efficacy of the influenza vaccine and 23-valent pneumococcal polysaccharide vaccine (PPV23) in the elderly with and without chronic obstructive pulmonary disease can be shown among recent epidemiological studies.

2. Important

Routine annual influenza vaccination is recommended for all persons aged 6 months and above (1,2). The elderly are considered a high risk group, because the risks for complications, hospitalizations, and deaths are higher among adults aged 65 years and older, in spite of rates of infection from seasonal influenza being highest among children. It should be considered that the elderly with poor physical and nutritional status tended to respond poorly to the influenza vaccination.

In addition to annual influenza vaccination, all persons should be vaccinated with PPV23 at age 65 years to prevent invasive pulmonary diseases in all-cause pneumonia or mortality (3). Even though it is said the immune response of the elderly is likely to be declined, almost all persons older than 65 years indicate antibody elevations above clinical effective response after vaccination of influenza and/or PPV23. The introduction of the 7-valent pneumococcal conjugate vaccine (PCV7) in children may alter the vaccine-preventable disease burden in older adults and, correspondingly, the potential magnitude of the benefit of PPV23(4).

3. Information

3.1 Influenza

The elderly have been considered the priority group for influenza vaccination, but their influenza vaccine-induced antibodies were believed to decline more rapidly than young adults. Song et al. evaluated long-term immunogenicity of the influenza vaccine among the elderly [5]. Serum hemagglutinin inhibition (HAI) titers were determined at pre- and post-vaccination periods. Of the 1,018 subjects, 716 (70.3%) were followed up during a 12-month period. Seroprotection rates at 4 weeks post-vaccination ranged from 70.1% to 90.3% depending on the age group and influenza vaccine virus strain. At 6 months post-vaccination, seroprotection rates for all three strains had declined significantly in adults 65 years old or older ($P<0.01$) as compared to young adults.

Hara et al. also assessed the immune response and serum nutritional status of 153 elderly residents of nursing homes (mean age 84.4 years) to the influenza vaccine [6]. Post-vaccination of HAI titers to A/H1N1 and B were low compared to young adults. However, seroconversion rates, which indicated greater than or equal to a fourfold rise for A/H1N1 and A/H3N2, were unexpectedly high among the elderly. Among all subjects, lower age and higher serum concentrations of total protein, albumin, Vitamin E and folate were associated with an intact immune response, e.g., post-vaccination HAI titers showed greater than 40 for at least one vaccine strain. In an age-adjusted analysis limited to the elderly, only Vitamin E showed a significant association with the immune response. These results suggested that Vitamin E may play an important role in maintaining the immune response, especially among the elderly.

The other publication by Sagawa et al. has considered physical and nutritional factors [7]. Pre- and post-vaccination HAI titers were determined for 203 individuals aged 65 years or older residing in a nursing home. For the assessment of physical and nutritional status, information was retrieved from care records. The immune response to the vaccination was assessed as good in 122 subjects based on a fourfold rise or more in HAI titer after vaccination for at least one of three vaccine strains. In a univariate logistic regression analysis with poor versus good immune response, factors found to be significantly associated with a poor immune response were disability, a combination of body mass index (BMI) less than 18.5 and body weight loss in 6 months or 5% or more, mid-upper-arm circumference of less than 80%, arm muscle circumference of less than 80% and total protein of less than 6.5 g/dL (Table 1). Physical and nutritional indicators might be useful in identifying individuals who are unlikely to have a good immune response to the influenza vaccination. In a multivariate analysis, the association remained significant for a low level of daily activities and a combination of BMI less than 18.5 and body weight loss in 6 months of 5% or more. Elderly individuals with poor physical and nutritional status tended to respond poorly to the influenza vaccination compared to elderly with good status. A low level of daily activities and a combination of being underweight and having had recent body weight loss are good indicators of a poor immune response.

According to the review by Skowronski DM[8], seroprotection rates of 70%-100% were maintained not just at 4 months but also at 5 months and even at >6 months, for the A/H3N2 and A/H1N1 vaccine components. Seroprotection rates appeared less consistent for the B vaccine component, throughout the postimmunization period. Seroconversion appears to vary substantially and inversely with preimmunization titers but not with age. The historic concern that the influenza vaccine-induced antibody response in the elderly declines more rapidly and below seroprotective levels within 4 months of immunization should be reconsidered.

3.2 Pneumococcal pneumonia

Bacteremic pneumonia is the most common cause of invasive pneumococcal disease (IPD), accounting for 90% of all cases [9]. There are over 90 different serotypes of *S. pneumoniae,* some are highly invasive whereas others rarely cause disease. Although there is variation in the serotype distribution between age groups and across different geographical populations, mortality associated with pneumococcal pneumonia in adults has remained unchanged at 25% of all pneumonia deaths over the past 40 years [10].

Variable	Crude			
	n	(%)	OR	95% CI
Male	44	21.7	0.95	0.48–1.87
Age ≥89 years	93	45.8	1.19	0.68–2.10
Disability	178	88.0	0.25	0.07–0.69
BMI <18.5	92	45.3	0.70	0.40–1.23
Bodyweight loss in 6 months ≥5%	35	17.2	0.81	0.45–1.46
BMI <18.5 and bodyweight loss in 6 months ≥5%	23	11.3	0.46	0.24–0.88
AC <80%	33	15.8	0.45	0.21–0.97
TSF <80%	104	51.2	0.88	0.50–1.55
AMC <80%	21	10.3	0.37	0.14–0.92
Diabetes	33	16.3	0.57	0.27–1.20
Pulmonary disease	15	7.4	1.33	0.45–4.40
Total protein <6.5 g/dL	63	31.0	0.52	0.29–0.95
Albumin <3.4 g/dL	52	25.6	0.74	0.36–1.53
Zinc <54 µg/dL	54	26.6	1.03	0.58–1.83
HDL cholesterol <43 mg/dL	52	25.6	1.08	0.57–2.09
LDL cholesterol >156 mg/dL	52	25.6	0.65	0.37–1.15

Mean ± standard deviation. AC, mid-upper-arm circumference; AMC, mid-upper-arm muscle circumference; BMI, body mass index; HDL, high-density lipoprotein; LDL, low-density lipoprotein; TSF, triceps skinfold thickness.

Table 1. Odds ratios (OR) with 95% confidence intervals (CI) of a good immune response for each subgroup [7]

Since 1997, the Advisory Committee on Immunization Practices (ACIP) has recommended to prevent IPD, i.e., bacteremia, meningitis or infection of other normally sterile sites through use of the PPV23 among all adults aged above 65 years and those adults aged 19-64 years with underlying medical conditions that put them at greater risk for serious pneumococcal infection (11). The updated recommendations (3) in 2010 include the following changes from 1997 ACIP recommendations: 1) the indications for which PPV23 vaccination is recommended include smoking (12) and asthma (13,14), and 2) routine use of PPV23 is no longer recommended for Alaska natives or American Indians aged below 65 years unless they have medical or other indications for PPV23 (15).

It has been reported that the antibody concentration level rose more than 1μg/ml (so-called protective level for vaccine-related pneumonia) referring to one muscle (or subcutaneous) injection of PPV23 among almost all of the elderly subjects (16). As the antibody levels among 14 serotypes can be commercially measured as showing in Figure 1, some several serotypes showed a level of more than 1μg/ml even before vaccination in among the elderly.

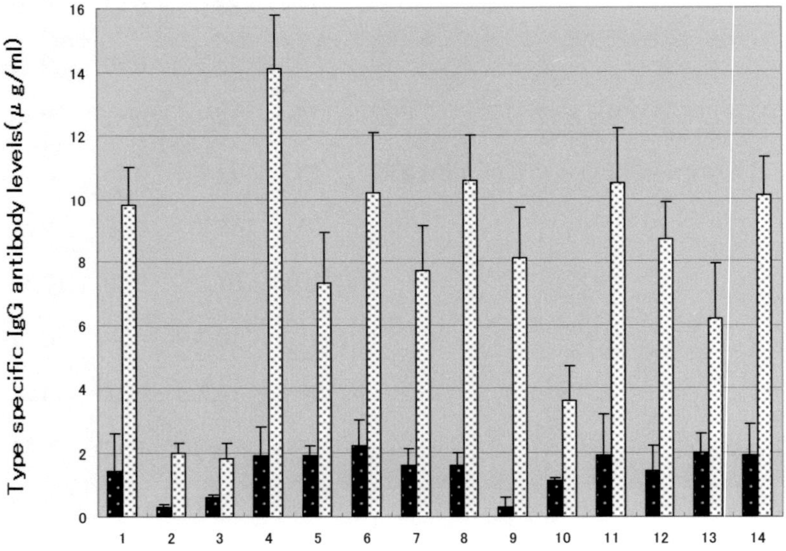

Type-specific IgG antibody levels to Streptococcus polysaccharide
Note: All types illustrated significantly (p<0.05) except type 3 and 4.

Fig. 1. The concentration of the type-specific IgG antibodies before and after PPV23 vaccination among elderly (mean±SE) (Before vaccination After vaccination) (16)

The Cochrane Collaboration supports the use of PPV23 to prevents invasive pulmonary diseases in all-cause pneumonia or mortality (17) by prospective, randomized controlled trials (RCTs) or quasi-randomised trials that compared PPV23 with placebo, control vaccines, or no intervention. The studies included participants at elevated risk of pneumococcal disease due to older adults aged 50 to 85 years with previous hospital admission for community-acquired pneumonia in Sweden (18) and community-based older adults in Finland (19).Ten studies involving 35,483 participants were included for outcome as IPD all causes with 15 events in the vaccinated group and 60 events in the control group, even though a subgroup analysis for the elderly was not performed. PPV23 reduced overall risk for IPD with was a pooled estimated odds ratio (OR) of 0.26 (95% confident interval (CI) 0.15 to 1.46; random-effects model). PPV23 was shown to be effective against all-cause pneumonia with a pooled estimated OR of 0.71 (95% CI 0.52 to 0.97) by a random-effects model. There was no evidence of protective efficacy against all-cause mortality, with a pooled estimated OR of 0.87 (95% CI 0.69 to 1.10; random-effects model). Enen though this meta-analysis has failed to demonstrate evidence for pneumococcal polysaccharide vaccination effectiveness against mortality (all cause or pneumococcal related), it demonstrates strong evidence of protection against IPD, with a correlate of efficacy from the RCTs of 74% (95% CI 56% to 85%) as shown in Fig 2.

	All studies	Vaccine	Control	Odds Ratio	Odds Ratio
invasive pneumococcal disease all causes	10	15/18132	60/17351		0.26[0.15, 1.46]
invasive pneumococcal disease vaccine	5	14/13889	140/17334		0.18[0.10, 0.31]
definitive pneumococcal pneumonia	10	15/18132	60/17351		0.26[0.15, 1.46]
presumptive pneumococcal pneumonia	8	86/9131	239/10198		0.47[0.23, 0.99]
definitive pneumococcal pneumonia (vaccine types only)	4	3/15583	30/14978		0.13[0.05, 0.38]
presumptive pneumococcal pneumonia (vaccine types only)	5	19/8755	130/9813		0.27[0.08, 0.87]
pneumonia all causes	13	835/21663	1350/24120		0.71[0.52, 0.97]
mortality all causes	11	899/23038	927/22571		0.87[0.69, 1.10]
mortality due to pneumonia	7	111/14699	182/14240		0.75[0.39, 1.43]
mortality due to pneumococcal infection	3	5/1221	1/1224		2.51[0.45, 14.13]

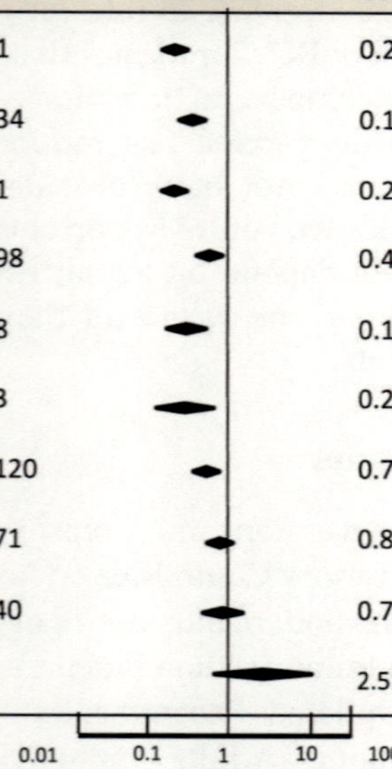

Fig. 2. Odds ratios (OR) with 95% confidence intervals (CI) of Comparison of RCTs of vaccination versus placebo for PPV23 vaccination (modified from article 17)

Observational studies have suggested effectiveness estimates ranging from approximately 50% to 80% for prevention of IPD among immunocompetent older adults and adults with various underlying illnesses, supporting the recommendations for using PPV23 to prevent IPD [20], although the effectiveness has not been demonstrated among immunocompromised persons or very old persons. A recent meta-analysis of 15 RCTs and seven non-randomized observational studies of PPV23 efficacy and effectiveness suggested an overall efficacy of 74% against IPD (CI = 56%-85%), based on pooled results of 10 of the RCTs [21]. Analysis of the results from the seven observational studies yielded a pooled vaccine effectiveness estimate of 52% (CI = 39%--63%). In contrast, a recent meta-analysis that included six RCTs estimated the combined PPV23 efficacy against pneumococcal bacteremia at only 10%, with a very wide CI (CI = -77%--54%) [13].

Regarding revaccination, ACIP recommendations for revaccination with PPV23 among the adult patient groups at greatest risk for IPD (i.e., persons with functional or anatomic asplenia and persons with immunocompromising conditions) remain unchanged. ACIP does not recommend routine revaccination for most persons for whom PPV23 is indicated. A second dose of PPV23 is recommended 5 years after the first dose for persons aged 19--64 years with functional or anatomic asplenia and for persons with immunocompromising conditions. ACIP does not recommend multiple revaccinations because of uncertainty regarding clinical benefit and safety.

It is said the changing epidemiology of IPD following the introduction of the 7-valent pneumococcal conjugate vaccine (PCV7) in children has altered the vaccine-preventable disease burden in older adults and, correspondingly, the potential magnitude of the benefit of PPV23 (22). Finally, newer vaccines, such as PCV7 (23,24) or those employing serotype-independent antigens, offer the potential to provide clinical protection against pneumococcal infection in the growing population of older adults in the 21st century. In summary, the decrease in rates of pneumonia (25) and IPD among young children after the introduction of PCV7 indicates that eliciting protective immunity against invasive and non-invasive pneumococcal infections by vaccination is a realistic goal. The unconjugated polysaccharide vaccine has reduced the risk of IPD among older adults, and protein-conjugated vaccines have provided substantial direct benefits to children and indirect benefits to adults. Future opportunities to further reduce the risk of pneumococcal infections in adults will depend on advances in our understanding of the mechanisms of protective responses to *S. pneumoniae* in the systemic and, particularly, in the respiratory mucosal compartments.

4. References

[1] CDC. Prevention and Control of Influenza with Vaccines. Recommendations of the Advisory Committee on Immunization Practices (ACIP), 2011/60(33); 1128-1132.

[2] CDC. Prevention and control of influenza: recommendations of the Advisory Committee on Immunization Practices [ACIP]. MMWR 2007 / 56(RR06);1-54.

[3] CDC. Updated Recommendations for Prevention of Invasive Pneumococcal Disease Among Adults Using the 23-Valent Pneumococcal Polysaccharide Vaccine (PPSV23)Weekly September 3, 2010 / 59(34); 1102-1106.

[4] Grijalva CG, Nuorti JP, Arbogast PG, Martin SW, Edwards KM, Griffin MR. Decline in pneumonia admissions after routine childhood immunisation with pneumococcal conjugate vaccine in the USA: a time-series analysis. Lancet. 2007;369:1179-1186.

[5] Song JY, Cheong HJ, Hwang IS, Choi WS, Jo YM, Park DW, Cho GJ, Hwang TG, Kim WJ. Long-term immunogenicity of influenza vaccine among the elderly: Risk factors for poor immune response and persistence. Vaccine. 2010 May 21; 28(23):3929-35.

[6] Hara M, Tanaka K, Hirota Y. Immune response to influenza vaccine in healthy adults and the elderly: association with nutritional status. Vaccine. 2005; 23(12):1457-63.

[7] Sagawa M, Kojimahara N, Otsuka N, Kimura M, Yamaguchi N. Immune response to influenza vaccine in the elderly: association with nutritional and physical status. Geriatr Gerontol Int. 2011; 11(1):63-8.

[8] Skowronski DM, Tweed SA, De Serres G. Rapid decline of influenza vaccine-induced antibody in the elderly: is it real, or is it relevant? J Infect Dis. 2008 Feb 15;197(4):490-502.
[9] Fedson D, Liss C. Precise answers to the wrong question: prospective clinical trials and the meta-analysis of pneumococcal vaccine in elderly and high risk adults. Vaccine 2004; 22:927-46.
[10] Pallares R, Linares J, Vadillo M, Cabellos C, Manresa F, Viladrich PF, et al. Resistance to penicillin and cephalosporin and mortality from severe pneumococcal pneumonia in Barcelona, Spain. New England Journal of Medicine 1995; 333:474-80.
[11] CDC. Prevention of pneumococcal disease: recommendations of the Advisory Committee on Immunization Practices (ACIP). Recommendations of the ACIP. MMWR 1997; 46(No. RR-8).
[12] Nuorti JP, Butler JC, Farley MM, et al. Cigarette smoking and invasive pneumococcal disease. Active Bacterial Core Surveillance Team. N Engl J Med 2000; 342:681--9.
[13] Talbot TR, Hartert TV, Mitchel E, et al. Asthma as a risk factor for invasive pneumococcal disease. N Engl J Med 2005; 352:2082--90.
[14] Lee TA, Weaver FM, Weiss KB. Impact of pneumococcal vaccination on pneumonia rates in patients with COPD and asthma. J Gen Intern Med 2007; 22:62-7.
[15] Singleton RJ, Butler JC, Bulkow LR, et al. Invasive pneumococcal disease epidemiology and effectiveness of 23-valent pneumococcal polysaccharide vaccine in Alaska Native adults. Vaccine 2007; 25:2288-95.
[16] Kojimahara N. Yamaguchi N. Antibody levels in response to influenza and pneumococcal polysaccharide vaccine in elder diabetes patients. Kansenshogaku Zasshi. 2007; 81(5):602-6 (in Japanese).
[17] Moberley S, Holden J, Tatham DP, Andrews RM. Vaccines for preventing pneumococcal infection in adults. Cochrane Database Syst Rev 2008; 1:CD000422.
[18] Ortqvist A, Hedlund J, Burman LA, Elbel E, Margareta H, Leinonen M. Randomised trial of 23-valent pneumococcal capsular polysaccharide vaccine in prevention of pneumonia in middle-aged and elderly people. Lancet 1998; 351:399-403.
[19] Koivula I, Sten M, Leinonen M, Makela PH. Clinical efficacy of pneumococcal vaccine in the elderly: A randomized, single-blind population-based trial. American Journal of Medicine 1997; 103:281-90.
[20] World Health Organization. 23-valent pneumococcal polysaccharide vaccine. WHO position paper. Wkly Epidemiol Rec 2008; 83:373-84.
[21] Huss A, Scott P, Stuck AE, Trotter C, Egger M. Efficacy of pneumococcal vaccination in adults: a meta-analysis. CMAJ 2009; 180:48-58.
[22] Lisa A. Jackson and Edward N. Janoff. Pneumococcal Vaccination of Elderly Adults: New Paradigms for Protection. Clin Infect Dis. 2008; 47 (10): 1328-1338.
[23] Jackson LA, Neuzil KM, Nahm MH, et al. Immunogenicity of varying dosages of 7-valent pneumococcal polysaccharide-protein conjugate vaccine in seniors previously vaccinated with 23-valent pneumococcal polysaccharide vaccine. Vaccine 2007; 25:4029-37.
[24] de Roux A, Schmoele-Thoma B, Siber GR, et al. Comparison of pneumococcal conjugate polysaccharide and free polysaccharide vaccines in elderly adults: conjugate

vaccine elicits improved antibacterial immune responses and immunological memory. Clin Infect Dis 2008; 46:1015–23.
[25] Grijalva CG, Nuorti JP, Arbogast PG, Martin SW, Edwards KM, Griffin MR. Decline in pneumonia admissions after routine childhood immunization with pneumococcal conjugate vaccine in the USA: a time-series analysis. Lancet 2007; 369:1179-86.

10

Beneficial Effect of Viscous Fermented Milk on Blood Glucose and Insulin Responses to Carbohydrates in Mice and Healthy Volunteers: Preventive Geriatrics Approach by "Slow Calorie"

Mari Mori[1], Atsumi Hamada[1], Satoshi Ohashi[2], Hideki Mori[1], Toshiya Toda[2] and Yukio Yamori[1]
[1]*Institute for World Health Development, Mukogawa Women's University,*
[2]*Fujicco Co.,Ltd.*
Japan

1. Introduction

WHO-coordinated Cardiovascular Disease and Alimentary Comparison (CARDIAC) Study covering over 61 populations of 25 countries in the world revealed the significant inverse association of the biomarkers of fish and soybean intakes in 24-hour urine with age-adjusted mortality rates of coronary heart diseases (CHD) (Yamori, 2006a; Yamori et al, 2006), indicating high fish and soybean consumptions might contribute to the No.1 average life expectancy of the Japanese with the lowest CHD mortality rates among developed countries (Yamori, 2006b). The mechanisms by which these food factors such as isoflavones and magnesium from soybeans as well as n-3 fatty acids and taurine from seafood could work as nutrients good for longevity have been studied experimentally and epidemiologically (Yamori, 2006c; Yamori, 2009; Yamori et al., 2010).

In contrast to soybeans and fish, fermented milk, yogurt is the common daily food consumed by some populations well-known for their longevity as Georgian and Uygur peoples studied by CARDIAC Study (Mori et al., 2006). However, the possible mechanisms for yogurt to contribute to their longevity have not been investigated. "Caspian Sea Yogurt" was introduced to Japan after CARDIAC Study for long lived populations in 1980's and this home-made fermented milk spread all over Japan due to its mild taste with less acidity and its smooth viscous character (Mori et al., 2006). Moreover, the health effects of this yogurt such as an improvement of defecation and the immunopotentiation of influenza vaccination were observed by a randomized placebo-controlled study (Toda et al., 2005; Mori et al., 2006). Therefore, in the present studies we investigated the effect of "Caspian Sea Yogurt" on the glucose absorption from simple and complex carbohydrates because our previous comparative studies on palatinose and sugar indicated slow absorption of glucose beneficially reduced risks of metabolic syndrome (Yamori et al., 2007; Matsuo et al., 2007; Holub et al., 2010; Okuno et al., 2010).

2. Caspian Sea Yogurt, its introduction and development in Japan

After the introduction of Caspian Sea Yogurt to Japan for nutritional analysis in CARDIAC Study, strains from the fermented milk were characterized (Ishida et al., 2005). Strain FC was Gram-positive, facultatively anaerobic cocci, and strain FA was Gram-negative, with aerobic rods. Phylogenetic analysis based on 16S rDNA sequences showed that strain FC formed a cluster with *Lactococcus (L) lactis* strains and was most closely related to *L. lactis* subsp. *cremoris*. Strain FA was included in the genus *Acetobacter* cluster and was most closely related to *A. orientalis*. Biochemical tests and DNA-DNA hybridization clarified that strain FC belongs to *L. lactis* subsp. *cremoris* and strain FA belongs to *A. orientalis*. Since the smooth viscous character of *L. lactis* subsp. *cremoris* is due to the bacterial exopolysaccharide (EPS), EPS non-producing variant (FC-EPS(-)) was isolated in order to clarify the effect of EPS by incubating the *L. lactis* subsp. *cremoris* FC-EPS(+) (stock strain of the Fujicco Co., Ltd. (Kobe, Japan)) in M17G broth at elevated, sublethal temperatures (37°C) for 72 hours. After growth on M17G agar at 25°C for 48 hours, colonies were isolated and maintained in the same medium. Thus, isolated non-ropy variant *L. lactis* subsp. *cremoris* FC-EPS(-) and the original ropy strain of *L. lactis* subsp. *cremoris* FC-EPS(+) were grown on M17G agar or broth (Difco) for 18 hours at 30°C. The existence of EPS forming was confirmed by Indian ink staining under microscopic observation (Figure 1).

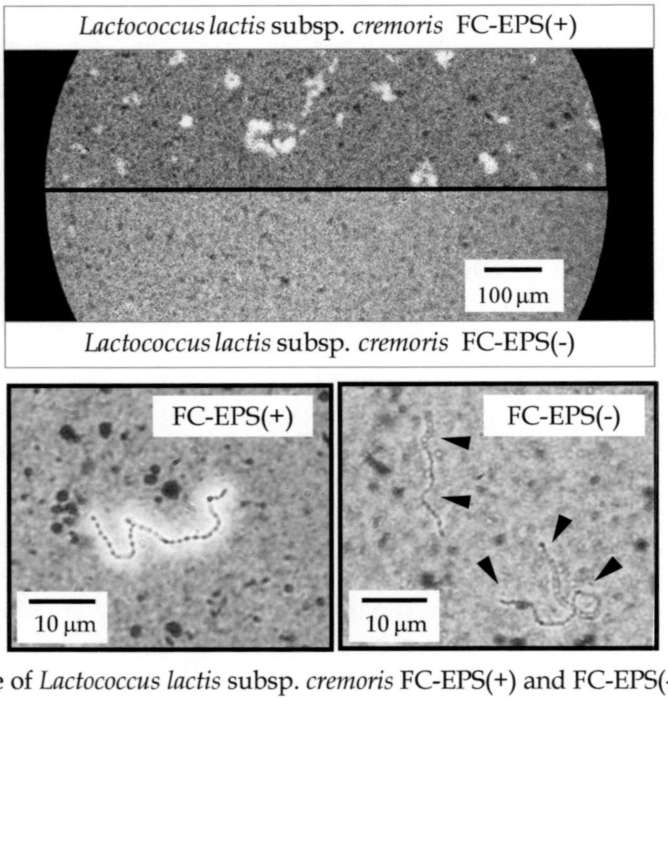

Fig. 1. The image of *Lactococcus lactis* subsp. *cremoris* FC-EPS(+) and FC-EPS(-) under the microscope.

Fig. 1 showed the photomicrograph of *L. lactis* subsp. *cremoris* EPS producing FC-EPS(+) and EPS non-producing variant FC-EPS(-) with Indian ink mixture. EPS was visible transparent white under the microscope. Fermented commercial milk with FC-EPS(+) or FC-EPS(-) was boiled at 85°C for 15 minutes and treated with protease at 37°C for 24 hours. Proteins were precipitated by addition of trichloroacetic acid (final concentration, 4%). After centrifugation and filtration, equivalent of acetone was added to the supernatant. The precipitated EPS from the yogurt fermented by FC-EPS(+) was 21 mg/kg, but was not detected from the yogurt by FC-EPS(-).

3. Caspian Sea Yogurt's effect on postprandial glycemia in mice

Since the viscous constituents derived from EPS of Caspian Sea Yogurt are supposed to affect glucose absorption, we compared in our animal studies the effect of non-fermented milk, the milk fermentation with *L. Lactis* subsp. *cremoris* FC (FC-EPS(+)) and the variant of *L. lactis* subsp. *cremoris* FC (EPS non-producing strain, FC-EPS(-)) on postprandial blood glucose levels by glucose tolerance tests.

3.1 Experimental animals and oral glucose tolerance test

Male ICR mice were purchased from Crea Japan, Inc. (Tokyo, Japan) and fed a commercial diet (MF; Oriental Yeast Co., Ltd., (Tokyo, Japan)) for a week. Mice were divided into a control group, milk group and two kinds of FC yogurt groups, and 7 mice with similar body weight in each group were housed in a plastic cage with controlled lighting (a 12-hour light/12-hour dark cycle), temperature (25 ± 1°C) and humidity (60 ± 5%) under conventional conditions. Yogurt materials were prepared by fermentation of pasteurized milk with *L. Lactis* subsp. *cremoris* FC-EPS(+) or EPS(-) at 30°C for 6 hours. Each of starter cultures were grown at 30°C for 8 hours and inoculated at 4% (wt/wt) concentration. After fermentation, they were stored at 4°C.

Postprandial blood glucose levels were evaluated using the oral glucose tolerance tests (OGTT). The tests were performed between 09:00 and 12:00h in a day. After fasting for 12 hours, the 30% glucose solution was given mixed with water, milk or fermented milk at the dosage of the glucose solution vs. water, milk or fermented milk for 1.5 g/kg vs. 5.0 g/kg of body weight of mice.

Blood samples were collected from tail vein at 0, 30, 60, 90 and 120 minutes after administration and allowed to stand at room temperature for 30 minutes. Serum was prepared by centrifugation at 800×g for 15 minutes at 4°C and applied to the assay of glucose. Serum glucose concentration was quantified using the glucose CII-test Wako (Wako Pure Chemical Industries, Ltd., Osaka, Japan).

All data are expressed as means ± S.D. The trapezoidal rule was used to determine the area under the curve (AUC). All areas below baseline were excluded from the calculations. Statistical analyses were performed using the Statcel2 (OMS publishing Inc., Saitama, Japan) and SPSS for windows package version 10.0J (SPSS Inc, Chicago, IL). P value below 0.05 was set as the level of significance. Differences between treatments at each time point were analyzed with a two-way repeated-measures ANOVA followed by *Tukey's-kramer test* or *Student's t-test*.

3.2 Postprandial hyperglycemia after fermented milk and milk administration

The blood glucose response 30 minutes after administration of milk fermented with *L. cremoris* FC-EPS(+) was significantly lower than the control. In the non-fermented milk group, the similar tendency was observed (Figure 2). However, after administration of milk fermented with FC-EPS(+), the curve of the blood glucose drew a slow arc and kept high value at 90 and 120 min.

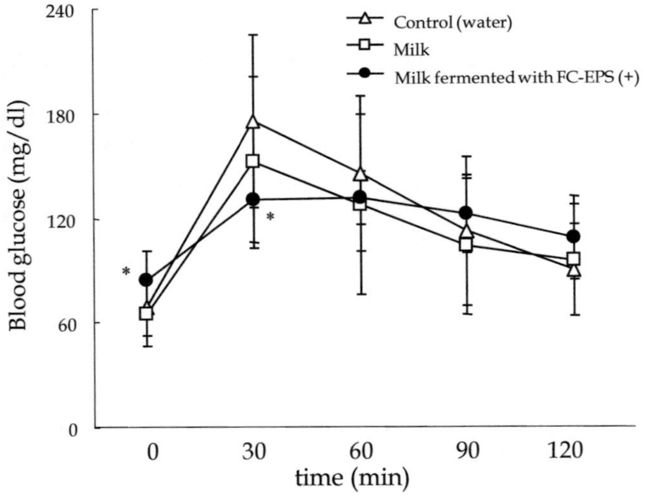

Fig. 2. Effects of fermented milk and milk on glucose tolerance test in ICR mice. Serum glucose concentrations were determined during the oral glucose tolerance test after the 30% glucose solution was administered at 1.5 g/kg body weight with 5.0 g/kg body weight of control (water), milk or fermented milk. *Significantly different from the response to control, $P<0.05$.

3.3 Differential effect on postprandial hyperglycemia by EPS-producing and –non producing fermented milk administration

The glucose levels were compared by glucose tolerance test after FC-EPS(+) and FC-EPS(-) fermented milk administration. FC-EPS(+) fermented milk group showed overall lower curve than FC-EPS(-) fermented milk group, and the levels at 60 and 90 minutes were significantly lower (Figure 3). The AUC of FC-EPS(-) fermented milk was significantly greater, over 1.5 times greater than that of FC-EPS(+) fermented milk (Figure 4). The elevation of blood glucose level was significantly suppressed and the AUC was decreased by the intake of FC-EPS(+) fermented milk, indicating EPS could attenuate postprandial hyperglycemia.

4. Caspian Sea Yogurt's effect on postprandial glycemia in humans

Based on the previous data obtained in mice, the effect of the Caspian Sea Yogurt fermented with FC-EPS(+) and of non-fermented milk on glucose tolerance was observed in healthy volunteer humans by a randomized crossover study.

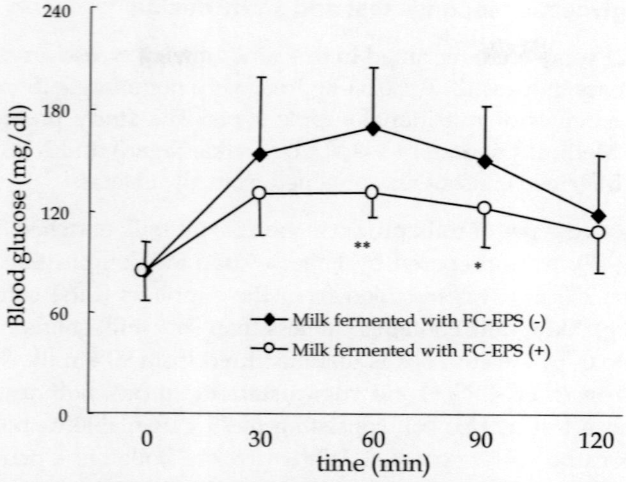

Fig. 3. Comparison of the effect of EPS producing (FC-EPS(+)) and non-producing (FC-EPS(-)) fermented milk on glucose tolerance test in ICR mice. Glucose responses were determined during the oral glucose tolerance test after the administration of the 30% glucose solution containing 1.5 g/kg body weight of glucose with 5.0 g/kg body weight of FC-EPS(+) or (-) fermented milk. Results are means ± S.D. (n=12-14). *Significantly different from milk fermented with FC-EPS(-) group, P<0.05 and ** P<0.01.

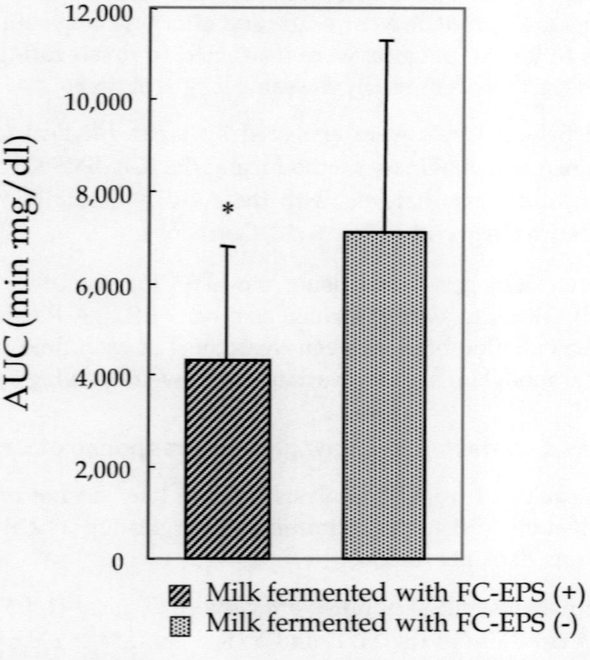

Fig. 4. Area under the curve for glucose (AUC), calculated using the trapezoidal rule by oral glucose tolerance test after FC-EPS(+) or (-) fermented milk administration. *Significantly different from milk fermented with FC-EPS(-) group, P<0.05.

4.1 Volunteers for glycemic response test and study design

Ten males aged 21-24 years were recruited in this randomized, crossover study. All subjects with normal body mass indexes (21.0 ± 0.83 kg/m^2) were not allergic to milk products and not taking either medicines or nutritional supplements. The study protocol was ethically approved by Japan Medical Laboratory Co., Ltd. (Osaka, Japan) and Mukogawa Women's University. Written informed consent was obtained from all subjects.

As for the test meals two types of milk products, normal fat milk enriched 5% skim milk (M) and fermented milk (F), were prepared by Fujicco Co., Ltd. Compositional information of normal fat milk (per 200 ml) was obtained from the suppliers (total carbohydrates 9.5 g, protein 6.6 g, fat 7.8 g). Skim milk contained no less than 95% milk-solids-nonfat, between 0-0.1% fat and between 0-0.5% water. F was manufactured from 90% milk, 5% skim milk and 5% *L. lactis* subsp. *cremoris* FC-EPS(+) and yogurt starter cultures. Both test meals, M and F, were served 180 g at a test. A rice ball consisting of 75 g available carbohydrates (R) was served as a complex carbohydrate product. White rice was boiled in a pan individually and made to be a rice ball. Trelan-G75 (T: 75 g/225 ml of glucose; Ajinomoto Pharma Co.,Ltd., Tokyo, Japan) was used for a simple carbohydrate source as a reference. For three tests, the combinations of meals were milk and Trelan (M/T), milk and a rice ball (M/R) and fermented milk and a rice ball (F/R).

Each participant was assigned to three treatments M/T, M/R and F/R on separate days at 7-day intervals. On each trial, after an overnight fast, blood samples were taken before and after a meal (0, 30, 60, 90, and 120 minutes) for analysis of glucose and insulin. The subjects were asked to eat up a milk product, M or F first and after finishing eating it, a carbohydrate product, T or R was followed. Subjects were instructed to finish eating within 10 minutes and asked to consume test meals in nearly the same length of time.

Plasma glucose and insulin levels were analyzed by Japan Medical Laboratory Co., Ltd. Glucose was determined by hexokinase method using the JCA-BM9020 analyzer (JEOL Ltd., Tokyo, Japan) and insulin was analyzed with the ADVIA Centaur immunoassay system (both Siemens Healthcare Diagnostics, Fernwald, Germany).

All statistical analyses were performed using the SPSS for windows package version 15 (SPSS Inc, Chicago, IL). Results were presented as means ± S.E. A P value of 0.05 was set as the level of significance. Differences between treatments at each time point were analyzed with the general linear model (analysis of variance) followed by *Tukey's post-hoc test.*

4.2 "Slow calorie" as a characteristic slow glycemic response of Caspian Sea Yogurt

Three subjects were excluded from all analysis because two did not meet the homeostasis model assessment-insulin resistance requirements in fasting (<2.5) and one did not complete the study for a personal reason.

The plasma glucose response at 30 minutes after the M/T meal (140.7 ± 20.7 mg/dl) was significantly higher than those of the M/R and Y/R meal (M/R; 108.6 ± 18.5, Y/R; 100.3 ± 8.2 mg/dl, respectively) (Figure 5-A). Peak glycemic responses appeared at 30 minutes after the consumption of M/T and M/R, whereas the peak delayed at 60 minutes after the consumption of Y/R (111.7 ± 17.5 mg/dl). Insulin response showed a similar pattern to glucose response; the peak occurred 30 minutes after the consumption of M/T and M/R (61.8 ± 23.6 and 46.6 ± 9.2 μIU/ml, respectively) (Figure 5-B), and 60 minutes after the consumption of Y/R (40.5 ± 18.2 μIU/ml).

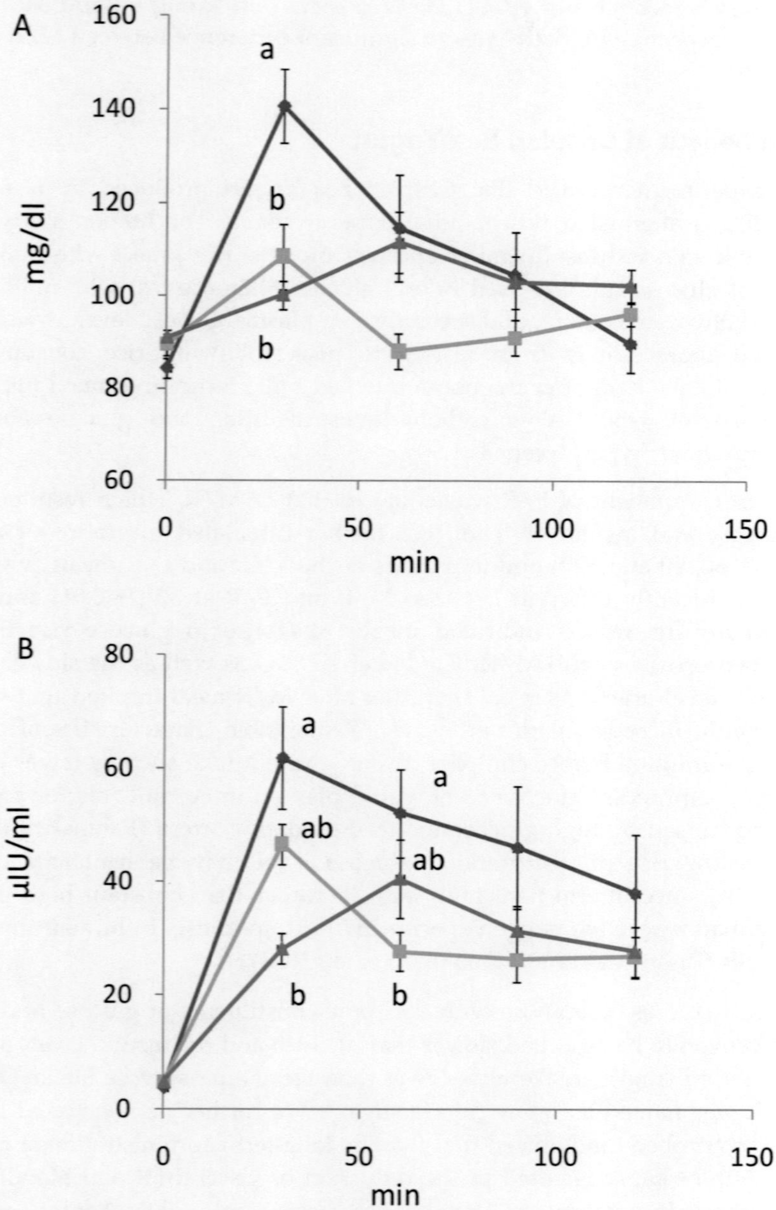

Fig. 5. Mean (± S.E.) plasma glucose (A) and insulin (B) concentrations after M/T (◆), M/R (■) and F/R (▲) meal. Values with different superscript letters are significantly different, P<0.05.

The area under the curve (AUC) for glucose (AG) and insulin (AI) responses were calculated using the trapezoidal rule from Figure 5. Although the AG and AI of M/T (13405.7 ± 887.8 min X mg/ml and 5424.6 ± 794.7 min X μIU/ml, respectively) were significantly different from those of M/R (11421.4 ± 312.5 min X mg/ml and 3486.6 ± 232.3 min X μIU/ml, respectively) or F/R (12355.7 ± 351.5 min X mg/ml and 3487.16 ± 297.9 min X μIU/ml, respectively), there was no significant difference between M/R and F/R in both AG and AI.

5. Potential benefit of Caspian Sea Yogurt

The animal experiment revealed that Caspian Sea Yogurt produced by *L. lactis* subsp. *cremoris* FC-EPS(+) attenuated postprandial hyperglycemia. The human study confirmed firstly lower glycemic and insulinemic responses after the rice intake with milk than after the ingestion of glucose solution used in oral glucose tolerance test with milk despite the equivalent carbohydrate content, and secondly that plasma glucose level as well as insulin level increased more slowly from fasting to peak following rice consumption after fermented milk intake than after the non-fermented milk, indicating much EPS-producing Caspian Sea Yogurt would slow carbohydrates digestion and glucose absorption to attenuate postprandial hyperglycemia.

The nutritional component of F/R was equal to that of M/R, which resulted in similar AUC for glucose and insulin of them. We further calculated the ratios of AI and AG (AI/AG) at 30, 60, 90 and 120-minute periods of the M/R and F/R meals (Figure 6). The ratios were significantly different between M/R and F/R at 30 ($P<0.01$) and 60-minute ($P<0.05$) periods. The results indicated insulin response to glucose rise in F/R was attenuated in comparison with M/R. The lower AI/AG as well as the slower increase of plasma glucose level after F/R meal than that after M/R meal implied that the Caspian Sea Yogurt would increase insulin efficiency. Remarkable characteristics of the Caspian Sea Yogurt consumption before complex carbohydrate intake such as lower AI/AG and peak delay in postprandial glucose level would play an important role for prevention of vascular aging caused by high glucose induced oxidative stress (Labinskyy et al., 2009). Furthermore, slow rise of postprandial glucose level may be beneficial on vascular endothelial cells, since intermittent high glucose rather than constant high glucose was revealed to enhance reactive oxygen species-induced apoptosis in human umbilical vein endothelial cells (Risso et al., 2001, Quagliaro et al., 2003).

By the previous studies, palatinose with the same constituents of glucose and fructose as sucrose was proven to be absorbed slower than sucrose and the insulin levels at 30, 60 and 90 minutes after palatinose intake were lower than those after sucrose intake (Kawai et al., 1985, 1989). It was named as "slow calorie sugar". We further demonstrated by a double blind placebo controlled randomized trial that the long-term administration of palatinose in comparison with of sugar resulted in the reduction of visceral fat and blood pressure in high-risk Japanese immigrants in Brazil (Moriguchi et al., 2006; Yamori et al., 2007). Therefore, it is speculated the daily consumption of Caspian Sea Yogurt with meals may attenuate postprandial hyperglycemia and be useful to manage blood glucose level for preventing from the insulin resistance, diabetes and cardiovascular diseases as previously proven in lower GI diets by epidemiologically (McMillan-Price et al., 2006; Chiu C-J. et al., 2011) and experimentally (Ludwig, D. S. 2002, van Schothorst et al., 2009).

Sedentary lifestyle generally associated with urbanization and aging weaken intestinal motility in the elderly suffering often from constipation. Since Caspian Sea Yogurt was so far proven for its beneficial effect on intestinal motility to improve constipation (Toda et al., 2005) and also for immunopotentiating effect on antibody titer elevation after influenza vaccination in the sedentary elderly (Mori et al., 2006), fermented milk popular in long-lived populations may be recommended for the prevention of communicable and non-communicable diseases from the scope of "preventive geriatrics".

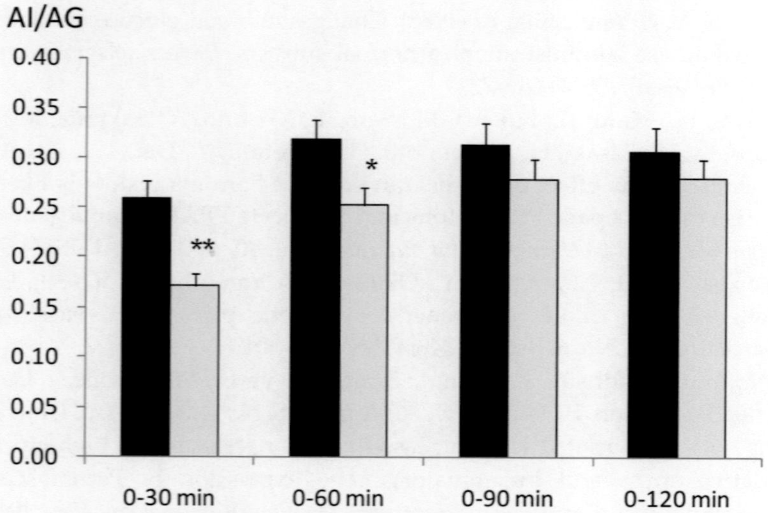

Fig. 6. Mean (± S.E.) ratios of areas under the curve for insulin (AI) and glucose (AG) calculated over 30-, 60-, 90- and 120-min periods after M/R (black column) and F/R (gray column) meal. *Significantly different from M/R group, P<0.05 and ** P<0.01.

6. Conclusion

After "Caspian Sea Yogurt" was introduced to Japan from the longevous population living in Georgia, the bacterial strains of this fermented milk was analyzed for the isolation into exopolysaccharide (EPS) producing and non-producing strains. Intestinal glucose absorption after the fermented milk ingestion, particularly the one from EPS producing strain was proven to be attenuated experimentally in mice as well as clinically in humans. Although it is needed to be tested if fermented milk may contribute to cardiovascular risk reduction as indicated in paratinose, the customary intake of fermented milk would contribute to health promotion in the elderly.

7. References

Chiu, C. J.; Liu, S.; Willett, W. C.; Wolever, T. M.; Brand-Miller, J. C.; Barclay, A. W. & Taylor, A. (2011). Informing food choices and health outcomes by use of the dietary glycemic index. *Nutrition Reviews*, Vol. 69, No. 4, pp. 231-242, ISSN 1753-4887

Holub, I.; Gostner, A.; Theis, S.; Nosek, L.; Kudlich, T.; Melcher, R. & Scheppach, W. (2010). Novel findings on the metabolic effects of the low glycaemic carbohydrate isomaltulose (Palatinose). *The British Journal of Nutrition*, Vol. 103, No. 12, pp. 1730-1737, ISSN 0007-1145

Ishida, T.; Yokota, A.; Umezawa, Y.; Toda, T. & Yamada, K. (2005). Identification and characterization of lactococcus and *Acetobacter* strains isolated from traditional Caucasian fermented milk. *Journal of Nutritional Science and Vitaminology*, Vol. 51, pp. 187-193, ISSN 0301-4800

Kawai, K.; Okuda, Y. & Yamashita, K. (1985). Changes in blood glucose and insulin after an oral palatinose administration in normal subjects. *Endocrinologia japonica,* Vol. 32, No. 6, pp. 93-96, ISSN 0013-7219

Matsuo, K.; Arai, H.; Muto, K.; Fukaya, M.; Sato, T.; Mizuno, A.; Sakuma, M.; Yamanaka-Okumura, H.; Sasaki, H.; Yamamoto, H.; Taketani, Y.; Doi, T. & Takeda, E. (2007) The Anti-Obesity effect of the palatinosebased Formula Inslow is likely due to an increase in the hepatic PPAR-alpha and adipocyte PPAR-gamma gene expressions. *Journal of clinical biochemistry and nutrition*, Vol. 40, pp. 234-241, ISSN 0912-0009

Kawai, K.; Yoshikawa, H.; Murayama, Y.; Okuda, Y. & Yamashita, K. (1989). Usefulness of palatinose as a caloric sweetener for diabetic patients. *Hormone and metabolic research,* Vol. 21, No. 6, pp. 338-340, ISSN 0018-5043

Labinskyy, N.; Mukhopadhyay, P.; Toth, J.; Szalai, G.; Veres, M.; Losonczy, G.; Pinto, J. T.; Pacher, P.; Ballabh, P.; Podlutsky, A.; Austad, S. N.; Csiszar, A. & Ungvari, Z. (2009) Longevity is associated with increased vascular resistance to high glucose-induced oxidative stress and inflammatory gene expression in Peromyscus leucopus. *American journal of physiology. Heart and circulatory physiology.* Vol. 294, No. 4, pp. H946-956, ISSN 0363-6135

Ludwig, D. S. (2002). The glycemic index: physiological mechanisms relating to obesity, diabetes, and cardiovascular disease. *JAMA*. Vol. 287, No. 18 pp. 2414-2423, ISSN 0098-7484

McMillan-Price, J.; Petocz, P.; Atkinson, F.; O'Neill, K.; Samman, S.; Steinbeck, K.; Caterson, I. & Brand-Miller, J. (2006). Comparison of 4 diets of varying glycemic load on weight loss and cardiovascular risk reduction in overweight and obese young adults: a randomised controlled trial. *Archives of internal medicine* Vol. 166, pp. 1466–1475, ISSN 0003-9926

Mori, M.; Kosaka, H.; Terai, M.; Mori, H.; Benno, Y.; Yamori, M.; Hirota, H.; Yamori, Y. & Toda, T. (2006). Effects of "Caspian Sea Yogurt" (Fermented milk with *Lactococcus Lactis* subsp. *Cremoris* FC) on the health of Japanese people –Lessons from traditional western food culture. *Proceedings of the International Symposium: Food Culture: Development and Education,* Paris, France, October 2005

Moriguchi, E.; Mori, M.; Mori, H.; Ishikawa, P.; Sakura, T.; Moriguchi, Y. & Yamori, Y. (2006). The effect of Palatinose on atherogenic index and visceral fat in male Japanese Brazilians. *Proceedings of the XIV International Symposium on Atherosclerosis,* ISSN 0021-9150, Rome, Italy, June 2006,

Okuno, M.; Kim, M. K.; Mizu, M.; Mori, M.; Mori, H. & Yamori, Y. (2010). Palatinose-blended sugar compared with sucrose: different effects on insulin sensitivity after 12 weeks supplementation in sedentary adults. *International journal of food sciences and nutrition,* Vol. 61, No. 6, pp. 643-651, ISSN 0963-7486

Quagliaro, L.; Piconi, L.; Assaloni, R.; Martinelli, L.; Motz, E. & Ceriello, A. (2003). Intermittent high glucose enhances apoptosis related to oxidative stress in human umbilical vein endothelial cells: the role of protein kinase C and NAD(P)H-oxidase activation. *Diabetes*. Vol. 52, No. 11, pp. 2795-2804, ISSN 0012-1797

Risso, A.; Mercuri, F.; Quagliaro, L.; Damante, G. & Ceriello, A. (2001). Intermittent high glucose enhances apoptosis in human umbilical vein endothelial cells in culture. *American journal of physiology. Endocrinology and metabolism.* Vol. 281, No. 5, pp. E924-930, ISSN 0363-6135

Toda, T.; Kosaka, H.; Terai, M.; Mori, H.; Benno, Y. & Yamori, Y. (2005). Effects of fermented milk with *Lactococcus lactis* subsp. *cremoris* FC on defecation frequency and fecal microflora in healthy elderly volunteers. *Journal of the Japanese Society for Food Science and Technology,* Vol. 52, No. 6, pp. 243–250, ISSN 1341-027X

van Schothorst, E. M.; Bunschoten, A.; Schrauwen, P.; Mensink, R. P. & Keijer, J. (2009). Effects of a high-fat, low- versus high-glycemic index diet: retardation of insulin resistance involves adipose tissue modulation. *The FASEB Journal,* Vol. 23, No. 4, pp. 1092-1101, ISSN 0892-6638

Yamori, Y. (2006a). Food Factor for Atherosclerosis prevention: Asian perspective derived from analyses of worldwide dietary biomarkers. *Experimental & Clinical Cardiology,* vol. 11, pp. 94-98, ISSN 1205-6626

Yamori, Y. (2006b). Nutrition for healthier aging -Two decades of world-wide surveys on diet and human life. *Proceedings of the International Symposium: Food Culture: Development and Education,* Paris, France, October 2005

Yamori, Y. (2006c). Soy for "Health for all": Message from WHO CARDIAC study and dietary intervention studies. In: *Soy in Health and Disease Prevention,* Sugano, M., pp. 107-121, Taylor & Francis, ISBN 978-0-8493-3595-2, Florida, USA

Yamori, Y.; Liu, L.; Mizushima, S.; Ikeda, K.; Nara, Y. & CARDIAC Study Group. (2006). Male cardiovascular mortality and dietary markers in 25 population samples of 16 countries. *Journal of Hypertension,* vol. 24, pp. 1499-1505, ISSN 0263-6352

Yamori, Y.; Mori, M.; Mori, M.; Kashimura, J.; Sakuma, T., Ishikawa, P. M.; Moriguchi, E. & Moriguchi, Y. (2007). Japanese perspective on reduction in lifestyle disease risk in immigrant Japanese Brazilians: a double-blind, placebo-controlled intervention study on palatinose. *Clinical and Experimental Pharmacology and physiology,* Vol. 34, pp. S5-S7, ISSN 1440-1681

Yamori, Y. (2009). Do diets good for longevity really exist? *Japan Medical Association journal* Vol. 52, No. 1, pp. 17-22, ISSN 1346-8650

Yamori, Y.; Taguchi, T.; Hamada, A.; Kunimasa, K.; Mori, H. & Mori, M. (2010) Taurine in health and diseases: consistent evidence from experimental and epidemiological studies. *Journal of biomedical science*, Vol. 17 Suppl 1: S6, ISSN 1021-7770

11

Health Education for the Elderly

Ayla Kececi and Serap Bulduk
Duzce University/ Vocational School of Health Services,
Turkey

1. Introduction

Health promotion and wellness are a great responsibility, particularly for all health care providers who work with elderly people. Some health care providers claim that because of their age, activities pertaining to prophylactic measures, health and wellness maintenance will not be helpful to elderly people. On the contrary, wellbeing should not be regarded as a concept specifically relevant to younger individuals. The wellness concept is applicable to every age from older adults to the young (Reicherter & Greene, 2005; Tabloski, 2010).

The world population on the whole is growing older and wellness and common diseases (infectious diseases, acute illnesses, chronic diseases and degenerative diseases, etc.) have been changing. Although many chronic diseases cause serious defects, some studies show that if a healthy life style is adopted and maintained, these defects can be delayed. Besides, these illnesses generally pose risk factors for individuals and their life styles. Studies on wellness and the prevention of diseases have been found effective, especially in providing lifelong behavioral change. Since the elderly population is at a huge risk of major diseases and defects, members of health care units should handle their education carefully. Through such education, benefits are provided regarding protective and wellness development for many elderly people (Reicherter & Greene, 2005; Tabloski, 2010).

Health education is a concept directly linked to health promotion in both clinical and educational preparation fields. Health promotion reform has developed an increasing interest in acute injuries and diseases from the mid-1980s. However, opportunities to promote health have generally been neglected (Choi et al., 2010).

Health education increases individuals' knowledge of health and health care and makes them informed about their health care choices. Prophylactic health behaviors (such as physical activities and having healthy food) keep older adults' lives active, delay going to nursing homes and increase satisfaction with life. Among the topics where elderly people need help most, a lack of knowledge comes first (Leung et al., 2006). World Health Organization (WHO) has emphasized the importance of health education to support health care needs and health promotion for elderly people (Rana et al., 2010).

Health education requires a careful handling of knowledge, attitude, objective, perception, social status, power structure, cultural practices and other social perspectives. Health education is not a concept about individuals or their families but can profoundly affect individuals' social status (Glanz et al., 2008).

An ageing population makes countries face many kinds of struggle in terms of health care and education. First of all, social support and care offered by elderly people's friends and family members can be inadequate (Hoving et al., 2010). If elderly people can afford health-protective and self-management behaviors in their daily lives, they can live more independently. However, a higher prevalence of chronic diseases like diabetes, cancer, heart diseases and dementia in this age group makes self-management of these illnesses and patient education more complicated. Educational programs for elderly people have complicated treatment plans because their age will increase their awareness level of medical treatment (Shen et al., 2006). Likewise, in studies conducted in different parts of the world, it was found that there is a need for serious educational programs related to old age (Liu&Wong, 1997; Kahn et.al., 2004; Doucette&Andersen, 2005; Koh, 2011; Vintila et.al., 2011).

Health care personnel's personal belief that elderly people have a poor understanding and learning ability has been an important obstacle in providing elderly people with an effective education. The myths about ageing have regarded elder people as unproductive, resistant to change, impotent and stereotyped individuals. In addition, health care personnel's lack of knowledge and skill may often prevent them from seeing all behavioral symptoms. For instance, behaviors of an elderly person who suffers from a mental disorder due to dementia can be seen as manipulative, or an older person with impaired hearing may respond intricately or inappropriately. In these situations, elderly people are considered "difficult" or "complicated" by health service providers (Smith, 2006). Many elderly people, however, do not experience biological, psychological and socially excessive negative effects. Instead, for those who are physically fit and extrovert, social and psychological abilities continue. On the other hand, experiencing some changes may disrupt learning in the health education process. Below are the commonly seen changes that may affect the learning process in elderly people (Tabloski, 2010; Cornett, 2011).

- **Physical changes:** The beginning, direction and order of the ageing process of elderly people depend physically and biologically on genetic and environmental factors. Degenerative changes may occur in hearing, seeing, feeling and responding skills. Spatial variability, mobility, and motor coordination may be spoilt. The working level may affect most body systems (Tabloski, 2010; Cornett, 2011).
- **Psychological changes:** The psychological aspect of ageing is related to a person's adaptation capacity. There might be changes in perception and memory, learning and problem solving, psychological state and attitude, sense of self and personality. Problems with memory in particular are common. The most declining cognitive skills are reported to be thinking with numbers and retention skills. The least decrease is seen in interpreting ideas and events, establishing relationships between events and ideas, generalizing, vocabulary and knowledge. Besides, regardless of a recession in their ability to learn, memory and intelligence, the rich life experience of elderly people makes their ideas valuable and health education should benefit from this experience. Another factor that can psychologically affect elderly people is losses. The loss of a former role and status, wife, friend, economical power and familiarity can be experienced. Due to these changes, self-respect diminishes and fulfillment decreases. Evaluating elderly people in terms of the losses they experience and the effects of these losses on their struggle is extremely important. Also, loss of confidence suppresses the ability or readiness to learn. However, preparing the person by strengthening self-

esteem with personal achievements and skills is an important strategy. Safety and safety needs are major anxiety factors for the elderly in a crisis situation. Unless these needs are satisfied, an active elderly person cannot actively participate in health education (Cornett, 2011).

- **Socio-Cultural Changes:** Social change and cultural factors affect self-care of the elderly as a personal component. Independency is a crucial purpose for most elderly people regardless of their health conditions. This is an expression of self-respect and pride. Elderly people seek help in gaining independency. The health education offered should contribute to their self-management skills. As their physical power decreases, elderly people move away from the activities that require mobility and much energy and prefer to choose more passive life styles. Especially the ones with poor education pass their time with limited activities. Yet, mentally and socially active elderly people face the limitations derived from ageing at a low level (Tabloski, 2010). An older adult's ability to cope with problems is closely related to health care and education. If an elderly person sees himself or herself as an experienced and wise individual, education can be built on these positive experiences and ways of adapting to the occurring inevitable changes can be sought. However, unrealistic goals and demands should be explained to the less adaptive people before the education (Cornett, 2011). In some countries, the fact that elderly people do not want to stay in their own houses or places specifically for elderly people is an obstacle in providing and maintaining health care. Additionally, physical, social and environmental liabilities cause problems regarding benefiting from services to maintain wellness. For this reason, all the liabilities that might affect elderly people's learning process should be determined and minimized prior to education (Reicherter & Greene, 2005).

2. Older adult learners

Knowing the learner is the key to successful teaching! Some features of adult and older adult learners constitute the key.

Self-concept: The self-concept of an adult learner is to be able to direct himself or herself and to be mature and positive in society. Adults want to make their own decisions and take the responsibility for the consequences of these decisions. They expect to be respected and regarded as unique beings (DeYoung, 2009; Cornett, 2011). Ericson mentioned some features of adulthood in the eighth phase of the human development period which he defines as "self-integrity." According to Ericson, in this phase, maturity and unity of the personality features gained in the previous phase are the most crucial task. Self-integrity is ego's having an order and meaning in itself. In other words, it is the acceptance of a life with all its positive and negative aspects. This prevents welcoming the future with fear and anxiety. However, the most important sign of lacking self-integrity is the idea that past days were not spent well, despair and fear of death. Especially in the process of health education for the elderly, educators must show respect for elderly people's needs, choices and their desire to manage their own lives. Creating an environment which makes them feel accepted, respected and trusted will encourage them to express their feelings and thoughts away from fear and pressure. For this reason, educators should ask elderly people how they would like to be called and call them that way. Adults are motivated to learn when they realize that they need to learn. Learners must be helped to express their feelings about their needs because they want to take the responsibility for their learning and management of their lives in the learning process. For this purpose, educators regard every interaction with elderly people as an opportunity to support their self-concept (Karaoz & Aksayan, 2009, Cornett, 2011).

Life Experiences: An older adult has considerable background information and life experiences in her/his lifetime. Life experiences are rich sources for learning. When an adult's experiences are supported and approved by others, positive feelings come into being since these experiences constitute her or his self-identity. If these experiences are not noticed, the person might feel rejected (Tabloski , 2010). Negative past experiences should be identified and dealt with since they might disrupt the learning process. For instance, an elderly person who has had bad experiences with "ageing and chronic diseases" might think that the education offered will not have any positive effect on him or her and because of this he or she may not learn. Positive experiences of adults should be used as an experimental teaching strategy. If new learning is related to a person's past experiences, they become more appropriate and meaningful. New self-management skills become more meaningful when a person adapts himself or herself to routine and a normal life style. Sharing their experiences with people having similar problems contribute to the problem-solving process among older adults (DeYoung, 2009; Cornett, 2011).

Being ready to learn: Before an effective education, adult learners should be ready for learning. When an individual is ready to learn, he or she will make the most of it (Gokkoca, 2001). People's attitudes and responses to a situation that threatens their wellness are mostly determined by an illness causing loss of control and self-confidence, disability and perceptions and experiences related to other factors. Readiness is strongly affected by individuals' social roles and developmental tasks. Some social roles and developmental roles after adulthood can be listed as an adaptation to decreasing physical strength and health, retirement and a decrease in income, and the death of a spouse and other family members (DeYoung, 2009; Cornett, 2011).

Readiness to learn and problem-solving skills can be enhanced by role-plays and group work with adults who have the same roles (Cornett, 2011). Previous achievements of elderly people have been an important motivating factor in the things that should be done and will be done in the future. Prompts like "......you can do it, you can achieve it" strengthen their belief in self-efficacy. Individuals' physical or mental conditions strengthen or weaken their belief in performing an expected task (Bikmaz, 2006).

Problem-oriented or Goal-oriented: Adult learners are motivated when there is a problem or crisis concerning them. In other words, they have a different point of view when compared to the young (Cornett, 2011, Gokkoca, 2001). They see learning as a way to overcome these problems and learn the things that are related to them and helpful to the fulfillment of responsibilities. Adult education is behaviorist oriented (how is it done?). However, in order to limit the education circumstances, minimum requirements such as "vital" or "good to know" must be known. Patients should be provided with practical solutions to their problems and should be immediately assisted with hands-on-practice and problem-solving sessions to practice new information. Unless patients require information on this issue and understand self-care, providing information on the illness process is not a priority. On the other hand, urgent needs should be prioritized. If potential problems patients might face are not known, questions about their concerns and aiming to know how to handle the situation should be asked. This gives an idea of the "rehearsal" situation or the possible response in case a problem occurs (DeYoung, 2009; Cornett, 2011).

From another point of view, elderly people's values and beliefs can be a facilitator or obstacle in caring for their health. For instance, elderly adult symptoms (e.g., tiredness, depression) are not taken seriously, requiring medical aid, and are regarded as an inevitable part of old age. Advanced age can affect the efforts of protecting health and self-management in a psychosocial context. For instance, due to changes in social relations (e.g., being divorced or losing a spouse), the amount and quality of social support might have changed. Following a balanced diet and positive sickness should be taken into consideration (Connell, 1999, Cornett, 2011). Since the results are related to support, elderly adults have more problems with their health and self-management (e.g., diet, exercise) compared to young and middle-aged adults. These examples are only a few of how health education will be affected in the context of physical and psychosocial changes. Age-related changes should always be taken into consideration, especially in the design, implementation and evaluation of health education programs.

3. Possible barriers to education of the elderly

Possible barriers that need to be considered during teaching should be known so that the learning potential of the elderly can be realized. These barriers can be mostly classified as sensory loses, mental illnesses and chronic diseases (Tabloski, 2010; Cornett 2011).

3.1 Sensory losses

The five senses tend to decline with advancing age. Sensory losses are problems with one or more senses (auditory, visual, tactile, olfactory, or taste). Hearing and vision changes affect communication while the other losses can affect thinking processes in the elderly (Tabloski, 2010; Smith, 2006).

3.1.1 Hearing deficiency

Individuals with hearing problems are people who either completely lost this sense or have decreased sensitivity to sounds. Individuals experience various obstacles related to communication in the process of patient education depending on their level of hearing loss. Individuals with hearing loss may be unable to speak or may have a limited verbal ability and a weak vocabulary. Just like other healthy people, these individuals will need health care or health education throughout their lives. Although the health educator offers support in different ways, individuals with hearing loss always have to use their other senses to get information (Bastable, 2008; Cornett, 2011). A general hearing loss may be the result of an illness, noise or bone changes while gradual hearing loss can bring about the loss of sounds like S, SH and CH or high frequency sounds (Smith, 2006). There are so many different ways of communication with individuals with hearing loss. First of all, educators should discover the individual's preference to communicate. Sign language, written information, lip reading and visual support are the most commonly used alternatives. In addition to these means, facial expressions, gestures and mimics should be included in the communication process for sharing information. During all education sessions, educators should be natural and not strict, speak clearly with simple sentences, adopt a way of asking for consent like a touch of the hand before starting to talk, set up face-to-face communication and maintain a distance of about 100 cm (6 feet). In conclusion, there is not just one way to communicate with individuals suffering from hearing deficiency. What matters is determining whether the messages are received correctly and if they are clear (Bastable, 2008; Tabloski, 2010; Cornett, 2011).

3.1.2 Visual deficiencies

Vision deficiencies are particularly common among older people. Most vision problems like glaucoma, cataracts and macular degeneration occur in the retina. Changes in vision can usually be seen in the form of a reduced ability to see distant objects, a loss of the ability to see objects on the side, and a loss of the ability to see very close (even faces) and some colors (peripheral vision) (Smith, 2006). Older people with reduced visual acuity may display behaviors such as dimming eyes, needing to touch, reluctance to communicate or withdrawal (Bastable, 2008; Cornett, 2011). The following are some recommendations for education of the elderly with a reduced visual ability:

- Education materials should be prepared in a format and size elderly people can easily see,
- Their other senses (touch, smell, hearing, taste) should be improved,
- It should be considered that especially hearing and touch are significant for sharing information,
- The procedures should be explained as descriptively as possible,
- Elderly individuals should be allowed to touch, hold and smell the related materials,
- Materials should be prepared in larger fonts for the elderly with visual deficiencies,
- Education materials should be prepared in black on a white background or in white on a black background,
- Contrasting colors should be preferred when using different colors,

Audio recording devices should also be included in the educational process, and Computers and texts using the Braille alphabet should be preferred if possible (Bastable, 2008).

3.1.3 Deficiencies of smell and taste

Formation of papillary atrophy in the tongue with ageing brings about losses in sensing sweet and salty tastes. Some chronic diseases (e.g., Alzheimer's disease, Parkinson's disease) can affect the sense of smell and taste. Similarly, drugs, surgical interventions and environmental factors contribute to losses in taste and smell senses. Elderly people need the same nutrients as young people but in different amounts. As a result of ageing due to factors that negatively affect nutrition, a lack of nutrients in the elderly is found more often.

Elderly people need the same nutrients as young people but in different amounts. Due to the factors that negatively affect nutrition as a result of ageing, a lack of nutrients is more prevalent in the elderly. For this reason, one should be more careful about consuming some nutrients in terms of energy, protein, folate, vitamin B12, calcium, vitamin D, iron, zinc, and riboflavin. All these elements, which are necessary for elderly individuals, act as catalysts for certain diseases that may affect their learning process. For this reason, the health educator should evaluate the levels of these substances, especially when assessing an individual's physical characteristics (Tabloski, 2010).

3.1.4 Deficiencies of sense of touch

Older adults may suffer from a reduction in feeling cold or hot and have pain due to the decrease in the thickness of the dermis of the skin in old age, vitamin D synthesis, its protection against micro-organisms, capillaries, collagen production, and senses of touch and pressure (Tabloski, 2010).

3.2 Mental illnesses

Individuals with mental disorders have possibly been existing in community mental health centers, in society, in the family or workplace environments for the last 25 years. People who work with such individuals should consider their feelings and thoughts about mental illnesses before the start of the teaching-learning process. Although there are some basic principles in the education of individuals with mental illnesses, there are still some specific instructional strategies that need to be considered. One of the first steps in any educational attempt is mental diagnostics. Firstly, in order to diagnose the anxiety level of an individual, it is necessary to determine whether the individual has any mental incapability or insufficiency. When there is an emotional threat depending on the mental illness, the individual's anxiety level will increase and the level of readiness will decrease. While working with an aged individual with a mental illness, the following points must be considered:

- Training must be organized according to their needs.
- Learning desire and the joy of life should be kept alive.
- Teaching should be performed by using short and simple words and information must be repeated as often as possible. Important pieces of information should be written on cards, certain techniques such as drawing one of the cards which is appropriate for them should be used and plain symbols and drawings must be used.
- Sessions should be kept short and frequently repeated. (Four fifteen-minute sessions instead of a one-hour session, etc.)
- All possible sources for the individual and his or her family should be used, all appropriate learning styles for the individual must be sought and training must be organized in this direction, and training should be supported by visual tools such as computers and videos.
- Assistance from the individual's family members, relatives, neighbors and volunteers must be accepted.
- Instead of an authoritarian attitude, a calm and understanding approach must be adopted in communication (Smith, 2006; Bastable, 2008; Kurt, 2000).

In addition, since individuals with mental illness face stigma both in society and in the family, it is crucial to determine appropriate instructional strategies. Motivation of individuals with mental illness is quite an important issue. After completing the program, giving a certificate to participants will increase the motivation of each individual. However, it is necessary to give useful information to increase the quality of life of elderly individuals with mental illnesses. As for healthy individuals, achieving and maintaining the independence and self-government of such individuals are extremely important (Smith, 2006; Bastable, 2008; Cornett, 2011).

3.3 Chronic diseases

The learning process of individuals with chronic diseases is full of difficulties. Many diseases have many phases that may affect the educational needs of the individual patients and their families. Therefore, there is no unique approach to provide the most appropriate teaching-learning. What matters is the start of the disease, its progress and intensity. The perception and the reaction of these individuals' families to the learning-teaching process are also very important. Families are in need of education and information on the limitations related to the changes and limitations in the lives of individuals. Usually, these individuals experience conflicts between their needs to become dependent or independent in their lives. Maintaining energy and independence could sometimes be physically and emotionally repressing. Living with a chronic disease often causes a loss of role and some other changes. When a loss of role and a decrease in self-respect appear, the situation affects readiness for learning. Thus, it will be right to take the following actions:

- Prevent medical crises and problems before they happen.
- Take control of symptoms.
- Apply the existing treatment plan and provide the management of self-care-related problems.
- Prevent their social isolation from other people.
- Help them balance their living standards and their relations with other people.
- To provide changes related to illness, adjust yourself.
- Provide funding for treatment if necessary.
- Prevent psychological, marital and family problems from happening (Tabloski, 2010; Cornett, 2011).

4. Health education process for the elderly

People offering health education have many responsibilities to determine the needs of the elderly and to take actions according to their needs (Kulakçı & Emiroğlu, 2011). The main objective of health education is to provide individuals and society with assistance so that they can lead a healthy life through their own efforts and actions. Therefore, health education supports and develops all kinds of individual learning processes. Similarly, it makes changes in the beliefs and value systems of individuals, their attitudes and skill levels; in other words, it changes their lifestyles (Tabak, 2000).

The role of health educators is to apply education to develop responsibilities for the self-care of individuals who are incompetent, which is also what they are supposed to do. Families increasingly become more involved in the work of self-care-incompetent individuals' rehabilitation, and individuals with poor self-care are expecting to become a part of life in the community. In addition, health educators have responsibilities to determine the learning needs of patients in cooperation with families, to plan appropriate educational initiatives and to provide a supportive environment (Bastable, 2008).

At the beginning of this education, the problems of patients, short and long-term consequences of their deficiencies, the effectiveness of coping mechanisms, and their needs related to the sensorimotor, cognitive, perceptual and communicational inadequacies need to be defined. Patients' level of knowledge related to their inadequacies, the amount and the kinds of information that may affect the needed behaviors and the readiness level for providing learning should also be determined separately. In order to determine the readiness levels of the patients, the following questions should be asked (Bastable, 2008):

- *Are other individuals and family members interested in patients' learning, do they ask questions about problem solving, or do they take patients' needs into consideration?*
- *Is there insufficient information, vision or hearing problems that prevent learning?*
- *If there are any sensory or motor changes, will the people around the patients be participative and supportive towards instructional activities? What is the most appropriate learning style that is applicable to the patient's self-care activities?*
- *Is there compatibility between the patient's and family's goals?*
- *Does the patient have learning values and skills for the purpose of functional development?*

After determining the level of readiness of the elderly, educational activities should be structured in accordance with the models of health education. These models are described below.

4.1 Health behavior models

Health behavior models and theories are inherently associated with health behavior measurements because they explain *what* they are to assess. The models used most in elderly individuals in articles published in the 2000s in education, health and behavioral sciences in the field of a theoretical framework are the Health Belief Model, the Theory of Reasoned Action/Planned Behavior, the Social Cognitive Theory and the Transtheoretical Model. These four health behavior models, which can be utilized in planning the health education process for the elderly, are summarized below.

4.1.1 Health belief model

The Health Belief Model (HBM) is the oldest of all the theories examined here. The Health Belief Model holds that people are more likely to take action to prevent disease when they realize that

- they can catch the disease themselves,
- the disease can have serious consequences,
- preventive behavior effectively will prevent disease, and
- benefits of reducing the dangers of the situation clearly outweigh the damages of taking action.

Affected by mediating variables, these four factors have an influence on the expectations of the known dangers and consequences of the disease. Therefore, they indirectly affect the possibility of exhibiting preventive health behavior.

Health Belief Model health screening is used to intervene in the disease, disease role and protective behaviors. This model has been subject to a number of changes since its development. Table 1 shows the four constructs model, the most common description of the Health Belief Model. The four main constructs of the model are perceived susceptibility, perceived severity, perceived benefits (efficacy), and perceived barriers (harms) (Champion & Skinner, 2008).

Constructs	Explanations
Perceived susceptibility	An individual's assessment of his or her risk of getting the condition
Perceived severity	An individual's assessment of the seriousness of the condition, treatment of the condition and its potential consequences
Perceived benefits	An individual's assessment of the positive consequences of adopting the promoted behavior
Perceived barriers	An individual's assessment of the influences that facilitate or discourage adoption of the promoted behavior or its psychological and physical consequences
Clues to action	Experiences and strategies promoting the desired behavior
Self-efficacy	An individual's self-assessment of ability to successfully adopt the desired behavior

From Redding, C.A., Rossi, J.S., Rossi, S.R., Velicer, W.F., & Prochaska, J.O. (2000). Health Behaviour Model. *The International Electronic Journal of Health Education*, Vol. 3 (Special Issue), pp. 180-193. http://www.iejhe.siu.edu

Table 1. Health Belief Model Constructs

4.1.2 Theory of reasoned action/planned behavior

The Theory of Reasoned Action (TRA) is a socio-psychological approach aimed at understanding and predicting the determinants of health behavior and is a widely-used theory of prediction. The Theory of Reasoned Action has been applied to many health-related behaviors in the elderly including weight loss, smoking, excessive alcohol consumption, HIV risk behaviors and mammography screening, etc. According to the Theory of Reasoned Action, the intention of adopting a behavior is closely associated with realization of that behavior. The Theory of Reasoned Action is based on two main assumptions: behavior is controlled by will and people are rational. The Theory of Reasoned Action holds that individuals believe: *We do something because we have chosen to do so and go through a logical decision-making process when we choose and plan our behavior.*

Designed to predict behavior by looking at the intention, the Theory of Reasoned Action claims mathematical relationships between beliefs, attitudes, intensions and behavior. A modified version of the Theory of Reasoned Action adds perceived behavioral control to the theory. It is called the Theory of Planned Behavior (TPB) (Montano & Kasprzyk, 2008). Table 2 describes the main concepts of the Theory of Reasoned Action and the Theory of Planned Behavior.

Concepts	Explanations
Behavioral intention	Possibility of undertaking the perceived behavior
Attitudes	The sum of beliefs about a particular behavior, weighted by evaluations of these beliefs
Behavioral belief	An individual's belief about consequences of a particular behavior
Evaluation of behavioural belief	An individual's positive or negative evaluation of self-performance of the particular behavior
Subjective norm	The sum of normative beliefs and motivation to comply with
Normative belief	An individual's perception of the particular behavior, which is influenced by the judgment of others
Motivation to comply	Every personal contact, an individual's drive to engage
Perceived behavioral control	The sum of control beliefs and perceived power
Control beliefs	Possibility of the presence of factors that may facilitate or impede performance of the behavior
Perceived power	The effect of each situation that may facilitate or impede performance of the behavior

From Redding, C.A., Rossi, J.S., Rossi, S.R., Velicer, W.F., & Prochaska, J.O. (2000). Health Behaviour Model. *The International Electronic Journal of Health Education*, Vol. 3 (Special Issue), pp. 180-193. http://www.iejhe.siu.edu

Table 2. Theory of Reasoned Action/Planned Behavior

The ultimate goal of the Reasoned Action Theory is to predict. The theory holds that the intentions of the behavior affect the behavior. The three main variables that affect the intention are subjective norms, attitudes and self-efficacy. Subjective norms involve an individual's assessment of what significant others think of his or her ability to undertake a behavior. For example, an elderly person with a cardiac condition tries to prevent complications from the condition by taking his or her medication on a regular basis and has regular medical checks. The intention of this individual is partly determined by the idea of his or her spouse or a friend who could be a role model: "What would he or she do if he or she were me?" Attitudes can be conceptualized in terms of values. In other words, a set of values can be developed in relation to behaviors. For instance, "healthy eating is a good way to prevent heart disease and/or cancer" (Redding et al. 2000; Montano & Kasprzyk, 2008).

4.1.3 Social cognitive theory

This theory goes far beyond individual factors to explain health behavior change and also utilizes environmental and social factors. Indeed, this theory is the most comprehensive model of human behavior proposed so far. Bandura's Social Cognitive Theory (SCT) is a behavioral theory of prediction that has a neutral approach to health behavior change. This theory is widely applied in health care in terms of health behaviors in prevention, health promotion, and improving the living conditions of unhealthy behavior. The Social Cognitive Theory emphasizes what people think and its impact on behavior. Based on triadic reciprocality of behavior, the Social Cognitive Theory suggests that behavior can be described using three key concepts, each of which serves as a determinant of one another. The basic regulatory principle of the Social Cognitive Theory is reciprocal determinism. This important concept represents a continuous and dynamic interaction between the individual, the environment and behavior. Hence, a change in any of these factors will affect the other two. The Social Cognitive Theory includes several auxiliary concepts for each of the three main concepts in order to explain the theory. Table 3 explains all the key concepts of the Social Cognitive Theory (Redding et al., 2000).

Concepts	Explanations
Environmental	Environmental factors other than the person
Situation	Individual's perception of the environment
Behavioral Capability	The knowledge and skills of an individual in performing a behavior
Expectations	The prospects of an individual performing a behavior
Expectancies	An individual's assessment of how the results could be good or bad
Self-control	Regulation of one's own behavior
Observational Learning	Observing behaviors of other people to acquire new behaviors
Reinforcements	Reaction to the individual's behavior that affects the possibility of repetition
Self-efficacy	An individual's self-belief in achievement in performing a behavior. Emotional coping
Emotional Coping Responses	An individual's emotional strategies to cope with provocative ideas, events and experiences
Reciprocal Determinism	Dynamic interaction of individual, behavior, and environment

from Redding, C.A., Rossi, J.S., Rossi, S.R., Velicer, W.F., & Prochaska, J.O. (2000). Health Behaviour Model. *The International Electronic Journal of Health Education*, Vol. 3 (Special Issue), pp. 180-193. http://www.iejhe.siu.edu

Table 3. The Concepts of Social Cognitive Theory

Bandura conceptualized the effects on human behavior including the concept of human in terms of basic human capacities that are cognitive by their nature. Key concepts associated with the person include: personal characteristics, emotional arousal/coping, behavioral capacity, self-efficacy, expectation, expectancies, self-regulation, observational/experiential learning, and reinforcement. The Social Cognitive Theory also highlights the importance of cognitive and behavioral skills in building health behavior changes. For this reason, smokers who want to quit smoking but lack the necessary cognitive and behavioral skills to cope with stressful situations without smoking in the future are less likely to be successful in changing smoking behavior, no matter how enthusiastic they are (Redding et al., 2000).

4.1.4 Transtheoretical model

In the last 20 years, research based on the Transtheoretical Model has revealed that there are some common principles of behavior changes that can be applied to several health behaviors. Examples of these behaviors are smoking cessation, exercise acquisition, sun protection, dietary fat reduction, condom use, supporting mammography screening, the spread of medicine use, coping with stress, and cessation of substance use. These problem behaviors are very important in regards to both clinical and public health, as they are closely related to an increase in the rate of illness and death and a decrease in the quality of life. The Transtheoretical Model is a model of intentional behavior change that provides a large volume of research and services in the field of problem behaviors. This model describes the relationships among: stages of change; processes of change; decisional balance, or the pros and cons of change; situational confidence, or self-efficacy in the behavior change; and situational temptations to relapse. (Prochaska et al., 2008). Table 4 explains the concepts that make up the Transtheoretical Model.

This model has some advantages over the other models. First of all, this model considers behavioral change as a process rather than an event. Then, by dividing the change process into phases and investigating which variables are associated with the improvement and the extent of their association, it presents important clues both in research and intervention development areas. The second advantage is that its emphasis on measuring concepts constituted a rigid base for the model. Among different problematic behaviors, different variables are associated with phase behaviors in each change phase. The Transtheoretical Model studies report significant similarities among different types of behavioral change. In the same way, it was found that phases of change had a predictable relationship with positive and negative aspects of behavioral changes, confidence in behavioral changes, the tendency to recur and processes of change (Redding 2000; Prochaska et al., 2008).

4.2 Health education process

The health education process consists of some elements such as data collection, diagnosis, planning and implementation.

4.2.1 Data collection/diagnosis

The data collection step is an important part of the education process. For example, in education that targets elderly individuals, it is essential to determine the real needs in detail at first in order to establish the needs and to meet those needs. Determination of the needs also helps us to see whether the educational program meets the real needs or not (Demirel, 2000). In needs analysis studies, the individual's and the related group's needs have to be determined. Determination of the needs that are peculiar to the individual or the group will enable us to determine the goals that are appropriate to the health education program to be prepared and will enable the individual to be more integrated with the society by showing self-managing behaviors. What does the society expect an elderly individual to accomplish basically? The program should be constructed with the regulations related to the answers to this question at first (Demirel, 2000; Gokkoca 2001).

	Concepts	Explanations
Stages of change	**Pre-contemplation**	The absence of any intention to take action within the following six months
	Contemplation	Intention to begin the healthy behavior within the next six months
	Preparation	Being ready to act within the next 30 days and passing some behavioral stages
	Action	Having a clearly-changed behavior for less than six months
	Maintenance	Individuals at this stage changed their behavior more than six months ago
Decisional Balance	**Pros**	The benefits of change
	Cons	The losses of change
Self-efficacy	**Confidence**	Trust in individuals' ability to perform healthy behavior in spite of temptations
	Temptation	Encouragement to perform unhealthy behavior in various tempting situations
Change Processes	**Consciousness Raising**	Gathering new facts, thoughts and tips that support healthy behavior change
	Dramatical Relief	Having negative emotions (fear, worry, anxiety) that are part of the unhealthy behavioral risks
	Selfreevaluation	Being aware of the fact that behavior change is an important part of an individual's personality
	Environmental Reevaluation	Becoming aware of the negative effect of the unhealthy behavior and the positive impact of healthy behavior on their proximal social and /or physical environment
	Self-liberation	Full commitment to change
	Helping Relationships	Searching and using social support for healthy behavior change
	Counterconditioning	Replacement of unhealthy behaviors or cognition with more healthy alternatives
	Reinforcement Management	Rewarding positive behavior change more and /or reducing the award to unhealthy behaviors
	Stimulus Control	Eliminating clues or reminders to unhealthy behavior or using clues or reminders to promote healthy behavior
	Social Liberation	Becoming aware of the fact that social norms have changed in the direction of supporting healthy behavior change.

From Redding, C.A., Rossi, J.S., Rossi, S.R., Velicer. W.F., & Prochaska, J.O. (2000). Health Behaviour Model. *The International Electronic Journal of Health Education*, Vol. 3 (Special Issue), pp. 180-193. http://www.iejhe.siu.edu

Table 4. The Concepts of the Transtheoretical Model

While determining the educational needs, and in the data collection step, the knowledge, attitudes and behaviors that will be acquired by the target group are taken into consideration. In order to learn this, it is necessary to live together with the target group, establish meetings, to know them, to get information from their social leaders, to benefit from the data of the related literature, and to examine their health records (Hacıalioglu, 2009). While determining educational needs, the following questions have to be answered:

1. *What is the general situation?:* There should be sufficient information about the characteristics, number and the level of success of the educational programs for the elderly; the economic resources of these educational programs, the proficiency level of educators, and educational materials and the technologies.
2. *What is known about the participants?:* The participants' cognitive, affective, and physical abilities, their previous experiences, their perceptions of themselves and the society can be evaluated (Demirel, 2000). In order to achieve this, an examination HBDH (REALM-Rapid Estimate of Adult Literacy) can be implemented to determine the cognitive level of the individual and his or her knowledge level in the treatment process in a short time like one or two minutes. In addition, individuals can be asked how they feel while filling out the documents (Rojda & George, 2009).
3. *What is the content of the educational materials like?:* The material to be prepared should be checked for their suitability and consistency with the aims of the education and for legibility for the elderly (Demirel, 2000). In order to evaluate the material, a checklist can be prepared and implemented to see whether the material is consistent and suitable and can easily be read. In addition, with some tools like Fleisch-Kincaid Grade Level and SMOG (Simple Measure of Gobbledygook), the number of the sentences and the words can be counted and the suitable material can be decided on (Rojda & George, 2009).

4.2.2 Planning

While planning the health education plan, elderly individuals' socio-economic level and cultural background should be taken into consideration. Therefore, the material to be used in the education should be chosen carefully. The level of instruction should be parallel to the understanding level of the individuals. In addition, the place and the duration of the implementation must be indicated in the plan (Hacıalioglu, 2009).

Who will train?/ The trainer	The trainer
Who will get the education? / The target group	The elderly individuals who cannot feed themselves properly in a nursing and rehabilitation center
What to teach? /The subject	Eating habits
Why to teach? /The aim	To inform – the acquisition of the behavior

How to teach/ The methodology →	Instruction – modeling- doing-discussing, and etc.
Where to implement / The place →	The classroom, etc.
The time of the education/The date →	Month – day - hour
The duration of the education →	E.g., twice a day, or three times a week.

A health education plan must be designed based on some principles. These principles are:

- *Functionality:* The plan must have the qualities and the content to achieve the educational goal or goals. And it must consist of the goals that can be measured, beneficial, action-based, and valid for real life.
- *Flexibility:* The plan must be creative and flexible, be able to answer the individuals' changing needs and be open to new developments.
- *Realistic:* The health education plan must not include over-idealistic and utopic aims.
- *Practicability:* Not only the people who prepared the plan but also other people can use the health education plan easily at different times.
- *Being Scientific:* The health education plan should include scientific qualities in terms of the knowledge and the behavior to be gained.
- *Suitability to the social values:* The plan shouldn't contradict the life philosophy, ideals, beliefs and the values of the society where it is implemented.
- *Being Economical:* The costs of the implementation steps of the health education plan and the behaviors to be acquired should be affordable (Tabak, 2000).

Another factor to be considered in the planning is the determination of learner-centered objectives. The objectives are defined as the changes in the behaviors of the individual or the group. The objectives have priority in the determination of the target group and the content of the educational program. Besides, the objectives should be determined first in order to decide on the methodology and the techniques to be used in the program. The goals can be determined as the short and long-term (Demirel, 2000; Tabak, 2000). For example, teaching an elderly individual with type II diabetics how to inject insulin is a short-term objective. On the other hand, it is a long-term objective for the same individual to manage the illness effectively.

The objectives to be determined in health education can be developed for individuals' cognitive, affective and psychomotor skills. The cognitive field is related to the knowledge and the mental abilities that are derived from knowledge (Demirel, 2000; Tabak, 2000). The cognitive domain objectives related to an elderly individual's health education can be written as follows:

While preparing an educational program, the trainer, the target group, the aim of the education, the methodology to be used in the education, and the place and time of the education should be clearly determined (Demirel, 2000; Hacıalioglu, 2009). For example, a health education plan for the elderly individuals who cannot feed themselves properly can be as follows.

Knows the complications of Type II diabetics. Knows the normal blood glucose level.	Tells the normal blood pressure values. Interprets the relation between hypertension and salt.
Plans his/her dietary program.	Tells the associations related to the hypertension.
Evaluates his/her diet's effects on the type II diabetics.	Evaluates the effects of regular health controls for the effective management of hypertension.
Knows the complications of Type II diabetics Knows the normal blood glucose level.	Tells the normal blood pressure values. Interprets the relation between hypertension and salt.

The affective domain target behaviors are related to the emotion and value systems. Interest, attitude, appreciation, belief, etc. include behaviors that are difficult to measure (Demirel, 2000; Tabak, 2000). Affective domain objectives can be written as follows:

Believes in the importance of measuring the blood glucose at regular intervals.	Is careful about keeping the blood pressure at correct levels.
Is willing to participate in the scientific and social activities related to diabetics.	Is willing to follow the up-to-date resources about hypertension.
Accepts the new diet special to him or her.	Accepts being an active member of the associations related to hypertension.
Cares about the continuation of the regular physical exercises.	Believes in the importance of regular health controls for the effective management of hypertension.
Believes in the importance of measuring the blood glucose at regular intervals.	Is careful about keeping the blood pressure at correct levels.
Is willing to participate in the scientific and social activities related to diabetics.	Is willing to follow the up-to-date resources about hypertension.

Finally, the psychomotor domain includes skills that require the individual's muscle and mind coordination (Demirel, 2000, Tabak, 2000). Psychomotor domain objectives can be written as follows:

Follows the stages of the measurement in the blood glucose meter.	Follows the stages of blood pressure measurement.
Measures the blood sugar level alone.	Measures blood pressure properly.
Performs a proper physical preparation for the measurement of blood sugar.	Takes a proper position when blood pressure rises.
Applies a self-insulin injection.	Prepares hypertension drugs properly.

Some programming approaches should be utilized so that the content can be managed consistent with the objectives. These can be summarized as linear, spiral and modular programming approaches. The linear programming approach is used to arrange the topics, which consist mainly of learning that is successive, closely related or a prerequisite for each other. Spiral approach programming involves addressing issues over and over when necessary. Finally, in the modular programming approach, the subjects to be learnt are divided into modules, modules are connected to each other and each module gains meaning within itself. The content should be offered after determining the most appropriate programming approach for the elderly. What programming approach to choose should be decided by considering factors such as learning preferences, cognitive-affective and psychomotor skill levels of the target elderly population, qualifications of the educator and available sources (Demirel, 2000). After organizing the content based on the appropriate programming approach, the next step is to decide with which method, technique, material, etc. to present that content. The group's characteristics, size, target learning domains, duration of education, funds, available educational resources, the educator's qualities and so on have to be taken into account when choosing educational methods tailored for the elderly (Demirel, 2000; Tabak 2000).

Methods such as lectures, discussions, questions and answers, demonstrations, role-plays, etc. can be used according to the goals and objectives in the process of education. However, no matter what method is used, there should be active participation of the elderly, feedback and a supportive communication style (Tabak, 2000). Therefore, educational environments should be designed in a way that allows everyone to see each other easily, have eye contact with each other comfortably, and should be free of hierarchy. Common seating arrangements are U-type, team style, circle, and work units seating orders; arrangements can be shaped according to the educational method chosen.

In order to determine the location and time for health education, educators and the target group should take the decision jointly. It would be appropriate to choose convenient times and places (Tabak, 2000). In addition, the place of education must have efficient acoustic features; enough space for writing activities and tools like wheelchairs, sticks and walkers; a suitable temperature; non-slip stairs and a floor, and comfortable chairs with back support on which individuals of different physical sizes can comfortably sit (Grandal, 2008).

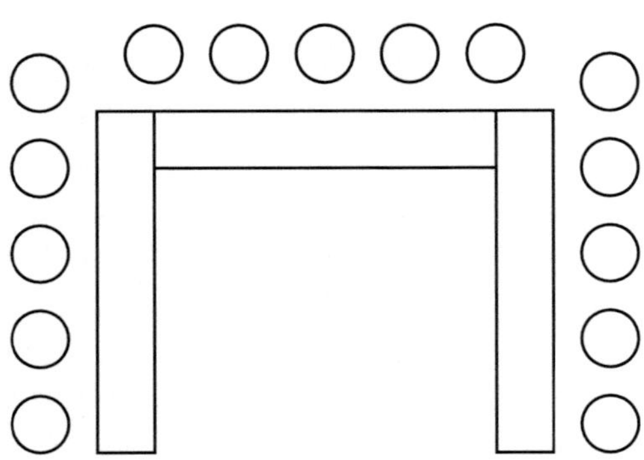

Fig. 1. U Seating Order

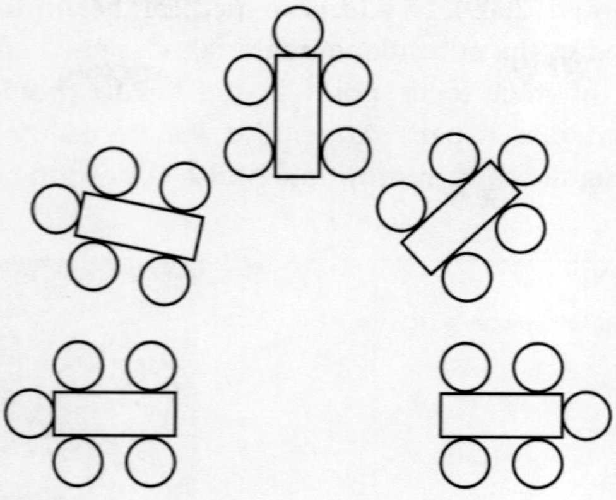

Fig. 2. Team Seating Order

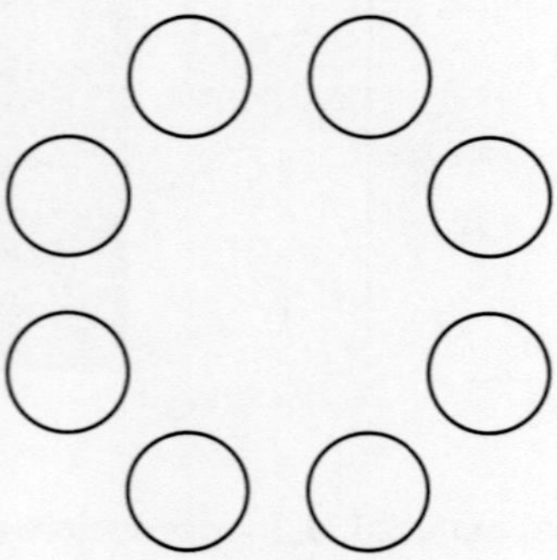

Fig. 3. Circle Seating Order

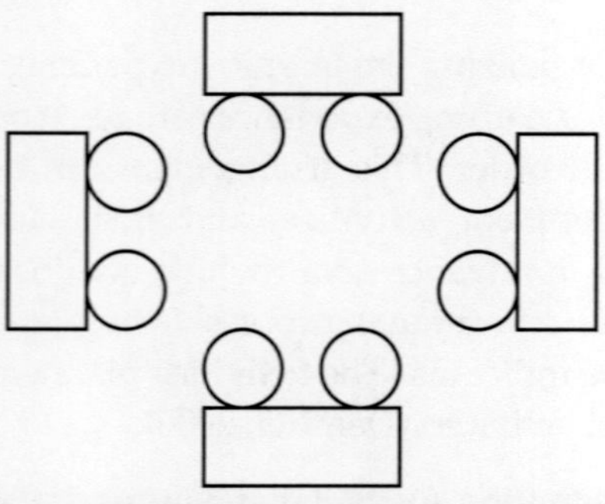

From Demirel, Ö (2000). *Learning Art*. Ankara, Turkey: Pegem A Publishing.

Fig. 4. Working Units

Another component of this educational process is materials; the answer to the following question is important when choosing educational materials: Are the font of these materials large enough for the elderly to read easily? The font of educational materials should be large enough and the background should contain white areas because it is easier to read when the background largely consists of white areas. Also, images and graphics should be preferred as they make the message clearer. Words and posters should be used instead of long paragraphs (Rojda & George, 2009). In addition, medical/health terminology (i.e., medical jargon) should be avoided in the educational materials designed specifically for the elderly (Figure 5 a, b). Finally, another focus point in the health promotion for the elderly is encouraging health promotion experts to acquire the necessary skills so that they can develop culturally and linguistically appropriate health education materials (Wallace, 2004).

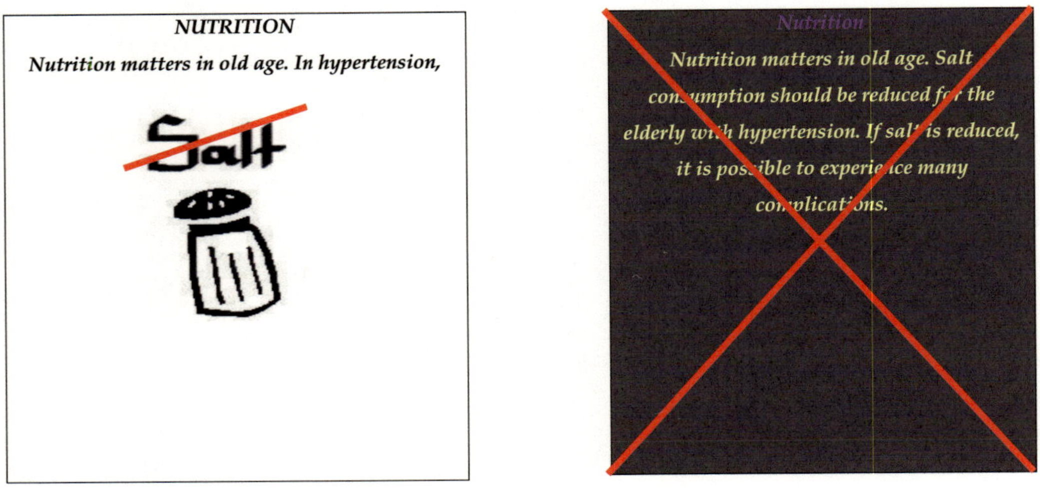

a. b.

Fig. 5. a. Appropriate educational material. b. Inappropriate educational material

4.2.3 Implementation

It is the phase that involves organizing the learning experiences that enable the individuals to gain the targeted behaviors. Learning experiences are to be oriented to the individual, and must be arranged in a specific order. This arrangement can be ordered as introduction or preparation activities, development activities, and final activities (Demirel, 2000). The individual must be informed in advance about which qualities and competences he or she will have by the end of the educational process. Afterwards, the necessary content to achieve these goals should be indicated. The activities planned to be implemented must be assessed during improvement activities (Demirel, 2000).

It is crucial to pay specific attention to the language used and communication when you apply the health education process. The essential strategies to communicate effectively with elderly individuals can be summarized as follows:

Improving communication with an elderly individual

1. *Using the principles of individual-centered care*
- Knowing the person to be educated: An educator that works with elderly individuals is required to be able to use his or her tone of voice, facial expressions, gestures, and the words correctly, and have the ability to listen without expressing criticism, sadness, or complaint.

- Applying the principles of gentle listening: The educator must listen what is being said without interrupting the person, or "tuning out" his or her words. The educator should understand what the real problem is.
- Allowing time to "right" (positive aspects of their lives) things as well as talking about problems: The individual's positive qualities/strengths must be stressed while talking about problems. Emphasizing "wrong" things can create a bad feeling. Listen to personal stories and experiences properly. What does the person say? What is the individual doing to improve his or her power and abilities?
- Slow down and focus on the individual: What is he saying? What is he conveying? The educators shouldn't have a hasty or duty-based approach. Attention should be paid not only to what they say about their health but also to other things they mention. Think about being an old person, he or she has lived a long life. What is the meaning of the current situation for him or her?

2. *Arrange the environment and the routines*

- Adjust changes in seeing: An older adult can see you better in bright light. Avoid standing too close in order not to being seen blurred. You should stand in front of the person to be seen easily. Yellow and red or green and blue colors should be used for signs and markers.
- Adjust to changes in hearing: Make sure that the individual can read your lips. If it is necessary to speak out, a low tone of voice should be used. Ear wax accumulation ought to be checked as it can prevent hearing. Hearing aids and batteries should be checked.
- Pay attention to environmental effects: in educational environments, the noise must be prevented. Rooms must be lit enough to see them and let them read your lips. Elderly individuals mustn't worry about others' hearing what they say (privacy respected).
- Evaluate the personal comfort level of the individual: They should be physically comforted.

Hunger, thirst, pain, or the need for the toilet must be eliminated. What they think and feel should be evaluated for their effects on learning.

3. *Adjust your interaction with the elderly*

- Think about the approach and the language: They should be given time to respond to your questions, or ask questions (Note: The reaction time slows down). Familiar and understandable words should be used, and medical terminology or slang should be avoided. The educator should be clear and understandable, and should not use long explanations or instructions.
- Adapt to changes in responses: If you need to improve participation, yes/no questions should be used. Important points should be written in large fonts. Use physical gestures to enhance verbal communication. Questions with only two options may be used in order to promote success.
- Help them think by giving clues like "When?" or "How long ago?" Apologize for misunderstandings and provide an explanation.

4. *Adapt your approach to accommodate changes in EXPRESSION:* Listen for meaningful words and ideas, trying to identify the main theme or goal. Respond to the person's emotional tone and validate feelings (e.g., understandable to feel frustrated, angry). Accept/understand cursing or other foul language as an expression of distress and discomfort – not an "insult" to you. Using guessing (e.g., trying to replace words the

person is having difficulty saying) based on how well you know the person and the relationship you have; guessing can been annoying to the person and may further increase confusion (Smith, 2006; Cornett, 2011).

4.2.4 Evaluation

The success of health promotion can be evaluated by measuring to what extent the intended objectives can be achieved. What were the individual's knowledge, attitudes and skills on the subject before the education? What have they accomplished after the training? How much lack of information has been fixed? Has an attitude change been provided? Have the skills been gained? How much have they gained? What more skills should be gained? The correct answers to these questions, etc. are obtained by measurement and evaluation (Hacıalioglu 2009).

Evaluation processes are usually performed with qualitative and quantitative assessment techniques. The knowledge level of elderly individual/individuals participating in a health education program can be estab;ished only through post-training tests. During the evaluation process, qualitative methods such as observation and interviews can also be used. Qualitative evaluation includes the views and expectations of educational program participants and other people related to the program and provides a much broader perspective than quantitative assessment (Tabak, 2000). In recent years, however, these two types of assessment have been used together in a holistic approach to minimize the disadvantages of both methods.

5. References

Bastable, S.B (2008). *Nurse as an Educator* , Jones & Bartlett Learning, pp. 1-667.

Bikmaz, F.H. (2006). Self-efficacy Beliefs, In: *Individual Differences in Education*. Y. Kuzgun, D. Deryakulu (Eds), Ankara, Turkey.

Champion, V.L. & Skinner, C.S. (2008). Health Belief Model, In: *Health Behavior and Health Education*, K. Glanz, B.K. Rimer, K., Viswanat (Eds.), 45-62, Jossey-Bass, ISBN 978-0-7879-9614-7, San Francisco, USA.

Choi, W.H.H., Hui, G.K.H., Lee, A.C.K. & Chui, M.M. L. (2010). Student Nurses' Experiences and Challenges in Providing Health Education in Hong Kong. *Nurse Education Today*, Vol.30, pp. 355–359.

Connell, C.M. (1999). Older Adults in Health Education Research: Some Recommendations. *Health Education Research Theory & Practice*, Vol. 14, No.3, pp. 427–431.

Cornett S. (August 2011). Teaching the Elderly. 20.08.2011. Available from http://medicalcenter.osu.edu/patiented/materials/pdfdocs/employee/elderly.pdf

Demirel, O. (2000). *Learning Art.* Ankara, Turkey: Pegem A Publishing.

DeYoung, S. (2009). Learning Theory. In: *Teaching Strategies for Nurse Educators*, 23-30. New Jersey, USA: Pearson Education.

Doucette, W.R., Andersen, T.N.(2005). Practitioner activities in patient education and drug therapy monitoring for community dwelling elderly patients. *Patient Education and Counselling*.Vol.57, pp.204-2010.

Glanz, K., Rimer, B.K. & Viswanat, K. (2008). Theory, Research, and Practice in Health Behavior and Health Education. In: *Health Behavior and Health Education*, K. Glanz,

B.K. Rimer, K. Viswanat (Eds.) 23-38, Jossey-Bass, ISBN 978-0-7879-9614-7, San Francisco, USA.

Gokkoca, F.Z.U. (2001). Adult Education in Relation to Health Education. *STED*, Vol. 10, No.11, pp. 412-414.

Grandal, K. (August 2011). Class Acts: A+ Educational Activities for the Elderly in Healthcare Facilities. 02.08.2011. Available from www.recreativeresources.com

Hacıalioglu N. (2009). Health Education. In: *Public Health Nursing*, B. Erci (Ed.), 166-181. Turkey: Göktug Publishing.

Hoving, C., Visser, A., Mullen, P.D. & Borne, B. (2010). A History of Patient Education by Health Professionals in Europe and North America: From Authority to Shared Decision Making Education. *Patient Education and Counseling*, Vol. 78, pp. 275–281.

Kahn, M.H., Goto, R., Sonoda T., Sakauchi F., Washio M., Kobayashi K., Mori M. (2004). Impact of health education and screening over all-cause mortality in Japan: evidence from a cohort study during 1984–2002. *Preventive Medicine*. Vol.38, pp.786-792.

Karaoz, S. & Aksayan, S. (2009). Ageing and Nursing. In: *It's called September - Ageing in Health Sciences*. MN. Gacar (Ed.), 463-537. Istanbul, Turkey: Nobel Medical Publishing.

Koh, L.C. (2011). Student attitudes and educational support in caring for older people - A review of literature. *Nurse Education in Practice*.pp.1-5.

Kurt, İ. (2000*). Adult Education*. Istanbul, Turkey: Nobel Medical Publishing.

Leung, A., Chi, I. & Lui, Y.H. (2006). A Cross-Cultural Study in Older Adults' Learning Experience. Asian J Gerontol Geriatr, Vol. 1, pp. 78–83.

Liu, E., Wong, E. (1997). Health Care For Elderly People. Research and Library Services Division Provisional Legislative Council Secretariat's Document, Hong Kong.

Montaño, D.E. & Kasprzyk, D. (2008). The theory of reasoned action, theory of planned behavior, and Integrated Behavioral Model. In: *Health Behavior and Health Education*. K. Glanz, B.K. Rimer, K. Viswanat (Eds.), 67-92, Jossey-Bass, ISBN 978-0-7879-9614-7, San Francisco, USA.

Prochaska, J.O., Redding, C.O. & Evers, K.E. (2008). The Transtheoretical Model and Stages of Change. In: *Health Behavior and Health Education*, K. Glanz, B.K. Rimer, K. Viswanat (Eds.), 97-117, Jossey-Bass, ISBN 978-0-7879-9614-7, San Francisco, USA.

Rana, A.K.M.M., Kabir, Z.N., Lundborg, C.S. & Wahlin, A. (2010). Health Education Improves Both Arthritis-related Illness and Self-rated Health: An Intervention Study Among Older People in Rural Bangladesh. *Public Health*, Vol.124, pp. 705-712.

Redding, C.A., Rossi, J.S., Rossi, S.R., Velicer, W.F. & Prochaska, J.O. (2000). Health Behaviour Model, *The International Electronic Journal of Health Education*, Vol.3 (Special Issue), pp. 180-193. Available from http://www.iejhe.siu.edu

Reicherter, E.A. & Revenda-Greene, R. (2005). Wellness and Health Promotion Educational Applications for Older Adults in the Community. *Topics in Geriatric Rehabilitation*, Vol. 21, No. 4, pp. 295–303.

Rojda, C. & George, N. M. (2009). The Effect of Education and Literacy Levels on Health Outcomes of the Elderly. The Journal for Nurse Practitioners (JNP), pp. 115-119.

Shen, Q., Karr, M. , Ko, A., Chan, D.K.Y., Khan, R. & Duvall D. (2006). Evaluation of a Medication Education Program for Elderly Hospital In-Patients. *Geriatric Nursing,* Vol.27, No.3, pp.184-192.

Smith, M. (2006). Getting the Facts: Communicating with the Elderly. *The Geriatric Mental Health Training Series,* for the Hartford Center of Geriatric Nursing Excellence, College of Nursing, University of Iowa. Available from http://www.nursing.uiowa.edu/hartford/nurse/effective_communication/Commun-Support-Mat.pdf

Tabloski, P.A. (2010). Challenges of Aging and Cornerstones of Excellence in Nursing Care. In: *Gerontological Nursing,* 87-343, Pearson Education, ISBN 978-0-13-503810-9, New Jersey, USA.

Tabak, R.S. (2000). *Health Education.* Ankara, Turkey: Somgür Publishing.

Wallace L. S. (2004). The Impact of Limited Literacy on Health Promotion in the Elderly. *Californian Journal of Health Promotion,* Vol.2, No.3, pp. 1-4.

Vintila, M., Marklinder, I., Nydahl, M., Istratı, D. & Kuglisı, A. (August 2011). Health behavior of the elderly: Between needs and reality: A comparative study, 02.08.2011, Available from www.community-health.eu/.../Article%20Revista%20de%20psihologie%20aplicata.pdf

Part 3

End of Life Care

12

Expanding the Time Frame for Advance Care Planning: Policy Considerations and Implications for Research

Jeffrey S. Kahana, Loren D. Lovegreen and Eva Kahana
Case Western Reserve University, USA

1. Introduction

This paper addresses the policy challenge of comprehensive advance care planning in late life. It envisions end-of-life decision making as promoting meaningful living, even for individuals with end stage diseases. We first review the current state of end-of-life decisions based on a personal autonomy model. This is followed by a summary of our prior research about attitudes of community dwelling aged toward end-of-life decision making. Based on this data we developed a proactive and collaborative approach to end-of-life planning. This is built upon patient preferences, physician and family partnerships, and best practices regarding advance care. Expanding the time frame from advance care to future care planning (FCP) empowers patients to be better advocates for their own care. It also supports a dynamic planning orientation that focuses on living as well as possible, while providing direction for immediate end-of-life needs.

The recent literature on end-of-life care emphasizes advance directives as the central feature of end-of-life care (De Boer et al., 2010; Perkins, 2007). These studies have also raised concerns about the current state of end-of-life care. They show that advance directives may not reflect the patient's desires near the end of life, and don't guarantee that directives will be implemented by family and/or health care providers (Lynch et al., 2008; Perkins, 2007). There is concern, too, about the appropriateness of hospitals as the settings where many individuals die, and the limited access of patients to different end-of-life care locations (Detering et al., 2010; Hallenbeck, 2008; Miller & Han, 2008). This literature also recognizes that options for end-of-life care are enhanced where there is coordination between patients, health care providers and family members (Cartwright et al., 2009; Engelberg et al., 2010).

The emphasis on the final days that patients live is consistent with the current policy focus on advance directives for end-of-life care. However, this tends to draw attention away from the period that precedes the immediate end-of-life. Our paper seeks to emphasize this time frame that is between the individual's knowledge that he/she has life-limiting illness, recognition of the nearness of the end of life, and the actual death. We believe that end-of-life decision making should encompass health care planning for this more extended time frame – which is so critical to ensuring that the individual can live as well as possible

(Berzoff & Silverman, 2004). Such planning is entirely consistent with promoting the goals of personal autonomy that animates end-of-life public policy (Tauber, 2005).

2. The law and end-of-life decision making

In the United States, federal law cedes authority to states and every state has statutory provisions for preparation of advance directives (Pollack et al., 2010). Generally these laws call for naming a single person as a proxy decision maker, should the patient no longer be competent to make decisions in his or her own behalf. The Patient Self -Determination Act of 1990 requires all hospitals in the U.S. to inform adult patients, on admission, about their rights regarding advance directives (Yates & Glick, 1997).

The principle of personal autonomy has guided end-of-life legal policy. Based on the broad concept of a "right to privacy," American courts have presumed that individuals - and not the state or medical professionals - are the ultimate decision-makers with respect to their own lives. This solicitude for personal autonomy applies whether the decisions being made are beneficial or injurious. Indeed, in case after case, the law has sustained decisions by competent individuals to end medical treatments, notwithstanding the impact on the patient.

While the principle of autonomy has deep roots in Anglo-American law, practical considerations also support this principle as applied to end-of-life legal policy. The organizational needs of hospitals, long-term care facilities and the physicians, who operate within them, are advanced when patients have clearly stated plans for when they would like treatments to end. Without patient direction - made when the individual was competent - these difficult choices must be made by others, and may cause conflict with family members. The lack of direction can lead to greater financial costs involved in prolonging life with extraordinary treatments. It can generate fears of lawsuits by health care organizations and providers, and can result in unnecessary suffering and undignified deaths.

For these reasons, the use of advanced directives for end-of-life decisions are necessary and should be encouraged as a matter of public policy. By statute, living wills are recognized as the basic model for providing advance directives - and seek to avoid issues presented when a patient is no longer competent to make decisions. These statutes make provision for relieving physicians or health care organizations from liability if they follow the patient's wishes as stated in the living will.

Another mechanism for advanced planning is the durable power of attorney. This allows the patient to transfer authority to an agent who becomes a health care decision maker. This authority is considered "durable" in that the incapacity of the patient does not extinguish the authority of the agent. This represents a modification to the common law "powers of attorney" that would end with the incapacity of the principal, and was provided by statutes (e.g., Uniform Probate Code) beginning in the 1970s to accommodate the needs of the aged. It should be noted that these powers can be withdrawn by the principal, amended, and cannot be utilized where the patient has the competence to provide informed consent.

The responsibility for following patient wishes is not vitiated if the patient lacks a living will or durable power of attorney. An effort must be made by the physicians and health care organization to ascertain what the wishes of the patient would have been if he were competent. Thus it is recommended that those treating the patient consult with family members. Nevertheless, under the law the ultimate decision must be in alignment with the wishes of the patient – which at times may not be consistent with those of the family.

The utility and need for formalized end-of-life directives cannot be minimized, even as complementary models, like those advocated in this paper, are explored. These serve a crucial purpose at the very last stage of life. But the role of social support, caring interventions, and community based involvement are not central features of the current legal model of end-of-life decision making. Indeed, the model at present puts little emphasis on planning for living, and the husbanding of family and community resources. These can greatly enhance quality of life during a prolonged period of life that many individuals experience when dealing with a terminal illness.

Putting aside criticisms pertaining to the existing advance directive orientation (George & Harlow, 2011; Fried & Drickamer, 2010), the following sections explore the enhanced quality of life framework we are proposing. We do not weigh in on the questions related to percentages of adults who in fact prepare advance directives, or the controversy surrounding cost savings by patients who forego end-of-life treatments. Rather, we explore the attitudes of the aged population toward advance planning, and consider the possibilities for them to build capacity to enhance the remaining period of their life. To do so, we also recognize that health care professionals, social workers, and families are critical to improving care during the prolonged end-of-life period (Stein & Sherman, 2005).

3. Expanding the time frame for future care planning

We aim to expand advance care planning by focusing on the multiple care needs that emerge in the final years of life (Penrod et al., 2011). Few people face death in the absence of disabling health conditions. Individuals of advanced age, who have experienced some form of chronic illness and disability, make up the vast majority of those facing end-of-life decisions. Nevertheless, these individuals strive for, and often experience, a good quality of life during extended periods prior to death. The information obtained from these older individuals – which will be discussed in the section below – provides a useful template for understanding the challenges faced by people of all ages near the end of life (Thomas, 2007).

Understanding of the maintenance of good quality of life, in the time frame prior to the end of life, has been limited by lack of systematic theoretical attention (Conway, 2011). In order to improve care, and promote policies that further caring, we must synthesize orientations from the fields of gerontology, nursing, social work, psychology, and sociology. Approaches we find useful include recent developments from the palliative care movement (Lorenz et al., 2008), as well as long standing frameworks relating to stress models (Pearlin, 1989).

The palliative care movement has called for systemic changes in health care delivery to decrease the suffering of seriously ill and dying patients. These changes are advocated across care settings ranging from hospitals to nursing homes (Abbey et al., 2006; Chochinov et al., 2007). This movement endorses caring for patients in the period leading up to death. During this time-frame careful judgments must be made to ensure that life of the impaired is valued and respected (Kastenbaum, 2004). The social stress model captures the normative nature of health related stressors and social losses (Folkman, 2010). Individuals, under this model, must adapt proactively to ensure that they can maintain a good quality of life even as they face disability due to chronic illness, encounter acute health events, and deal with a shrinking social network (E. Kahana & B. Kahana, 2002; Kelley-Moore et al., 2006).

Drawing on ideas from the palliative care movement and social stress models - in addition to our empirical work in the field of aging - leads us to conclude that enhancing capacity for "care-getting" is crucial to end-of-life planning. This entails marshaling informal and formal support to help individuals maintain comfort, experience psychological well-being and feel that others are caring for them (E. Kahana et al., 2010; Nolan & Mock, 2004).

The ability of an individual near the end of life to draw on a variety of social resources and to secure advocates who can represent their values is a crucial component of planning. This will assist individuals in obtaining responsive home care, if this is possible, as well as ensure that their medical and longer term care needs are considered fully. For many individuals, and especially seniors, this also entails mobilizing community resources within the broader aging network (Force et al., 2010; Gelfand, 2006).

In the United States, Area Agencies on Aging (AAAs) can serve important roles in offering transportation, caregiver support and health promotion resources for frail elders (J. Kahana & Force, 2008, Force et al., 2010). This broader vision of services is consistent with emerging approaches to health promoting palliative care delivered in a community context that is becoming prevalent in Australia (Rosenberg &Yates, 2011). Indeed, for seniors, planning that includes "care getting" can be vital to aging in place and completing one's final years living independently. Nevertheless, a growing number of elders live out their final years in nursing homes (E. Kahana, et al., 2011). These facilities are not well equipped to address the care needs of seriously ill and of dying patients (Wetle, et al., 2005). The current set-up of long term care facilities - and reimbursement patterns - creates obstacles to offering individualized and dignity-conserving care to patients.

Ethical dilemmas are presented "inside the world of the nursing home" that impinge on patient autonomy (Moody, 1992, p. 109). Paternalistic policies on the one hand, and lack of adherence to informed consent principles on the other, leave patients with little control over the final period of their lives. Patient autonomy is further compromised by the assumption that those with cognitive deficits are lacking in the capacity for self-determination (Small et al., 2008). Public policies that support caring for seniors within long term care facilities - especially in the period leading up to death - are needed to protect the welfare of these individuals. Utilizing the existing resources of long-term care ombudsmen can help achieve these objectives (J. Kahana, 1994).

4. Attitudes of the aged toward end-of-life care and planning

Gerontologists have paid relatively little attention to end-of-life issues. The emphasis on productivity in aging, health in advanced years, and continuing to make social contributions has made "successful aging" the dominant model (Rowe & Kahn, 1998). The medical literature addresses end-of-life issues in the context of chronic illness. It does so based on illness categories such as cancer, dementia and heart disease (Keating et al., 2007; Selman et al., 2007; Van der Steen & Deliens, 2009). The nursing community has shown a greater interest in the subject of care for older individuals at the end of life (Hansen et al., 2009).

Watson's notion of being "cared for" is particularly relevant to the service needs of those at the end stage of life (Watson, 1996).

The Elderly Care Research Center has conducted several funded studies to inform our approaches to end-of-life care (E. Kahana & B. Kahana, 2002; E. Kahana, 2010). These studies include Adaptation to Frailty among Dispersed Elders, a National Institutes of Health 20-year study of healthy older adults. More recently, the National Institute of Nursing Research funded a study about attitudes and behaviors of diverse community dwelling elders regarding planning for advance care (E. Kahana & B. Kahana, 2010).

Our interest in end-of-life research has been a natural outgrowth of the aging of our original research sample. As respondents in our longitudinal study were increasingly lost to mortality, we became interested in perspectives on the end of life among representative samples of older adults. Our review of the literature on end-of-life issues revealed that knowledge about the end of life is based on the health care literature focusing on terminally ill patients (Thomas & Lobo, 2011). We realized that much could be learned about the end of life by considering perspectives of older adults who confront varying trajectories as they approach this period of life.

These studies have shown that, as older adults get closer to the end of life, they do not seem to fear death. They do, however, fear suffering close to the end of life (E. Kahana & B. Kahana, 2010). Thus, 85.6% of our respondents are in favor of obtaining effective medications that relieve pain close to the end of life. Attitudes of respondents regarding death and dying may be characterized by the adage "hope for the best and prepare for the worst" (E. Kahana, et al., in press).

Attesting to valuation of social relations close to the end of life, 90.3% want to be surrounded by friends and family, and 91.8% want to have others pray for them as they near the end of life. The vast majority of respondents prefer to die at home (92.3%). Our findings thus reveal that social connections remain salient to older adults as they contemplate the end of life. These concerns can best be addressed by meaningful dialogue between patients, their family members and their health care providers. Such dialogue can result in anticipating responsive care (E. Kahana et al., 2010).

Important themes that emerged from elders' narratives include lack of fear by the very old about impending death, and a strong desire to remain connected to significant others in their lives. In discussing preparations for the end of life, the focus was not as much on their preferences, fulfillment or comfort, but on their desire to care for the people they felt close to or responsible for. Respondents reported making plans for end-of-life care so that their families would not be burdened. They also made funeral arrangements to leave their loved ones with minimal worry of financial responsibility (Casarett, 2010).

5. The role of providers, community, and family in advance care planning

The role of doctors, patients and family in care of the aged close to the end of life has been the subject of our research. We sought to understand the health care partnerships that emerge as older adults encounter the cascade of disability reflected in increasing chronic illnesses, physical impairments, and functional limitations (Verbrugge & Jette, 1994). We conducted interviews with older adults, their primary care physicians and family members who played a major role in their health maintenance. We inquired about advance directives based on questions posed to elders, their primary care doctors and family members.

A majority of 231 respondents, whose physicians and family participated in this study, prepared advance directives (60%). Those who discussed end-of-life issues most often did so with family, and particularly, spouses. Among different types of advance directives, the most common was a living will (84%), followed by durable power of attorney (32%). It is notable that about one-quarter (24%) of the sample made no end-of-life care plans

Few respondents (15%) discussed their advance directives with their physicians. Primary care physicians whom we interviewed confirmed this pattern, as they were generally unaware of advance directives prepared by their patients. Only 28% of physicians whose patients reported having made advance directives were informed about their patient's wishes. Furthermore, about a third of physicians whose patients did not provide advance directives, were under the mistaken impression that such plans existed. In contrast, family caregivers were far more likely to be well informed about their relative's advance directives.

Findings suggest insufficient communication between elders and health care professionals. There is little evidence of effective health care partnerships close to the end of life (B. Kahana et al., 2004). It is also important to recognize that different factors may be salient to patients, family and health care providers near the end of life (Steinhauser et al., 2000).

Our research has investigated health communication relevant to the very old, including those close to the end of life. In our ongoing study we explored respondents advance care planning in terms of traditional indices of living wills, power of attorney of health care, and conversations with family and with health care providers about end-of-life issues. Based on data from 514 community-dwelling respondents, less than one third of our sample reported having had conversations with family members (28%). An even smaller proportion reported conversations about advance care plans with physicians (14.7%). Elderly respondents indicated that discussions were generally initiated by the patient, rather than the doctor.

The subject of physician initiated discussion generally focused on preparation of documents such as living wills. Our findings indicate that advance care plans were typically undertaken to protect family members from being burdened. In response to the question, "Is there anything that you would like your health care providers and family to know about your wishes for end of life care?" there was a notable lack of specificity. Only 21% stated specific wishes. Among those expressing wishes the most frequently noted were the desire to avoid extreme measures (20%), such as life support. These data raise provocative questions about the absence of motivation and/or opportunities for meaningful end of life conversations for elderly persons who are nearing the end of life (B. Kahana et al., 2004).

Our findings based on relatively healthy older adults who are able to live in the community in spite of multiple chronic illnesses, have helped us take a broader view of older adults' attitudes and preferences regarding planning for the end of life. Nevertheless, we recognize that, with aging and the cascade of disability (Verbrugge & Jette, 1994), there may be greater interest in end-of-life planning focused on maintenance of personal comfort and management of the dying process.

6. Practice implications

What are the implications of these research findings for consideration of the needs of elders close to the end of life? Educational interventions may benefit such elders to enhance their competence and confidence in communication with families and health care providers (E. Kahana et al., in press). It is particularly important as part of an expanded end-of-life planning program to enhance communication skills among seniors, and especially minority, underserved, and disabled older adults (Elder et al., 2009).

Theorizing about maintenance of the self in late life underscores the abiding desire of human beings to maintain their long established identity, retain autonomy, and garner respect from their social environment for their values, preferences, and cultural diversity (George, 1999). Throughout much of adult life and well into healthy old age, this identity can be autonomously maintained. The final years of life pose a challenge to this self-reliant, autonomous identity, as aged persons facing frailty and social losses must increasingly be cared for by others (Wykle et al., 2005). This developmental challenge and its successful resolution present the basis for a care-getting model we developed (E. Kahana et al., 2010).

The final stage of life is often characterized by severe symptoms, and dependence on others (Twycross & Lichter, 1996). It is at this point that sensitivity and responsiveness of health care providers to patient preferences and needs becomes most challenging and important. While advance directives may reflect personal patient preferences, health care providers must also remain sensitive to the cultural values of patients and their families and to subtle communications about changing needs (Nolan & Mock, 2004).

During the final stage of life, care is focused on comfort, while 'cure' remains primarily the focus of medical therapy. For older adults suffering from many co-morbidities, treatment may have to be continued even while comfort needs increase in priority. Care in the final stage focuses on understanding psychological needs and providing optimal comfort to the patients. Supportive care emphasizes the individual's wishes and needs. At the same time, for some older adults, life extension can remain an enduring desire (Singer et al., 1999).

In this paper we argued for expanding the temporal context of end-of-life care. It is important to note that decisions relevant to the end of life may be legitimately made long before the final days or months of living. A second important point relates to the paradigm shift away from leaving the responsibility for advocacy and communication near the end of life to physicians and other health care professionals. Given the failures of the current health care system, it is important for patients and their family advocates to be informed, and to take initiatives toward ensuring responsive health care close to the end of life. We propose that formal health care advocates and agencies support both patient education and provider education efforts, to improve care close to the end of life. Empowerment, involvement and participation by patients, families and communities are increasingly called for in public health and public policy approaches to improve end-of-life care (Kumar, 2011).

We support recommendations for expanding the definition and time frame for palliative care. This can result in removing unnecessary stigma and expanding substantive benefits to patients regarding comfort and a more hospitable health care environment. To make progress in improving lives of elders close to the end of life we must think outside the box regarding empowerment of patients during the final period of their lives. This involves risk-taking by presenting patients with real choices in areas that are meaningful to them.

We must also re-examine our orientation to diversity in order to ensure that patients can define culturally meaningful practices related to the final period of their lives (Elder et al., 2009). We must acknowledge potential differences in desires and value orientations of those facing long term, sudden or gradual disability in late life. The concept of "inherent dignity" (Robinson et al., 2006) is useful for achieving a synthesis between concerns of disability advocates and perspectives of older adults who are latecomers to the disability community and may not identify themselves as persons with disabilities, even close to the end of life.

7. Lived experience: A challenge to prevailing practices

We distilled these perspectives from up-close observations of the final years of "Sari", a close relative of the two senior authors. Sari died at the age of 85 in a high quality, not-for-profit nursing home. Her struggles and experiences are quite typical of the challenges faced by many older adults as they approach the end of life. They also call into question many of our current practices in caring for patients close to the end of life. Her reactions to prevailing treatment practices illustrate the need for a paradigm shift in offering "caring," rather than just medical care, close to the end of life (Watson, 1996).

Our initial anecdote aims to emphasize the complexities of advance directives. It is generally agreed upon that advance directives are a necessary and desirable way to influence and possibly curtail medical care close to the end of life. Recent literature has demonstrated that in spite of mandated efforts to obtain advance directives, especially from patients in long-term care facilities, such directives are not regularly implemented (Lynch et al., 2008; Perkins, 2007). It is only very recently that more fundamental questions have been raised about the value and meaning of advance directives.

Sari was diagnosed as a diabetic at age 75. She developed circulatory problems and required amputation of her leg at age 80. She refused to give permission for the amputation, arguing that her life would not be worth living as an amputee. She made it clear that she was ready to die. At the time, she was a distraught, cognitively intact, bright and opinionated woman. Her family concluded that her wishes expressed both verbally and in writing should be honored. We do not know what transpired in the operating room, but after many frantic phone calls and psychiatric consults Sari's leg was amputated below the knee. The physician who had known her for a number of years indicated that he was convinced that she really wanted to live but could not accept the specter of becoming a disabled amputee.

After her amputation, Sari was in a good frame of mind and thanked profusely everyone who did not listen to her. She felt she survived in spite of herself and that she had much to live for. While still in the hospital, she decided that she did not want the home health services offered that were predicated on her being homebound. Instead, in the spirit of the Americans with Disabilities Act, she called the Hungarian church and asked to find a personal aide who could take her shopping and help her cook for her family from her wheelchair. In many subsequent conversations, Sari explained that prior to being faced with the prospect of amputation and permanent disability, she could not know that life could be worth living in the aftermath. She was convinced that she was at the end of life. Of course it is important to realize the distinction between prospects of living as an amputee, where a meaningful life is still possible, from the prospects of living in a vegetative state. Nevertheless, the question is still unanswered regarding the knowledge of what we would want in a future situation that we cannot fully comprehend in advance of its occurrence.

Our next relevant encounter involved advance directives regarding end-of-life issues. Sari lived a very meaningful life sharing a home with her family for three years after her initial amputation. She did suffer a number of mini strokes during this time and exhibited relatively mild signs of dementia. Her circulatory problems continued and she required a second amputation that resulted in her placement in a nursing home. Sari was given about three months to live at the time of her admission. To everyone's amazement she lived for two more years. Once again, estimates of when the end of life would occur were inaccurate.

Close to the end of her life, Sari left us with one more lesson to ponder. Her condition was generally deteriorating as her dementia progressed. One day, when her daughter came to visit, she was in bed and running a fever. The daughter was told that the doctor wanted to talk with her. The doctor, a kindly older geriatrician, came by and standing at Sari's bedside, noted that Sari had a severe urinary tract infection and that he was hesitant to transfer her to the hospital. He felt that based on her poor quality of life this might be a good time to "let go" and protect her from further, ultimately futile interventions. The doctor was persuasive and the family agreed. At this point, totally unexpectedly, Sari opened her eyes and announced in a clear voice "I want to get better, take me to the hospital".

How does this incident inform our understanding of the recent literature on end of life? One of the clear recommendations in this literature relates to not transferring demented elders from nursing homes to acute care hospital settings (Van der Steen & Deliens, 2009). This is framed as diminishing the suffering at the end of life and seldom referred to as a cost-saving measure. Sari's story points to the complexity of this picture. The three days that Sari spent at the hospital treating her infection became the highlight in her life near the end of her life. She enjoyed the attention of the nurses, the dignity with which she was treated and the fact that they did not treat her as an incontinent patient as they did in the nursing home. During this hospital visit we discovered that, in fact, she was not incontinent, but required a great deal of effort to be toileted. The hospital made the accommodations to provide her access to the toilet. Her infection cleared up and she did not want to go back to the nursing home. She lived three more months after this end-of-life hospitalization.

Looking at the situation in an unimpassioned way, a reasonable argument could be made that funds would have been saved by the health care system had she been allowed to die three months earlier without this final hospitalization. But it would be hard to argue that she would have been better off. Sari's lived experience reflects on current controversies in the end-of-life literature. It raises important questions regarding individuals' ability to predict at earlier points in their lives what would be in their best interest during critical periods when decisions about their end of life are being made. It also calls into question whether the effort to limit hospital placements for elderly disabled and demented patients at the end of life always benefit the patient. These are just some of the questions that illustrate the complexity involved in bureaucratizing end-of-life care and decision making.

8. Policy considerations

This paper has considered expanding end-of-life decision making, beyond advanced directives, to include care planning for meaningful living even when individuals are confronting life-threatening illnesses. Public policies, and funding mechanisms within existing social programs (Medicare, Medicaid, Area Agencies on Aging), can support individuals and families who are facing chronic and disabling illnesses during the final years of life (Binstock & Post, 1991).

Our approach to planning as a distinctive policy goal for end-of-life decision making and care builds upon the palliative care movement and existing stress models. Research has shown that planning can minimize suffering and enhance opportunities for fulfilling social relationships (Jackson, 2002). Conflict between professionals, family members and those at the end of life can be reduced through planning efforts (Burck & Lapidos, 2002). It is also likely that substantial cost savings can be achieved when individuals remain in their communities longer and avoid expensive hospitalizations or admission to skilled nursing facilities. Even when more intensive care is needed, planning is an effective mechanism for limiting legal liability on the part of health organizations and providers.

The effectiveness of planning is dependent upon the partnerships and collaborations of all those interested in the well-being of the person nearing the end of life. Patients, family members, health care providers and institutions will make planning more effective when they are able to be proactive rather than responsive to upcoming medical events, including those psychological challenges facing individuals at the end of life (Steinhauser et al., 2000). Planning seeks solutions to upcoming challenges, and affords opportunities for joint discussion and decision making. In this respect it is an appropriate strategy for individuals who are in skilled nursing facilities and for their families (Kahana, 1994).

The growth of the aged population makes policy choices concerning planning especially timely. The "longevity revolution" is associated with more elderly also living and dying from chronic diseases (Roszak, 2001). Older individuals can expect to live with serious chronic illness during a period of several years prior to their ultimate death (Lynn & Adamson, 2003). Longer life spans and chronic illnesses for seniors increasingly occur in an environment where children and relatives live away from those in need of care. Thus, patterns of end-of-life care have also changed from being provided primarily by families in earlier times to being subsidized by Medicare/Medicaid and delivered by professional caregivers in long-term care facilities or in acute care hospitals (Wilner, 2000).

These demographic and social changes with respect to our senior population call for a public policy response that encourages planning. It must also be understood – as the research we presented earlier shows - that few individuals at present are comfortable with communicating ideas about planning, both within the family and between providers and patients. Without planning, especially for those with chronic illnesses such as cancer, stroke, diabetes and heart disease, medical events are likely to become crises, at which point too little time is available to properly consider all options relating to care (Pinquart et al., 2005).

The use of community resources, and policies that make these resources more accessible, are pivotal to enabling individuals to plan for likely medical events. Organizations like Area Agencies on Aging (AAAs) are a valuable resource for seniors and their families to find information about community programs (J. Kahana & Force, 2008). These include home care services, opportunities for socialization, and nutrition programs through senior centers or home delivered meals (Grande et al., 1998). Those who qualify can also obtain support from case workers who can help with management of care. It is crucial, however, for family members to engage with such organizations prior to a medical crisis, as this affords the best chance for appropriate planning.

Health care providers and social workers within hospital settings must be encouraged through policy initiatives to help those at the end of life with planning (Stein & Sherman, 2005). Reimbursement protocols that fund such planning would achieve cost savings, as planning would emphasize utilizing community and family resources. When such information is provided by individuals perceived as medical authorities, older individuals will be more likely to marshal support from family and community service organizations.

9. Research implications

Future research on advance care planning will benefit from linking planning in late life in general to domain-specific planning relevant to health care and end-of-life care (Sorensen & Pinquart, 2001). The elderly patient's perspectives on health care options in times of serious illness must also be better understood. This is related to knowledge of diagnosis, prognosis and medical procedures. Additionally, we must have a better understanding of alternative orientations and needs of older adults, their family advocates, and of health care providers. There are many situations where conflicts of interest exist between older patients' desire for comfort and independence, and caregivers' concerns about patient safety (McCollough et al., 2002). Quantitative and qualitative studies that help us compare congruence and discordance in these stakeholders' perspectives, can offer guidelines for improving patient care during the final years of life. At present there is only very limited information about older adults' values and preferences about obtaining responsive care close to the end of life. Having a broad understanding of these processes before specific crises arise, positions elderly patients to make meaningful plans for future and advance care.

The role of communication between older adults, family caregivers, and health care providers represents a fruitful area for future research (E. Kahana & B. Kahana, 2003). While prior work has documented the limited communication between older patients and physicians, particularly related to advance directives, the nature of barriers to communication is not well understood. Research is also needed on the relationship between patient initiatives and the influence of consumer behavior on care received (E. Kahana et al., 2010). Better understanding of care needs and opportunities for future care planning among low health literacy and disadvantaged elders will also illuminate health care needs of an increasingly diverse population of frail older adults (Institute of Medicine, 2004). There is also a need for qualitative research that moves beyond assessments of the preparation of legal documentation such as power of attorney for health care and withholding life-sustaining procedures at the very end of life. This research should focus on a broader array of concerns, wishes, values and preferences for how older patients wish to be cared for and live out their final period of life.

Future research can also benefit from exploring perspectives of diverse health care providers who may be involved in caring for patients in the final years of life. Direct care of elderly patients has benefited, as well as suffered, from introduction of technology in health monitoring, home health care delivery and care provision in acute and long term health care settings (Thomas, 2003). More research is needed on the impact of electronic health care records, health communication and self-care close to the end of life.

Although the benefits of mixed methods research are increasingly recognized in the complex arena of health services research, our understandings for integrating perspectives based on alternative value orientations is limited. Finally, consistent with the focus of our discussion on policy perspectives, surveys of public attitudes regarding sponsorship, financing and delivery of high quality and responsive end-of-life care would be useful.

10. Conclusion

This paper helps articulate a vision of advance care that is consistent with emerging trends in palliative medicine. It seeks to enlarge the scope of caring for patients, and particularly for the elderly who are living with life-limiting illness. We thus advocate for educational interventions to help older patients marshal responsive care during the extended period of service needs during the final years. We discuss the role of responsible and creative policy initiatives that can help patients avail themselves of the best services their communities can provide. Recognizing the theoretical underpinnings of advance directives on the one hand, and of marshaling responsive care on the other, enables us to integrate perspectives of autonomy and stress. Accordingly, effective advocacy can be assumed by patients and families to make the final period of life more comfortable and livable. Health care providers can forge real partnerships with patients who have planned for future care and who can articulate their values and preferences early in their illness trajectory.

11. References

Abbey, J., Froggatt, K.A., Parker, D., & Abbey, B. (2006). Palliative care in long-term care: A system in change. *International Journal of Older People Nursing,* Vol. 1, No. 1, pp. (56-63), ISSN 17483743.

Berzoff, J. & Silverman, P. (2004). *Living With Dying: A Handbook for End-Of-Life Healthcare Practitioners,* Columbia University Press, ISBN 978023112743, New York, NY.

Binstock, R.H., & Post, S.G. (1991). *Too Old for Health Care? Controversies in Medicine, Law, Economics, and Ethics,* Johns Hopkins University, ISBN 0801842481, Baltimore, MD.

Burck, R., & Lapidos, S. (2002). Ethics and cultures of care, In: *Ethical Patient Care: A Casebook for Geriatric Health Care Teams,* M.D. Mezey, C.K. Cassel, M.M. Bottrell, K. Hyer, J.L. Howe, & T.L. Fulmer (Eds.), pp. (41-66), Johns Hopkins University Press ISBN 0801867703, Baltimore, MD.

Cartwright, J., Miller, L., Volpin, M. (2009). Hospice in assisted living: Promoting good quality care at end of life. *The Gerontologist,* Vol. 49, No. 4, pp.(508-516), ISSN0169013.

Casarett, D. (2010). *Last Acts,* Simon & Schuster, ISBN 1416580379, New York, NY.

Chochinov, H.M., Kristjanson, L.J., Hack, T.F., Hassard, T., McClement, S., & Harlos, M. (2007). Burden to others and the terminally ill. *Journal of Pain and Symptom Management,* Vol. 34, No. 5, pp. (463-471), ISSN 10966218.

Conway, S. (Ed). (2011). *Governing Death and Loss: Empowerment, Involvement, and Participation,* Oxford University Press, ISBN 9780199586172, New York, NY.

De Boer, M.E., Hertogh, C.M.P.M., Droes, R.M., Jonker, C., & Eefsting, J.A. (2010). Advance directives in dementia: issues of validity and effectiveness. *International Psychogeriatrics,* Vol. 22, No., pp. (201-208), ISSN 10416102.

Detering, K.M., Hancock, A.D., & Reade, M.C. (2010). The impact of advance care planning on end of life care in elderly patients: randomized controlled trial. *British Medical Journal,* Vol. 340, pp. (1-9), ISSN 17592151.

Elder, J.P., Ayala, G.X., Parra-Medina, D., & Talavera, G.A. (2009). Health communication in the Latino community: Issues and approaches. *Annual Review of Public Health,* Vol. 30, pp. (227-251), ISSN 01637525.

Engelberg, R.A., Downey, L. Wenrich, M.D., Carline, J.D., Silvestri, G.A., Dotolo, D., … Curtis, J.R. (2010). Measuring the quality of end-of-life care. *Journal of Pain and Symptom Management,* Vol. 39, No. 6, pp. (951-971), ISSN 08853924.

Folkman, S. (2010). Stress, coping, and hope. *Psycho-Oncology,* Vol. 19, pp. (901-908), ISSN 10991611.

Force, L. Kahana,J. S. & Capalbo,V. (2010). The role of AAAs in promoting health for seniors: A preliminary research report. *Open Longevity Sci,* Vol. 4 pp. (30-35), ISSN 1886326X.

Fried, T. R., & Drickamer, M. (2010). Garnering support for advance care planning. *Journal of the American Medical Association, Vol.* 303, No. 3, pp. (269-270), ISSN 00987484.

Gelfand, D. (2006). *Aging Network: Programs & Services*. Springer, ISBN 0826102069, NY, NY.

George, L. K. (1999). Life-course perspectives on mental health. In: *Handbook of the Sociology of Mental Health,* C. S. Aneshensel & J.C. Phelan (Eds.), pp. (565-585), Kluwer Academic/Plenum Publishers, ISBN 100387325166, New York, NY.

George, R., & Harlow, T. (2011). Advance care planning: Politically correct but ethically sound? In: *Advance Care Planning in End of Life Care,* K. Thomas & B. Lobo (Eds), pp. (55-72), Oxford University Press, ISBN 10019956163X, New York, NY.

Grande, G.E., Addington-Hall, J.M., & Todd, C.J. (1998). Place of death and access to home care services: Are certain patient groups at a disadvantage. *Social Science and Medicine, Vol.* 47, No. 5, pp. (565-579), ISSN 02779536.

Hallenbeck, J. (2008). Access to end-of-life care venues. *American Journal of Hospice & Palliative Medicine, Vol.* 25, No. 3, pp. (245-249), ISSN 10499091.

Hansen, L., Goodell, T.T., Dehaven, J., & Smith, M. (2009). Nurses' perceptions of end-of-life care after multiple interventions for improvement. *American Journal of Critical Care,* Vol. 18, No. 3, pp. (263-271), ISSN 10623264.

Institute of Medicine. (2004). *Health Literacy.* IOM, ISBN 0309091179, Washington D.C.

Jackson, C. (2002). Classifying local retail property markets on the basis of rental growth rates. *Urban Studies, Vol.* 39, pp. (1417-1438), ISSN 00420980.

Kahana, J. (1994). Reevaluating the nursing home ombudsman role with a view toward expanding the concept of dispute resolution. *Journal of Dispute Resolution, Vol.* 2, pp. (217-232), ISSN 10522859.

Kahana, E., Cheruvu, V.K., Kahana, B., Kelley-Moore, J., Sterns, S., Brown, J.A., … Stange, K.C. (2010). Patient advocacy and cancer screening in late life. *Open Longevity Science,* Vol. 4, pp. (20-29), ISSN 1876326X.

Kahana, E. & Kahana, B. (2002). Contextualizing successful aging: new directions in age-old search. In: *Invitation to the Life Course: Toward New Understandings of Later Life,* J.R. Settersten (Ed.), pp. (225-255), Baywood Pub., ISBN 0895032694, Amityville, NY.

Kahana, E. & Kahana, B. (2003). Patient proactivity enhancing doctor-patient-family communication in cancer prevention and care among the aged. *Patient Education & Counseling,* Vol. 2075, pp. (1-7), ISSN 07383991.

Kahana, B., Dan, A., Kahana, E., & Kercher, K. (2004). The personal and social context of planning for end-of-life care. *Journal of the American Geriatrics Society,* Vol. 52, pp. (1163-1167), ISSN 15325415.

Kahana, J .S. & Force, L.T. (2008). Toward inclusion: A public centered approach to promote civic engagement by the elderly. *Public Policy & Aging Report, Vol.* 18, No. 3, (29-34), ISSN 10553037.

Kahana, E. (October 2010). What the aged can teach us about the final years of life. Presentation to Inaugural Meeting of the *NIH Special Interest Group on Palliative and End of Life Care.* Baltimore, MD.

Kahana, E., & Kahana, B. (2010). Stress and agentic aging: A targeted cancer adaptation model. In: *Handbook of Social Gerontology,* Dannefer, D. & Phillipson, C. (Eds.), pp. (280-293), Sage Publications, ISBN 101412934648, Thousand Oaks, CA.

Kahana, E., Kahana, B., & Wykle, M. (2010). "Care-Getting": A conceptual model of marshaling support near the end of life. *Current Aging Science,* Vol. 3, pp. (71-78), ISSN 18746098.

Kahana, E., Lovegreen, L. D., & Kahana, B. (2011). Long term care: tradition and innovation. In: *Handbook of Sociology of Aging,* R. Settersten & J. Angel (Eds.), pp. (583-602), Springer, ISBN 1441973737, New York, NY.

Kahana, E., Kahana, B., Lovegreen, L. Kahana, J., Brown, J., & Kulle, D. (in press). Health care consumerism and access to health care: educating elders to improve both preventive and end-of-life care In: *Health Care Consumerism and Access to Health Care,* J. Kronenfeld (Ed), Emerald Group Publishing, Bingley, UK.

Kastenbaum, R. (2004). *On Our Way: The Final Passage through Life and Death.* University of California Press, ISBN 0520218809, Los Angeles, CA.

Keating, N.L., Landrum, M.B., Guadagnoli, E., Winer, E.P., & Ayanian, J.Z. (2007). Care in the months before death and hospice enrollment among older women with advanced breast cancer. *J of General Internal Medicine,* Vol. 23, No. 1, pp. (11-18), ISSN 08848734.

Kelley-Moore, J.A., Schumacher, J.G., Kahana, E., & Kahana, B. (2006). When do older adults become disabled? *J Health Social Behavior,* Vol. 47, No. 2, pp.(126-141), ISSN 00221465.

Kumar, S. (2011). Neighborhood network in palliative care: A public health approach to the care of the dying. In: *Governing Death and Loss: Empowerment, Involvement, and Participation,* S. Conway (Ed.), pp. (109-118), Oxford, ISBN 0199586172, NY, NY.

Lorenz, K.A., Lynn, J., Dy, S.M., Shugarman, L.R., Wilkinson, A., Mularski, R.A., …Shekelle, P.G. (2008). Evidence for improving palliative care at the end of life: A systematic review. *Annals of Internal Medicine,* Vol. 148, No. 2, pp. (147-159), ISSN 00034819.

Lynch, H.F., Mathes, M., & Sawicki, N.N. (2008). Compliance with advance directives: Wrongful living and tort law incentives. *The Journal of Legal Medicine, Vol.* 29, pp. (133-178), ISSN 01947648.

Lynn, J., & Adamson, D.M. (2003). *Living Well at the End of Life: Adapting Health Care to Serious Chronic Illness in Old Age,* Rand, ISBN 0833034553, Santa Monica, CA.

McCollough, L., Wilson, N., Rhymes, J., & Teasdale, T. (2002). Conflicting interests: Dilemmas of decision making for patients, families, and teams. In: *Ethical Patient Care: A Casebook for Geriatric Health Care Teams,* Mezey, et al. (Eds), pp. (119-135), Johns Hopkins Press, ISBN 0801867703, Baltimore, MD.

Miller, S.C., & Han, B. (2008). End-of-life care in U.S. nursing homes: Nursing homes with special programs and trained staff for hospice or palliative/end-of-life care. *Journal of Palliative Medicine, Vol.* 11, No. 6, pp. (866-877), ISSN 10966218.

Moody, H. (1992). *Ethics in an Aging Society.* Johns Hopkins University Press, ISBN 0801853974, Baltimore, MD.

Nolan, M.T., & Mock, V. (2004). A conceptual framework for end-of-life care: A reconsideration of factors influencing the integrity of the human person. *Journal of Professional Nursing,* Vol. 20, No. 6, pp. (351-360), ISSN 87557223.

Pearlin, L.I. (1989). The sociological study of stress. *The Journal of Health and Social Behavior,* Vol. 30, pp. (241-256), ISSN 00221465 .

Penrod, J., Hupcey, J.E., Baney, B.L., & Loeb, S.J. (2011). End-of-life caregiving trajectories. *Clinical Nursing Research,* Vol. 20, No. 1, pp. (7-24), ISSN 10547738.

Perkins, H.S. (2007). Controlling death: The false promise of advance directives. *Annals of Internal Medicine,* Vol. 147, pp. (51-57), ISSN 00034819.

Pinquart, M., Sorensen, S., & Peak, T. (2005). Helping older adults and their families develop and implement care plans. *Journal of Gerontological Social Work,* Vol. 43, No. 4, pp. (3-23), ISSN 01634372.

Pollack, K.M., Morhaim, D., & Williams, M.A. (2010). The public's perspectives on advance directives: Implications for state legislative and regulatory policy. *Health Policy,* Vol. 96, No. 1, pp. (57-63), ISSN 01688510.

Robinson, E.M., Phipps, M., Purtilo, R.B., Tsoumas, A., & Hamel-Nardozzi, M. (2006). Complexities in decision making for persons with disabilities nearing end of life. *Topics Stroke Rehabilitation,* Vol. 13, No. 4, pp. (54-67), ISSN 10749357.

Rosenberg, J., & Yates, P. (2011). Transition from conventional to health-promoting palliative care: An Australian case study. In: *Governing Death and Loss: Empowerment, Involvement, and Participation,* S. Conway (Ed.), pp. (99-108), Oxford University Press ISBN 019958612, New York, NY.

Roszak, T. (2001). *Longevity Revolution: As Boomers Become Elders.* Berkeley Hills Books, ISBN 1893163504, Berkeley, CA.

Rowe, J., & Kahn, R. (1998). *Successful Aging.* Random House, ISBN 0440508630, NY, NY.

Selman, L., Harding, R., Beynon, T., Hodson, F., Coady, E., Hazeldine, C., … Higginson, I.J. (2007). Improving end-of-life care for patients with chronic heart failure. *Heart,* Vol. 93, No. 8, pp. (963-967), ISSN 13556037.

Small, N., Froggatt, K., & Downs, M. (2008). *Living and Dying with Dementia: Dialogues about Palliative Care.* Oxford University Press, ISBN 0198566878, New York, NY.

Stein, G.L., & Sherman, P.A. (2005). Promoting effective social work policy in end-of-life and palliative care. *J of Palliative Medicine,* Vol. 8, No. 6, pp. (1271-1281), ISSN 10966218.

Singer, P.A., Martin, D.K., Kelner, M. (1999). Quality end-of-life care: Patient's perspectives. *Journal of American Medical Association,* Vol. 281, pp. (163-168), ISSN 00987484.

Sörenson, S., & Pinquart, M. (2001). Developing a measure of older adults' preparation for future care needs. *International Journal of Aging and Human Development*, Vol. 53, pp. (137-165), ISSN 00914150.

Steinhauser, K., Christakis, N., Clipp, E., McNeilly, M., McIntyre, L., & Tulsky, J. (2000). Factors considered important at the end of life by patients, family, physicians, and other care providers. *Journal of the American Medical Association*, Vol. 284, No. 19, pp. (2476-2482), ISSN 00987484.

Tauber, A. (2005). *Patient Autonomy and the Ethics of Responsibility.* The MIT Press, ISBN 0262201607, Cambridge, MA.

Thomas, J. C. (2003). Commentary: Social aspects of gerontechnology. In *Impact of Technology on Successful Aging,* N. Charness & K. Schaie, (Eds), pp. (162-176). Springer, ISBN 0826124038, New York.

Thomas, C. (2007). *Sociologies of Disability and Illness.* Palgrave MacMillan, ISBN 1403936366, New York, NY.

Thomas, K., & Lobo, B. (Eds.). (2011). *Advance Care Planning in End of Life Care.* Oxford, ISBN 019956163X, New York, NY.

Twycross R, & Lichter, I. (1996). *The Terminal Phase. Oxford Textbook of Palliative Medicine,* Oxford University Press, ISBN 0192626280, New York, NY.

Van der Steen, J.T., & Deliens, L. (2009). End-of-life care for patients with Alzheimer's disease. In *Self-Management of Chronic Disease,* S. Bährer-Kohler & E. Krebs-Roubicek (Eds.), pp. (114-120). Springer Publishing Company, ISBN 3642003257, NY, NY.

Verbrugge, L.M., & Jette, A.M. (1994). The disablement process. *Social Science & Medicine*, Vol. 38, No. 1, pp. (1-14), ISSN 02779536.

Watson, J. (1996).Watson's theory of transpersonal caring. In: *Blueprint for Use of Nursing Models: Education, Research, Practice, and Administration,* P. Walker & B. M. Neuman (Eds.), pp. (141-184), National League for Nursing, ISBN 0887376568, NY, NY.

Wetle, T., Shield, R., Teno, J., Miller, S.C. & Welch, L. (2005). Family perspectives on end-of-life care experiences in nursing homes. *Gerontologist, Vol.* 45, No. 5, pp. (642-650), ISSN 00169013.

Wilner, M.A. (2000). Toward a stable and experienced caregiving workforce. *Generations, Vol.* 24, No. 3, pp. (60-65), ISSN 07387806.

Wykle, D.M., Whitehouse, P.J., & Morris, D.L. (2005). *Successful Aging through the Life Span.* Springer, ISBN 0826125646, New York, NY.

Yates, J., & Glick, H.R. (1997). The failed patient self-determination act and policy alternatives for the right to die. *Journal of Aging & Social Policy*, Vol. 9, No. 4, ISSN 08959420.

13

End of Life Care: Attitudes Toward Autonomy and Legal Instruments

Arthur Oscar Schelp
Department of Psychology, Neurology and Psychiatry,
Botucatu Medical School,
São Paulo State University – UNESP,
Brazil

1. Introduction

The World Health Organization describes healthy life expectancy (World Health Organization, 2011) as a statistic related to life expectancy, which estimates the equivalent years in full health that a person can expect to live based on the current mortality rates in a population. This statement opens up discussion concerning the boundaries between full health and compromise of the same, including the competence of the individual to make their own decisions. Determining the ethical standards for services provided to older individuals with serious illnesses that impair their own understanding of their state, requires an understanding of aspects such as autonomy and the capacity to preserve the best interests of patients and their relatives or guardians.

Respect of a patient's autonomy for decision making, with the preservation of choice, is essential to guarantee an ethical stance in relation to the individual and society. The imposition of "negative" options, which include restriction of movement, the right to drive a vehicle, and other daily activities, and at advanced stages of a disease, injunctions, lead to curtailment and loss. Enhancing the narrow line between restriction of autonomy and legal incapacity is imperative, but the matter is multidimensional, affecting specific patient groups with different civil capacities that have to be taken into consideration. The question is not just medical; it includes many social, cultural, religious, and economic aspects. The medical aspect includes the identification of disturbed competences and the expected duration and grade of incapacity, all confronted with the patient's disease prognosis. Another discussion point is the kind of test or examination that will assure the proper diagnosis of capacity and what is the correct time and form to submit and inform the patient, their relatives and designated curators about the necessity and the risks of non-liability attitudes. The clinical and neuropsychological examination must achieve both the expectations of the elderly patient and their relatives as well as the legal requirements of the eventual injunction. Personnel, who in any form were responsible for the health care of older patients and with impairment decision-making, must be aware that not revealing the prognosis and possible consequences of the loss of ability to make proper and independent choices could make them legally responsible for this attitude. Participation by people involved in supporting patients who are incapacitated or on the way to being incapacitated, have an important role to play in designating guardians, curators, and others. The decision to accept proposed treatments in the terminal stages of a disease is another subject for discussion. Some of the advanced directives manifested by older individuals could be out-of-date when confronted with new and emerging medical technologies. The society must ensure safeguard measures to avoid the over or sub-interpretation of elderly wishes.

2. Competency impairment and incapacity in older people

Elderly patient autonomy can be understood as their capacity to make decisions. Even though the term competency has been used with the same significance as capacity (Dekkers, 2001), some authors prefer to use the term capacity as a broad designation for global ability impairment (Appelbaum, 2007) which could be applied to legal matters the same as to medical questions. It seems to be appropriate and useful to use the expression mental capacity when referring to the ability of someone to make decisions (Mental Capacity Act, 2005). The capacity or incapacity of an individual is an event that comes in parallel with civilization and includes moral, legal, and medical aspects. In the Middle Ages those with incapacities were not submitted to the death penalty, and until now the debate continues on questions like the autonomy of those sentenced (Harrington, 2004). Many authors discuss the capacity to consent to proposed treatments (Roth et al., 1997, Wendler & Rid, 2011, Karlawish et al., 2005) and nowadays the increasing number of older patients with dementia and other disabilities raise many worries about the autonomy of the ill elderly to decide about their life and others actions related to belongings, etc. (Moye & Marson, 2007, Defanti et al., 2007, Hughes et al., 2002).

References to end-of-life events are made in the context of the last part of an individual's life span. But when capacity is to be evaluated it could be associated to diseases where the incapacity to make decisions occurs over a short period of time with worsening symptoms affecting not only mental capacity but also motor autonomy with dependence on ventilators for breathing. This situation is associated with the terminal stages of cancer in many organs, and in these cases determination of incapacity is not considered by doctors, proxies, or others. The designation of "intermittent incompetency" proposed by Linda Ganzini (Ganzini et al., 1993), exemplifies the limitations of proposing capacity standards to patients who are burdensome, depressed, and unmotivated. It's clear that not just pathology itself is of consequence, but also the temporality characteristic of the disease, when considering the establishment of elderly incapacity, in the terminal phase of diseases which compromise cognition. The authenticity of decisions, or in other words, the evidence that the choices expressed by the affected person are consistent with his or her values, past history, and decision-making style (Collopy, 1988) must be also taken in account. Considering that the patient's answers are authentic does not mean that the decision-making is completely autonomous (Ganzini & Lee, 1993).

Individuals with diseases that evolve with dementia represent a particular group, as they will invariably present, during the evolution of the disease, varying levels of incapacity, even considering that there could be periods with some symptom remission or stability. The attempt to stratify patients according to incapacity level conflicts with the distinct evolution of different dementia profiles, which often preserve some competencies, without therefore compromising others, enabling the individual to develop some social functions while unable to perform others. In differentiating between Alzheimer´s disease/mixed dementia and multi-infarct dementia, the preservation of personality was strongly associated with the latter. Currently, emotional incontinence is associated with multi-infarct dementia, but not mixed dementia (Moroney et al., 1997). The so called sub cortical dementias, like dementia in Parkinson´s disease, display visual hallucinations and the impairment of memory and executive functions (Marinus et al., 2003, Galvin et al., 2006), and are associated with patient age and not related to disease duration (Mayeux et al., 1992). The differential cognitive features that distinguish fronto-temporal dementia from Alzheimer´s disease include a relative preservation of drawings and calculation performance (Mendez et al., 1996), abilities that could interfere in the interpretation of some structured cognitive tests for determining capacity.

The different attitudes of professionals from different medical specialties towards autonomy (Pioltini et al., 2010), and the family and physician´s views of surrogate decision making open a broad discussion about the role of different individuals in decision capacity assessment. The medical professional is more likely to listen to the patient and exchange ideas with colleagues, whereas the family tends toward consensus, assuming a shared position, which may or may not include the patient's wishes (Silberfeld et al., 1996). A systematic review conducted by Wendler (Wendler & Rid ,2011), found differences in the feelings and attitudes of surrogates on making decisions for other. Apparently, geriatricians and general practitioners have a better knowledge of issues related to maintaining autonomy. This is possibly due to the fact that these professionals have a broader view of the interaction disease/society. In another study, 28% of general physicians changed their competency diagnosis after a second opinion given by a psychiatrist (Markson et al., 1994), thus enforcing the need for educational programs about the limits and goals of decision-making assessment in clinical practice (Ganzini et al., 2003). Even so, doctors are often not prepared to solve problems that involve caregivers. In a study they admitted having little knowledge about support services offered elsewhere and did not see themselves as the answer to most caregiver´s problems (Yaffe et al., 2008).

The issue of inter-professional interaction seems to have assumed an increasingly important role regarding the approach towards the independence and capacity of elderly patients in deciding their own interests. In the last decade, numerous publications have emerged that are critical of certain postures and attitudes in bioethics, based on technological values, excessively focused on the physician and that are too reductive (McGrath, 1998). It is evident that all decisions to be taken must respect the free will of the patient (autonomy), with determination of their competence and ensuring confidentiality in dealings with them, their families, and legal representatives. These skills are best assessed if the objectives are based on the assertion that the patients, caregivers and close relatives of the patients should be heard. The ethical commitment that should be observed in the care of patients with possible limitations in understanding their own disease and its likely consequences should be shared with family members, caregivers, and trustees (attorney-in-fact).

It is also interesting to discuss the self-awareness, perceived knowledge, and perceived skills demonstrated by the general population, professionals from different disciplines, and the patient himself, in evaluating impaired capacity in older people. Different studies demonstrate that despite no significant differences have been shown between different categories; there is a need for continued educational programs to provide the patient, family and potential caregivers with a better understanding of the course of various diseases. (Schelp et al., 2008, Grey C & Barton S, 2011, Prince et al., 2007). The acquired knowledge will undergird the actions in end situations that interfere with the ability to express the free will, thereby avoiding false expectations and decreasing psychological distress. The awareness that some diseases could evolve to decisional incapability, enforce the preventive measures that should be taken by the individual and their representatives.

3. Legal implications of incapacity

In connection with the ideas of dignity, integrity, and respect for vulnerability of the individuals, the principle of autonomy contributes to the expression of the political morality of the medical and legal systems in modern society (Rendtorff, 2010).

Evidence exists that most individuals with dementia would like to receive information concerning their diagnosis (Karlawish et al. 2005, Marzanski, 2000). On the other hand, the question of when, to whom, and how to communicate information regarding a suspected diagnosis, with all its implications, including loss of the patient's memory of experiences, must take to account several aspects. However, the decision to inform the patient should consider the power of discernment that individual has of their illness. It has been demonstrated that even patients with moderate impairment are not competent to make decisions related to their illness (Karlawish et al., 2005). The decision to remain silent regarding disease prognosis and its implications, including the risk of suicide (Rohde et al., 1995, Maguirre et al., 1996), is justifiable under certain circumstances and should always consider the socio-cultural and religious context in which the patient is inserted. Any medical conduct which could result in physical damage or any kind of personal loss to a citizen should be referred to a judicial sphere and should be a matter for the punishment of those implicated.

The incapacity may be present for delimited social situations and, in many cases, restricted to the family sphere. The requirement of guardianship is a judicial matter and must be decided by a judge after the statement of functional incapacity. Moye (Moye & Marson, 2007), highlighted two capacity domains which require either cognitive or procedural skills; they are independent living and general financial management. Independent living is a general designation that could be applied in distinct situations. In many cases the elderly still have some dependence on their children and other relatives. They are already retired and take few responsibilities for common social obligations. The situation becomes critical when capacity impairment arrives at the point when the family and surrogates decide to institutionalize the elderly. However specific conditions could be imposed such as prohibiting the person to drive a car (Wild & Cotrell, 2003), walk alone, swim alone, or cook. All the activities in some way represent the independence to assume and execute individual and collective actions. The thin line between what should be called an independent life and the restriction to perform some actions is related to age, social role, personal values, and family structure. The broad spectrum of incapacitating diseases also plays a role in this evaluation. Recognizing signs of possible impaired financial capacity is another key question to assure independence in daily living activities (Widera et al., 2011). But the apparent loss of the ability to manage economic affairs could be masked by the personal limitations of older people to acquire the competency to deal with Internet banking services. Moreover, the normal aging process is almost invariably accompanied by auditory and visual impairment. The assumption that the older a person gets, the less education he or she manages to acquire (Bellak, 1976), is fully applicable to the fast changes and developments in Internet transactions. It will be difficult to guarantee that the individual has impaired judgment to take decisions about their finances, faced with the loss of a particular skill attribute. A decline in some executive functions is a common behavior in many normal aging people.

Even before the institution of the Mental Capacity Act in England in 2005, there was a concern that mental health and incapacity legislation separation could act as a source of discrimination and a limitation in the application of consistent ethical principles across medical law (Dawson & Szmukler, 2006). The fact that the majority of decisions related to establishing incapacity in the aged occurs outside the judicial sphere (Kapp, 2002), does not imply that the will of the patient will always be accepted, as in certain circumstances the opinion of the family as " natural guardians", or the physician's silent decision could be the appropriate decision (Strong, 1993, Whitney & McCullough, 2007). As in other contexts, when the decision is based on the values, convictions, and attitudes of the patient, expressed before a diagnosis of incapacity, it must be distinguished from the behaviors in relation to impediments, institution of treatment, and other issues related to that person. Into this scene we have the appearance of community representatives and social workers, further increasing the already complex network of people involved in assessing the capacity of individuals.

After establishing the incapacity state of the elderly individual, with an apparently irreversible prognosis, there are still considerations on the Kantian concept that we should never use people as mere means to other people´s ends. Mark Yarborough (Yarborough, 2002), uses this interpretation to discuss using elderly people with dementia in clinical research. The health professional has a fundamental role in suspecting incapacity, nevertheless he also performs a critical and decisive role in finding out the values and beliefs manifested when the individual still had a clear decision-making capacity.

The identification and appointment of a person of reference to receive orientation and patient information is fundamental to preserving the ethics of care for incapacitated elderly individuals. In the absence of a natural partner or legally recognized trustee (administratore di sostegno, tutore - Italian; legal administrator, trustee, guardian and other denominations - English), it is up to the professional to identify responsible relatives and potential caregivers, whether they are individuals close to the patient or hired for such work. In a study performed with elderly people, with a mean age of 78 years, there was a low prediction rate between patients, their surrogates, and the physician (Seckler et al., 1991). The process of indicating guardianship to an elderly patient has a better chance of success when the unit social worker makes the recommendation, rather than the physician or a nurse (Burrus et al., 2000). The family's ignorance about substitute indictment (appointment) process; diseases cognition compromise; and absence of a memorandum of the patient wishes, also play a role in this context. We would also like to highlight the finding that most families do not know that physicians tend to use hospital records when coming to their surrogate indictment, allied with direct observation of the patient (Silberfeld et al., 1996). The discrepancies seen in attitudes toward the start and development of the surrogate appointment process again shows the need to listen to all the people involved in the care of disabled elderly. The role of health personnel as an information staff is crucial in guaranteeing respect for the patient and preserving the principles manifested by him when healthy and able. In an inquiry presented to medical professionals from different specialties, only the geriatricians spontaneously called attention to the medical and legal aspects of patient injunction, highlighting the need for better disclosure of these aspects (Pioltini et al., 2010). Otherwise it will be no expectations that all older people are competent to take advanced procedure actions or directives to indicate a responsible person to assume decisions in their late moments of life. At this point, it must be assured that the elderly maintains full capacity to express the proper choices. The lack of teaching about what is the role different members of health services have in evaluating incapacity, as well as in how to work with surrogate decision-makers when taking decisions about handling incapacitated patients, is a highly relevant aspect (White et al., 2010).

4. The choice of tests to analyze capacity

The broad spectrum of clinical pictures, evolution duration, associated with relatively maintenance of some abilities, and the precluded notion that there are distinct ways to define what independent life is, together with unspecific means and perceptions of autonomy, opens up discussion as to what should be the appropriate way of evaluating capacity and capacity impairment, including the decision-making autonomy register. In this sense a need arose to establish a structured battery of tests to be applied in several situations where determining capacity is imperative to an individual's welfare.

Integrating the legal perspective of incapacity with clinical knowledge of the issue is essential to safeguard a just intervention process, which does not bring suffering, uncertainty, and moral and financial costs to the patient and his relatives. The use of Mini Mental Score Examination (MMSE); (Folstein & Folstein, 1975) in evaluating dementia pictures is very widespread. Even so, the great variability in cutoff scores for determining incapacity must be considered. Also, even considering that scores below 16 represent a high probability of an association with incapacity (Etchells et al., 1999); these values are much lower in illiterate patients who also belong to other social groups (Bertolucci et al., 1994) which limits the specificity and sensitivity of the test, whose aim is to determine incapacity to make decisions.

Until the beginning of the 90's, tests in the USA to evaluate the competence to make decisions were based on five categories 1) Evidencing a choice, 2) Reasonable outcome of choice, 3) Choice based on "rational" reasons, 4) Ability to understand, and 5) Actual understanding (Roth et al., 1977). In 1992, Bonnie (Bonnie, 1992) proposed a theoretical reform of competence parameters for criminal defendants, which was later restructured for clinical application by Grisso (Grisso & Appelbaum, 1995), as the MacArthur Assessment Test. This test analyzes four functional domains: 1) Capacity to communicate a choice; 2) Understand the Relevant Information; 3) Appreciate the situation and its consequences, and 4) Reasons about offered options. Since then, the MacSAC-CD (MacArthur Structured Assessment of the Competencies of Criminal Defendants) has been used to evaluate the capacity of public defendants in criminal trials, and has been well accepted. The MacSAC-

CD was designed to evaluate two major dimensions, namely adjudication and decisional competence (Cruise & Rogers, 1998). The authors draw our attention to the limitations of this test when analyzing aspects of malingering attitudes. Even so, Hoge (Hoge et al., 1997), argued that the test had solid foundations both from a legal aspect, and in psycho-legal assessment theory. Agreement rates between mental health professionals and court determinations have been found to exceed 90% (Freckelton, 1996), which refers to the "fitness" to stand trial. It is still rational to imagine that capacity tests, which can trigger a process of civil injunction, should be interchangeable and indiscriminately applied, both for legal ends, and for guiding daily activities. It is mandatory to avoid both malingering attitudes and pseudo incapacity diagnosis. A philosophical criticism of MacCAT-T (McArthur Competence Assessment Tool-Treatment), which is basically the same test that has been applied to evaluate competency to act in judging the capacity of others, is that the test does not analyze non-cognitive aspects of behavior, or rather emotional, socio-cultural, and other influences (Breden & Vollman, 2004). Accordingly, multiple tests must be considered which include evaluating emotional factors, including references to cultural, social, and religious values.

5. Attitudes towards inclusion of older people in research protocols

Increased research on diseases that affect the elderly and their treatment have added to the ethical aspects, both for their participation in protocols and in decisions regarding the indication and use of high-cost medications. An inquiry in Sweden demonstrated that women and laypersons were generally keener to preserve a patient's integrity and medical professionals were more willing than laypersons to permit individuals with dementia to participate in placebo-controlled trials (Peterson &Wallin 2003). Confidentiality in research is critically important, but it is not an absolute legal principle in either research or clinical settings (Stiles & Petrila, 2011). The informed refusal to participate in a research project is also a matter for surrogates of elderly patients with incapacitating diseases (Meisel & Kuczewski, 1996).

6. Autonomy of older patients in advanced stages of incapacitating diseases

One critical aspect to be considered is the location for end-of-life care for elderly incapacitated patients. One study showed that from a family perspective, elderly patients who received home care with hospital services were more likely to report a favorable dying experience (Teno et al., 2004). In this survey, among those suffering dementia, the largest group remained at home with nursing care. Only a small group died at home with hospital care, similar to those who died in hospital. In a questionnaire applied in Japan (Ikezaki & Ikegami, 2011), there were a relatively high number of dementia and severe cognitively impaired patients with "unknown" place of dying, with or without nursing support. The authors attribute the findings to the fact that life support treatment preferences of family members in Japan were ignored by most of the general public the same as for the bereaved of patients who died in hospital (Ikegami & Ikezaki, 2010). The results of those epidemiological evaluations exemplifies the fact that in some cultures, including Japan, some diseases, particularly when severe cognitive impairment is present, receives distinct attention in their late moments of life. There seems to be consensus that shared decisions have advantages when they refer to end-of-life care for terminally ill patients (Sittisombut et al., 2009; Lee JCY et al., 2003). The need to encourage this to happen not only regarding the place of death, but also the form of care, requires debate and should be looked at by health authorities.

There are no valid protocols or agreed norms for suspending medication or interrupting other support measures, (Parson et al., 2010, and Derse, 1999), confirming the difficulty in establishing standards. Medical professionals have not demonstrated a clear consensus on palliative measure to be used, including posture in relation to family and trustees (Schneiderman et al., 1993; Hinkka H et al., 2002; Richter J et al., 2001, and Eisemann M et al., 1999).

Another aspect, which can be embarrassing, is the notion that the cost factor (burden) influences the society's attitudes toward patient autonomy in end-of-life decision-making (Kwon et al., 2009). The authors highlight this "anxiety" and suggest an open and balanced discussion on burden with the family, with possible adequate welfare support. The actual patients themselves give the impression, when they are competent, that the family's values in relation to costs must be taken into account when dealing with end-of-life decisions (Doukas & Gorenflo 1993). The discussion about the burden with surrogates and the family must take into account the wishes and beliefs manifested by the patient when they were in full charge of their decision making capacity.

The start of palliative care with the suspension of ineffective and unnecessary care for elderly and incapacitated patients in the terminal and irreversible stage of the life is also recognized as orthothasia in Brazil and some other countries (Pinto, 1991; Asorta-Bilajac& Segota, 2010; Gutiérrez-Samperio, 2001). To guarantee comfort, respect, and autonomy in line with the wishes of patients in the end stage of life is the ethical obligation of health professionals. However the circumstances in which such measures will be applied, as well as the factors which determine the place, manner, and the diligence applied to the process, are complex and must be the combined opinions of the actual patient and their family and legal representatives.

The upward trend in life expectancy increases the chances that more elderly patients will attend intensive care units and receive breathing support and feeding assistance. To handle this situation, many professionals have assumed the assurance behavior, imposing additional unnecessary services. In most cases, a defensive stance is practiced based on the belief that the procedures are medically acceptable by professional expert panels, but the attitudes assumed by physicians are in many circumstances aimed at avoiding malpractice claims (U.S. Office Technology Assessment, 1994).

The decision to not resuscitate a terminally ill patient is generally limited to the health staff, that is, the nurse and the physician, with compliance from surrogates to medical recommendations (Eliasson et al., 1997). The option to start or withhold tube feeding or gastrostomy is controversial and includes the physician's perception of patient and family wishes and liability concerns (Bell et al., 2008). For some authors the evidence that dysphagia is always a terminal symptom in dementia rules out the recommendation to use gastrostomy (Regnad et al., 2010). It must be remembered, to consider the offering of taste pleasure or feeding sensation to older people with tube feeding or gastrostomy. The use of positive airway pressure machines (CPAP), to guarantee ventilatory support for incapacitate patients at the end phase of life instead of more sophisticated apparatus with volumetric control, is preferable.

Finally it is important to stress that determining incapacity with autonomy restriction for the patient is a step-by-step process, with moment-to-moment characteristics and should be implemented in accordance with the circumstances in which the diagnosis of incapacity is requested. It would be naïve to imagine that uniform protocols or norms could be established for application in all situations. Analysis must me multidisciplinary with flexible individualized instruments. Establishment of a legal injunction must take into consideration the clinical diagnosis of incapacity as well as the advance directives expressed by the patient, a matter that is receiving little attention from responsible authorities in many countries. Nevertheless, people can find support of non-governmental organizations, receiving information, guidance, and preparation to stressful moments in final stages of life (Burrel, 2008). In many situations, there are more concern with informed consent for treatment and procedures to be adopted than to the advance directives expressed by the patient in any form at prior to manifestations of incapacity.

Birth and death are two critical transitions in a life time. When a child is born, it receives a legal identification that ensures rights which must be guaranteed by parents, its family, and the rest of the society to which he or she belongs. On the other side, with the approach of death of older people, it should be assured that the moral and legal obligation to the values and beliefs of the elderly will be respected and applied. The decision to request relatives to take actions which guarantee the patient complete respect of his or her expressed wishes up to or before the onset of the state of incapacity is never related to the diagnosis or proposed therapeutic measures, but to an attitude towards maintaining the autonomy of old people in their final stage of life. The patient's wishes must be an obligation for descendants and guardians, not just a moral one but a legal one which must be taken in account by health personnel when dealing with older patients in their final moments of life.

7. References

Appelbaum, P.S. (2007). Assessment of Patient's Competence to Consent to Treatment. *New England Journal of Medicine,* Vol.357, No.18, (November 2007), pp. 1834-1840, ISSN 0028-4793

Asorta-Bilajac, I. & Segota, I. (2010). Is there a Death with Dignity in Today´s Medicine? *International Journal of Bioethics,* Vol.21, No.4, (December 2010), pp. 149-156, ISSN 1145-0762

Bell, C., Somogyi-Zalud, E., Masaki, K., Fortaleza-Dawson, T. & Blanchette, P.L. (2008). Factors Associated with Physician Decision-Making in Starting Tube Feeding. *Journal of Palliative Medicine,* Vol.11, No. 6, (July 2008), pp.915-924, ISSN 1096-6218

Bellak, L. (1976). Psychological Aspects of Normal Aging, In: *Geriatric Psychiatry,* L. Bellack & B.K. Toksoz, (Eds.), 21, Grune & Stratton, ISBN 0808909673, New York.

Bertolucci, P.H.F., Brucki, S.M.D., Campacci, S.R. & Juliano, Y. (1994). The Mini Mental Examination: Impact of Escolarity. *Arquivos de Neuropsiquiatria,* Vol.52, No.1, (March 1994), pp. 1-7, ISSN 0004-282X

Bonnie, R.J. (1992). The Competence of Criminal Defendants: a Theoretical Reformulation. *Behavioral Sciences and the Law,* Vol.10, No.3, (Summer 1992), pp. 291-316, ISSN 1099-0798

Breden, T.M. & Vollman, J. (2004). The Cognitive Based Approach of Capacity Assessment in Psychiatry: a Philosophical Critique of the MacCAT-T. *Health Care Analysis*, Vol.12, No.4, (December 2004), pp. 273-283, ISSN 1065-3058

Burrel, G.M. (2008). Websites and addresses page of organizations, In: *Freedom to Choose: How to make End-of-Life Decision on your Own Terms*, D.A. Lund (Ed.), 125, Baymond Publishing Company Inc., ISBN 978.0.89503-340-6, Amityville, New York

Burrus, J.W., Kunik, M.E., Molinari, V., Orengo, C.A. & Rezabek, P. (2000). Guardianship Applications for Elderly Patients: Why Do They Fail? *Psychiatrics Services*, Vol.51, No.4, (April 2000), pp. 522-524, ISSN 1075-2730

Collopy, B.J. (1988). Autonomy in Long Term Care: Some Crucial Distinctions. *The Gerontologist*, Vol.28, Suppl., (June 1997), pp. 10-17, ISSN 0016-9013

Cruise, K.R. & Rogers, R. (1998). An Analysis of Competency to Stand Trial: an Integration of Case Law and Clinical Knowledge. *Behavioral Sciences and the Law*, Vol.16, No.1, (Winter 1998), pp. 35-50, ISSN 1099-0798

Dawson, J. & Szmukler, G. (2006). Fusion of Mental Health and Incapacity Legislation. *The British Journal of Psychiatry*, Vol.188, (June 2006), pp. 504-509, ISSN 0007-1250

Defanti, C.A., Tiezzi, A., Gasparini, M., Gasperini, M., Congedo, M., Tiraboschi, P., Tarquini, D., Pucci, E., Porteri, C., Bonito, V., Sacco, L., Stefanini, S., Borghi, L., Colombi, L., Marcello, N., Zanetti, O., Causarano, R., Primavera, A. & Bioethics and Palliative Care in Neurology Study Group of the Italian Society of Neurology. (2007). Ethical Questions in the Treatment of Subjects with Dementia. Part I. Respecting Autonomy: Awareness, Competence, and Behavioral Disorders. *Neurological Sciences*, Vol.28, No.4, (August 2007), pp. 216-231, ISSN 1590-1874

Dekkers, W.J.M. (2001). Autonomy and Dependence: Chronic Physical Illness and Decision-Making Capacity. *Medicine, Health Care, and Philosophy*, Vol.4, No.2, (2001), pp. 185-192, ISSN 1386-7423

Derse, A.R. (1999). Making-Decision About Life-Sustaining Medical Treatment in Patients with Dementia. The Problem of Patient Decision-Making Capacity. *Theoretical Medicine and Bioethics*, Vol.20, No.1, (January 1999), pp. 55-67, ISSN 1386-7415

Doukas, D.J. & Gorenflo, W. (1993). Analyzing the Values History: An Evaluation of Patient Medical Values and Advance Directives. *The Journal of Clinical Ethics*, Vol.4, No.1, (Spring 1993), pp. 41-45, ISSN 1046-7890

Eisemann, M., Richter, J., Bauer, B., Bonelli, R.M. & Porzsolt, F. (1999). Phicisian´s Decision-Making in Incompetent Elderly Patients: a Comparative Study between Austria, Germany (East,West), and Sweden. *International Psychogeriatrics*, Vol.11, No.3, (September 1999), pp. 313-324, ISSN 1041-6102

Elliasson, A.H., Howard, R.S., Torrington, K.G., Dillard, T.A. & Phillips, Y.Y. (1997). Do-not-Resuscitate Decisions in the Medical ICU: Comparing Physician and Nurse Opinions. *Chest*, Vol.111, No.4, (April 1997), pp. 1106-1111, ISSN 0012-3692

Etchells, E., Darzins, P., Siberfeld, M., Singer, M., McKenny, J., Naglie, G., Katz, M., Guyatt, G.H., Molloy, D.W. & Strang, D. (1999). Assesment of Patient Capacity to Consent to Treatment. *Journal of General Internal Medicine*, Vol.14, No.1, (January 1999), pp. 27-34, ISSN 0884-8734

Folstein, M.F. & Folstein, S.E. (1975). Mini-Mental State a Practical Method for Grading the Cognitive State of Patients for the Clinican. *Journal of Psychiatric Research*, Vol.12, No.3, (November 1975), pp. 189-198, ISSN 0022-3956

Freckelton, I. (1996). Racionality and Flexibility in Assesment of Fitness to Stand Trial. *International Journal of Law Psychiatry*, Vol.19, No.1, (Winter 1996), pp. 39-59, ISSN 0160-2527

Galvin, J.E., Pollack, J. & Morris, J.C. (2006). Clinical Phenotype of Parkinson Disease Dementia. *Neurology*, Vol.67, No.7, (November 2006), pp.1605-1611, ISSN 0028-3878

Ganzini, L. & Lee, M.A. (1993). Authenticity, Autonomy, and Mental Disorders. *The Journal of Clinical Ethics*, Vol.4, No.1, (Spring 1993), pp. 55-58, ISSN 1046-7890

Ganzini, L., Lee, M.A., Heintz, T. & Bloom, J.D. (1993). Is the Patient Self-Determination Act Appropriate for Elderly Persons Hospitalized for Depression? *The Journal of Clinical Ethics*, Vol.4, No.1, (Spring 1993), pp. 46-50, ISSN 1046-7890

Ganzini, L., Volicer, L., Nelson, W. & Derse A. (2003). Pitfalls in Assessment of Decision-Making Capacity. *Psychosomatics*, Vol.44, No.3, (May-June 2003), pp.237-243, ISSN 0033-3182

Grey, C. & Barton, S. (2011). Severe Self-Neglect: When is Decision-Making Capacity Lost? *Journal of the American Geriatrics Society*, Vol.59, Suppl.1, (April 2011), pp. S170, ISSN 0002-8614

Grisso, T. & Appelbaum, P.S. (1995). The MacArthur Treatment Competence Study: III. Abilities of Patients to Consent to Psychiatric and Medical Treatments. *Law and Human Behavior*, Vol.19, No.2, (April 1995), pp. 127-148, ISSN 0147-7307

Gutierrez-Samperio, C. (2001). Bioethics in the Face of Death. *Gaceta Medica de México*, Vol.137, No.3, (May-June 2001), pp. 269-276, ISSN 0016-3813.

Harrington, C.L. (2004). Mental Competence and End-of Life Decision Making: Death Row Volunteering and Euthanasia. *Journal of Health Politics, Policy and Law*, Vol.29, No.6, (December 2004), pp.1109-1151, ISSN 0361-6878

Hinkka, H., Kosunen, E., Lammi, E.K., Metsanoja, R., Puustelli, A. & Kellokumpu-Lehtinen, P. (2002). Decision Making in Terminal Care: a Survey of Finnish Doctor´s Treatment Decisions in End-of-Life Scenarios Involving a Terminal Cancer and a Terminal Dementia Patient. *Palliative Medicine*, Vol.16, No.3, (May 2002), pp.195-203, ISSN 0269-2163

Hoge, S.K., Bonnie, R.J., Poythress, N., Monahan, J., Eisenberg, M. & Feucht-Haviar, T. (1997). The MacArthur Adjudicative Competence Study: Development and Validation of a Research Instrument. *Law and Human Behavior*, Vol.21, No.2, (April 1997), pp. 141-179, ISSN 0147-7307

Hughes, J.C., Hope, T., Savulescu, J. & Ziebland, S. (2002). Carers Ethics and Dementia: a Survey and Review of the Literature. *International Journal of Geriatric Psychiatry*, Vol.17, No.1, (January 2002), pp. 35-40, ISSN 0885-6230

Ikegami, N. & Ikezaki, S. (2010). Life Sustaining Treatment at End-of-Life in Japan: Do the Perspectives of the General Public reflect those of the Bereaved of Patients who Have Died in Hospitals? *Health Policy*, Vol.98, No.2-3, (December 2010), pp. 98-106, ISSN 0168-8510

Ikezaki, S. & Ikegami, N. (2011). Predictor´s of Dying at Home for Patients Receiving Nursing Services in Japan: a Retrospective Study Comparing Cancer and Non-Cancer Deaths. *BioMed Central Palliative Care*, Vol.10, (March 2011), pp. 3, ISSN 1472-684X

Kapp, M.B. (2002). Decisional Capacity in Theory and Practice: Legal Process Versus "Bumbling Through". *Aging and Mental Health*, Vol.6, No.4, (November 2002), pp. 413-417, ISSN 1360-7863

Karlawish, J.H.T., Casarett, D.J., James, B.D., Xie, S.X. & Kim, S.Y.H. (2005). The Ability of Persons with Alzheimer Disease (AD) to Make Decision about Taking an AD Treatment. *Neurology*, Vol.64, No.9, (May 2005), pp. 1514-1519, ISSN 0028-3878

Kwon, Y.C, Shin, D.W., Lee, J.H., Heo, D.S., Hong, Y.S., Kim, S.Y. & Yun, Y.H. (2009). Impact of Perception of Socio-Economic Burden on Advocacy for Patient Autonomy in End-of-Life Decision-Making: a Study of Societal Attitudes. *Palliative Medicine*, Vol.23, No.1, (January 2009), pp. 87-94, ISSN 0269-2163

Lee, J.C.Y., Chen, P.P., Yeo, J.K.S. & So, H.Y. (2003). Hong Kong Chinese Teacher´s Attitudes Toward Life-Sustaining Treatment in Dying Patients. *Hong Kong Medical Journal*, Vol.9, No.3, (June 2003), pp. 186-191, ISSN 1024-2708

Maguirre, C.P., Kirby, M., Coen, R., Coakley, D., Lawlor, B.A. & O'Neill, D. (1996). Family Member´s Attitudes Toward Telling the Patient with Alzheimer´s Disease their Diagnosis. *British Medical Journal*, Vol.313, No.7056 (August 1996), pp.529-530, ISSN 0959-8138

Marinus, J., Visser, M., Verswey, N.A., Verhey, F.R., Middelkoop, H.A., Stiggelbout, A.M. & van Hilten, J.J. (2003). Assessment of Cognition in Parkinson´s Disease. *Neurology*, Vol.61, No.9, (November 2003), pp. 1222-1228, ISBN 0028-3878

Markson, L.J., Kern, D.C., Annas, G.J. & Glantz, L.H. (1994). Physician Assessment of Patient Competence. *Journal of the American Geriatrics Society*, Vol.42, No.10, (October 1994), pp. 1074-1080, ISBN 0002-8614

Marzanski, M. (2000). Would You Like to Know What is Wrong with You? On Telling the Truth to Patients with Dementia. *Journal of Medical Ethics*, Vol.26, No.2, (April 1994), pp. 108-113, ISSN 0306-6800

Mayeux, R., Denaro, J., Hemenegildo, N., Marder, K., Tang, M.-X., Cote, L.J. & Stern, Y. (1992). A population-Based Investigation of Parkinsons-Disease with and without Dementia – Relationship to Age and Gender. *Archives of Neurology*, Vol. 49, No.5, (May 1992), pp. 492-497, ISSN 0003-9942

McGrath, P. (1998). Autonomy, Discourse, and Power: a Postmodern Reflection on Principalism and Bioethics. *Journal of Medicine and Philosophy*, Vol.23, No.5, (August 1998), pp. 516-532, ISSN 0360-5310

Meisel, A., Kuczewski, M. (1996). Legal and Ethical Miths About Informed Consent. *Archives of Internal Medicine*, Vol.156, No.22, (December 1996), pp. 2521-2526, ISSN 0003-9926

Mendez, M.F., Cherrier, M., Perryman, K.M., Pachana, N., Miller, B.L. & Cummings, J.L. (1996). Frontotemporal Dementia Versus Alzheimer´s Disease: Differencial Cognitive Features. *Neurology*, Vol. 47, No.5, (November 1996), pp. 1189-1194, ISSN 0028-3878

Mental Capacity Act (2005). In: *U.K. Legislation*, 15.08.2011, Available from: www.opsi.gov.uk/acts/acts20050009.htm

Moroney, J.T., Bagiella, E., Desmond, D.W., Hachinski, V.C., Mölsä, P.K., Gustafson, L., Brun, A., Fischer, P., Erkinjuntti, T., Rosen, W., Paik, M.C. & Tatemichi, T.K. (1997). Meta-analysis of the Hachinski Ischemic Score in Pathologically verified dementias. *Neurology*, Vol.49, No.4, (October 1997), pp. 1096-1105, ISSN 0028-3878

Moye, J. & Marson, D.C. (2007). Assessment of Decision-Making Capacity in Older Adults: An Emerging Area of Practice and Research. *The Journals of Gerontology. Series B, Psychological Sciences and Social Sciences*, Vol.62B, No.1, (May 2007), pp. 3-11, ISSN 1079-5014

Parsons, C., Hughes, C.M., Passmore, P. & Lapane K.L. (2010). Withholding, Discontinuing and Withdrawing Medications in Dementia Patients at End of Life. *Drugs Aging*, Vol.27, No.6, (June, 2010), pp. 435-449, ISSN 1170-229X

Peterson, G. & Wallin, A. (2003). Alzheimer's disease Ethics – Informed Consent and Related Issues in Clinical Trials: Results of a Survey Among the Members of the Research Ethics Committees in Sweden. *International Psychogeriatrics*, Vol.15, No.2 (June 2003), pp. 157-170, ISSN 1041-6102

Pinto, V.F. (1991). Between Life and Death, a Reason for Hope (an Ethical Assessment of Euthanasia, Dysthanasia and Orthothanasia). *Servir*, Vol.39, No.1, (January-February 1991), pp. 8-22, ISSN 0871-2379

Pioltini, A.B.M., Mendes-Chiloff, C.L., Schelp, A.O. & Marcolino, E.S. (2010). Distinct Attitudes of Professionals from Different Medical Specialties Toward Autonomy and Legal Instruments in the Assessment of Patients with Alzheimer's Disease. *Dementia & Neuropsychologia*, Vol.4, No.2, (June 2010), pp.104-108, ISSN 1980-5764

Prince, M., Livingston, G. & Katona, C. (2007). Mental Health Care for the Elderly in Low-Income Countries: a Health Systems Approach. *World Psychiatry*, Vol.6, No.1, (February 2007), pp. 5-13, ISSN 1723-8617

Rendtorff, J.D. (2010). The Limitations and Accomplishments of Autonomy as a Basic Principle in Bioethics and Biolaw. In: Autonomy and Human Rights in Health Care, D.N. Weisstub & G.D. Pintos (Eds), 75-76, Springer, ISBN 978.90.481.7453.9, The Netherlands.

Regnard, C., Leslie, P., Crawford, H., Matthews, D. & Gibson, L. (2010). Gastrostomies in Dementia: Bad Practice or Bad Evidence? *Age and Ageing*, Vol.39, No.3, (May 2010), pp. 282-284, ISSN 0002-0729

Richter, J., Eisemann, M. & Zgonnikova E. (2001). Doctor´s Authoritarianism in End-of-Life Treatment Decision´s. A comparison between Russia, Sweden and Germany. *Journal of Medical Ethics*, Vol.27, No.3, (June 2001), pp. 186-191, ISSN 0306-6800

Rohde, K., Peskind, E.R. & Raskind, M.A. (1995). Suicide in Two Patients with Alzheimer's Disease. *Journal of the American Geriatrics Society*, Vol.43, No.2, (February 1995), pp. 187-189, ISSN 0002-8614

Roth, L.H., Meisel, A. & Lidz, C.W. (1977). Tests of Competency to Consent to Treatment. *The American Journal of Psychiatry*, Vol.134, No.3, (March 1977), pp. 279-284, ISSN 0002-953X

Schelp, A.O., Nieri, A.B., Hamamoto Filho, P.D., Bales, A.M. & Mendes-Chiloff, C.L. (2008). Public Awareness of Dementia. *Dementia & Neuropsychologia*, Vol.2, No.3, (September 2008), pp. 192-196, ISSN 1980-5764

Schneiderman, J.L., Kaplan, R.M., Pearlman, R.A. & Teetzel, H. (1993). Do Physician´s Own Preferences for Life-Sustaining Treatment Influence their Perceptions of Patient´s Preferences? *The Journal of Clinical Ethics*, Vol.4, No.1, (Spring 1993), pp. 28-33, ISSN 1046-7890

Seckler, A.B., Meier, D.E., Mulvihill, M. & Paris, B.E. (1991). Substituted Judment: How Accurate are Proxy Predictions? *Annals of Internal Medicine*, Vol.115, No.2, (July 1991), pp. 92-98, ISSN 0003-4819

Silberfeld, M., Gundstein-Amadom, R., Stephens, D. & Deber, R. (1996). Family and Physician´s Views of Surrogate Decisions-Making: the Roles and How to Choose. *International Psychogeriatrics*, Vol.8, No.4, (Winter 1996), pp. 589-596, ISSN 1041-6102

Sittisombutt, S., Maxwell, C., Love, E.J. & Sitthi-Amorin, C. (2009). Physician´s Attitudes and Practices Regarding Advanced End-of-Life Care Planning for Terminally ill Patients at Chiang Mai University Hospital, Thailand. *Nursing and Health Science*, Vol.1, No.1, (March 2009), pp. 23-28, ISSN 1441-0745

Stiles, P.G. & Petrila, J. (2011). Research and Confidentiality: Legal Issues and Risk Management Strategies. *Psychology, Public Policy, and Law*, Vol.17, No.3, (August 2011), pp. 333-356, ISSN 1076-8971

Strong, C. (1993). Patients Should not Always Come First in Treatment Decisions. *The Journal of Clinical Ethics*, Vol.4, No.1, (Spring 1993), pp. 63-65, ISSN 1046-7890

Teno, J.M., Clarridge, B.R., Casey, V., Welch, L.C., Wetle, T., Shield, R. & Mor V. (2004). Family Perspectives on End-of-life Care at the Last Place of Care. *The Journal of the American Medical Association*, Vol.291, No.1, (January 2004), pp. 88-93, ISSN 0098-7484

U.S. Congress. (1994). *Defensive Medicine and Medical Malpractice*, OTA-H-602. Office of Technology Assessment, Washington, DC. , (July 1994), U.S. Government Printing Office.

Wendler, D. & Rid, A. (2011). Systematic Review: the Effect on Surrogates of Making Treatment Decisions for Others. *Annals of Internal Medicine*, Vol.154, No.5, (March 2011), pp. 336-346, ISSN 0003-4819

White, D.B., Malvar, G., Karr, J., Lo, B. & Curtis, J.R. (2010). Expanding the Paradigm of the Physician´s Role in Surrogate Decision-Making: an Empirically Derived Framework*. *Critical Care Medicine*, Vol.38, No.3, (March 2010), pp. 743-750, ISSN 0090-3493

Whitney, S.N. & McCullough, L.B. (2007). Physician´s Silent Decision: Because Patient Autonomy Does Not Always Come First. *The American Journal of Bioethics*, Vol.7, No.7, (July 2007), pp. 33-38, ISSN 1526-5161

Widera, E., Steenpass, V., Marson, D. & Sudore, R. (2011). Finances in the Older Patient With Cognitive Impairment "He Didn´t Want Me to Take Over". *The Journal of the American Medical Association*, Vol.305, No.7, (February 2011), pp. 698-706, ISSN 0098-7484

Wild, K. & Cotrell, V. (2003). Identifying Driving Impairment in Alzheimer´s Disease: a Comparison of Self and Observer Reports Versus Driving Evaluation. *Alzheimer´s Disease and Associated Disorders*, Vol.17, No.1, (January- march 2003), pp. 27-34, ISSN 0893-0341

World Health Organization (2011). Health Topics: Life Expectancy, In: *World Health Organization*,20.08.2011,Available from www.who.int/topics/life_expectancy/en/

Yaffe, M.J., Orzeck, P. & Barylak, L. (2008). Family Physician´s Perspectives on Care of Dementia Patients and Family Caregivers. *Canadian Family Physician*, Vol.54, No.7, (July 2008), pp. 1008-1015, ISSN 0008-350X

Yarborough, M. (2002). Adults Are Not Big Children: Examining Surrogate Consent to Research Using Adults With Dementia. *Cambridge Quarterly of Healthcare Ethics*, Vol.11, No.2, (Spring 2002), pp. 160-168, ISSN 0963-1801

14

Health Economics and Geriatrics: Challenges and Opportunities

Julie Ratcliffe[1], Kate Laver[2],
Leah Couzner[2] and Maria Crotty[2]
[1]*Flinders Clinical Effectiveness, Flinders University*
[2]*Department of Rehabilitation and Aged Care, Flinders University*
Australia

1. Introduction

1.1 The relationship between health economics and geriatrics

The fundamental economic problem of limited resources coupled with unlimited claims upon those resources holds particular resonance for geriatrics given the projected huge future growth in demand for health and aged care services for older people as a consequence of demographic change. Population ageing is a world-wide phenomenon which poses major challenges and opportunities for health economics and geriatrics. Currently approximately 2 million Australians, almost 10% of the total population, are aged 70 years and over and this figure is set to double during the next two decades. It is estimated that by 2045, one in four Australians will be aged 65 years or more and nearly one in ten will be 80 years or over [Productivity Commission, 2005]. This situation is not unique to Australia, population ageing forecasts in many countries and regions throughout the world mirror these statistics. In addition, factors other than an ageing population are creating new pressures and challenges for geriatrics, particularly in relation to how health and aged care services are provided in the future. The so called post-war "baby boomer" generation is generally expected to have much higher expectations for choice and responsiveness in the provision of health and aged care services relative to previous generations. Therefore, techniques for systematically engaging older people to establish their preferences in relation to the provision and configuration of geriatric services are likely to become more important. This chapter discusses the challenges and opportunities for the application of health economics and geriatrics from two main perspectives. Firstly, in relation to economic evaluation and the methods for assessing the cost effectiveness of new health care technologies and models of aged care service delivery. Secondly, in relation to methods adopted by health economists for measuring and valuing patient or consumer preferences in health care.

2. Health economics and economic evaluation

Health economics is a sub-discipline of economics, principally concerned with issues related to scarcity in the allocation of resources for health care expenditures for the promotion of health [Drummond et al, 2005]. It has long been recognized that the resources available for expenditure in geriatrics, as in all other areas of medicine, are constrained and unfortunately difficult decisions must be made about which services are to be provided, to whom, where and when. Any decision to introduce new geriatric services or expand existing services will inevitably have resource and cost implications and will be associated with lost opportunities (otherwise known as opportunity costs) in terms of foregone health benefits [Brazier et al 2007]. For example, making more resources available for secondary care services e.g. expansion of diagnostic geriatric neurology services for older people means that fewer resources will be available to provide services in the community e.g. incontinence assessment and management. Inevitably, therefore, there will be opportunity costs and such decisions will potentially have major implications for health.

A recent influential policy report by the National Health and Hospital Reform Commission, established by the Australian Federal Government to develop a long-term health reform plan for a modern Australia, highlighted the need for greater evaluation in the provision of geriatric services [National Health and Hospital Reform Commission, 2009]. Health care policy makers within the United Kingdom, Canada and the United States have also called for greater evaluation of health, social and aged care services for older people, suggesting that this will lead to improvements in efficiency by targeting scarce resources towards interventions which promote the health, independence and well-being of older people [Department of Health, 2001; Glendinning, 2003; Kodner, 2006; MacAdam, 2009].

2.1 Economic evaluation and its role in promoting efficiency

Economic evaluation is an evaluation tool that can be used to facilitate resource allocation decision-making. There has been an increasing use of economic evaluation to inform health care policy making over the last decade through the establishment of organisations such as the National Institute for Health and Clinical Excellence in the UK and similar agencies in other countries. The overall aim of health economic evaluation methodology is to aid decision-makers to make efficient and equitable decisions about the allocation of scarce resources via a systematic and transparent comparison of the costs and benefits of competing interventions [Drummond et al, 2005]. In many instances, a new intervention will be more costly but will also result in increased health benefits relative to existing alternatives. Therefore the decision problem concerns whether the increased costs represent good value for money.

2.2 Types of economic evaluation

There are four main types of economic evaluation: cost minimisation, cost-effectiveness, cost-utility and cost-benefit analyses [Brazier et al 2007]. Cost-minimisation analysis seeks to establish which is the least cost alternative, but is only an appropriate technique of economic evaluation if it can be shown that the alternatives under consideration achieve identical outcomes. However, in practice this is very rarely achieved since there is always uncertainty around the measure of outcome. Cost-effectiveness analysis determines what is the best method of achieving a given objective, usually measured in clinical or 'natural' units, and presents results in terms of cost per unit of effect (e.g. cost per positive cancer detected or cost per symptom free day). Cost-utility analysis compares the costs of alternative health care programmes with their utility, usually measured in terms of quality adjusted life years (QALYs). QALYs combine survival and quality of life into a single measure of value and are discussed in detail in sections 3 and 4 of this chapter. Cost-benefit analysis compares the benefits with costs of a health care programme, where all the benefits are valued in money terms including health improvement. The most widely applied technique of economic evaluation is cost-utility analysis. Many regulatory authorities including the National Institute of Health and Clinical Excellence [NICE, 2008] in England and Wales and the Pharmaceutical Benefits Advisory Committee in Australia [Commonwealth Department of Health and Ageing, 2002] routinely require the presentation of a cost utility analysis alongside information relating to the clinical safety and efficacy of a new health technology as part of their reimbursement decision-making process.

2.3 Economic evaluations in geriatrics

Economic evaluations in geriatrics are rare in comparison with other medical specialties. A recent review of the National Institute for Health Research Centre for Reviews and Dissemination databases (which contain abstracts of published journal articles from around the world relating to the effectiveness and cost-effectiveness of health care interventions) recorded a total of 8428 abstracts relating to economic evaluations from all medical fields of which only 48 (<1%) were classified as relating to the field of geriatrics. Of these 37 (77%) were defined as cost effectiveness analyses and the remaining 11 studies (23%) were defined as cost utility analyses. Examples of recent cost effectiveness studies undertaken in geriatrics include a study by Jowett and colleagues which examined the cost effectiveness of warfarin versus aspirin in patients older than 75 years with atrial fibrillation [Jowett et al 2011] and a study by Holman and colleagues which examined the cost effectiveness of cognitive behavior therapy versus talking and usual care for depressed older people in a primary care setting [Holman et al 2011]. Both of the studies were undertaken in the UK. The study to assess the cost effectiveness of warfarin comprised an economic evaluation alongside a randomized controlled trial in 973 patients aged 75 years and over with atrial fibrillation randomized to receive either warfarin or aspirin. Patients were followed up for a mean of 2.7 years. The costs of thrombotic and hemorrhagic events, anticoagulation clinic visits and primary care utilization were determined. Clinical benefits were expressed in terms of a primary event avoided including fatal or non-fatal disabling stroke, intracranial hemorrhage, or systemic embolism. It was found that total costs over the four year study period were lower in the warfarin group (difference, -£165; 95% CI -£452 to £89). This difference was primarily driven by the difference in primary event costs as the primary event rate over 3 years was lower in the warfarin group (0.049 versus 0.099). With lower costs and a higher clinical benefit (characterized by a lower primary event rate) warfarin is the dominant treatment and the authors therefore concluded that warfarin represents a highly cost effective intervention compared with aspirin in atrial fibrillation patients aged 75 years and over. The aim of the study for older people with depression was to compare the cost effectiveness of cognitive behavior therapy (CBT) a talking control (TC) and treatment as usual (TAU) delivered in a primary care setting. The study presented cost data generated from a single blind randomized controlled trial of 204 people aged 65 years and over who were offered only TAU or TAU plus up to 12 sessions of CBT or a TC. The main outcome measure was the Beck Depression Inventory II. The primary analysis was focused upon the cost-effectiveness of CBT compared with TAU at 10 months follow up. It was found that total costs per patients were significantly higher in the CBT group compared with the TAU group (difference £427; 95% CI £56 to £787). Reductions in the Beck Depression Inventory II scores were significantly greater in the CBT group (difference 3.6 points, 95% CI: 0.7-6.5 points). It was therefore found that CBT is associated with an incremental cost of £120 per additional point reduction in the Beck Depression Inventory II score. The authors concluded that CBT is likely to be recommended as a cost effective treatment option for this patient group provided that the value placed on a unit reduction in the Beck Depression Inventory II score is greater than £115 since CBT is significantly more costly than TAU alone or TAU plus TC but more clinically effective.

All 11 studies categorised as cost utility analyses by definition included cost per QALY as the main measure of outcome and reflected a wide range of topics including an assessment of the impacts of aggressive treatment strategies (including mechanical ventilation and intensive care) for older people [Hamel et al 2001], a systematic review to assess the impact of falls prevention strategies in community and residential aged care [Church et al 2011], hip protector use in community [Honkanen et al, 2006] and nursing home settings [Colon-Emeric et al, 2003] and the impact of universal versus selective bone densitometry for osteoporosis [Ito et al 2009; Schousboe et al 2005]. The methods used to estimate QALYs (see section 3 below) varied considerably across these studies as did the reported cost per QALY ratios; ranging from $106 (AUS) per QALY for Vitamin D supplementation for older people living in residential aged care to $100,000 per QALY for ventilator support and intensive care for high risk patients (defined as those with a ≤ 50% probability of surviving at least two months) in the 65-74 years age group with acute respiratory failure.

3. The measurement and valuation of health

In order to conduct a cost utility analysis, there is a need to collect and present data relating to the measurement and valuation of health in addition to the presentation of data relating to the measurement and valuation of resource use (costs). Traditionally health related utility measures, principally the quality adjusted life year (QALY), have been utilised to value the benefits of health care services and programs within cost utility analysis [Weinstein et al, 2009]. To calculate QALYs it is necessary to represent health on a scale where death and full health are assigned values of 0 and 1 respectively. Therefore, states rated as better than dead have values between 0 and 1 and states rated as worse than dead have negative scores which, in principle, are bounded by negative infinity. Table 1 provides a simple hypothetical illustration of how the benefits of health care services and programs can be estimated using QALYs. This table compares medical and surgical management for treating coronary artery disease. Health in each year is approximated by the mean health state value for two groups of patients, the first group receiving medical management and the second group receiving surgical management. It can be seen that for those patients receiving medical management life expectancy is 5 years on average whereas for those patients receiving surgical management life expectancy is longer, 9 years on average. The total QALY gain for each group of patients is calculated using area under the curve methods, by summing the mean health state values for each period of time (in this case each year) [Drummond et al, 2005]. Medical management is associated with a total QALY gain of 4.068 QALYs whereas the total QALY gain from surgical management is somewhat higher, 7.614 QALYs.

Year	Medical management	Surgical management
1	0.856	0.850
2	0.856	0.850
3	0.856	0.850
4	0.800	0.850
5	0.700	0.850
6	Dead	0.850
7		0.850
8		0.832
9		0.832
10		Dead
Total	**4.068**	**7.614**

Table 1. Calculation of QALY's gained for treatment of coronary artery disease

There are a number of approaches which can be used to generate health state values for the calculation of QALYs including direct valuation of their own health status by older people using an established utility elicitation technique or indirect valuation through the utilisation of generic preference based measures of health [Brazier et al, 2007].

3.1 Direct valuation of health

An example of the direct valuation of health by older people is a study which was undertaken within the context of a randomised trial of external hip protectors for older women at risk of hip fracture [Salkeld et al 2000A]. The main objective of this study was to use an elicitation technique known as time trade off (TTO) to estimate the utility associated with hip fracture and fear of falling among older women. The TTO derives an estimate of preference for health by finding the point at which respondents show no preference between a longer period of time in impaired health versus a shorter period of time in full health. Respondents were asked to rate three health states; fear of falling, a "good" hip fracture, and a "bad" hip fracture on the 0-1 QALY scale using TTO. A "bad" hip fracture which results in admission to a nursing home was valued at 0.05; a "good" hip fracture resulting in the maintenance of independent living in the community was valued at 0.31, and fear of falling was valued at 0.67. In addition, 80% of the women surveyed indicated that they would rather be dead (utility = 0) than experience the loss of independence and quality of life that results from a bad hip fracture and subsequent admission to a nursing home. Thus the study authors concluded that older women place a very high marginal value on their health and a loss of ability to live independently in the community has a considerable detrimental effect on their quality of life.

3.2 Indirect valuation of health

In practice, examples of the direct valuation of health are less commonly found within economic evaluations, both within geriatrics and in other medical specialities. Indirect valuation through the utilisation of generic preference based measures of physical and mental health such as the AQoL (Assessment of Quality of Life), the EQ-5D (EuroQol) and the SF-6D have become the most popular mechanisms for the estimation of quality adjusted life years or QALYs for cost utility analyses [Brazier et al 2007]. Generic preference based measures of health comprise two main elements: a descriptive system for completion by patients or members of the general population comprising a set of items with multiple response categories covering the different dimensions reflecting health related quality of life and an off the shelf scoring algorithm which reflects society's strength of preference for the health states defined by the instrument. The scoring algorithms are typically generated from large general population surveys to elicit health state values for a selection of health states described by each descriptive system [Brazier et al, 2007]. Statistical modelling techniques are then employed to infer health state values for all health states described by each descriptive system. The scoring algorithms are anchored on the numerical scale required to construct QALYs, where full health is one and zero is equivalent to death. For some instruments eg.EQ-5D particularly severe health states are associated with negative values, reflecting the average general population view that these states are considered worse than death.

An example of the indirect valuation of health in older people is provided by a cost utility analysis of an outpatient geriatric assessment with an intervention to increase adherence undertaken in the USA by Keeler and colleagues [Keeler et al, 1999]. This study employed the SF-6D scoring algorithm [Brazier et al, 2002] in subjects aged 65 years and over to devise a single preference based measure of health-related quality of life from individual responses to the SF-36 at various time points throughout the five year time horizon of the randomised controlled trial. The algorithm generates an index value where 0 represents death and 1 perfect health, with intermediate values for all remaining health states. The valuations are based upon the preference weights obtained for a series of health states defined by the SF-6D from a sample of 611 members of the UK general population. The area under the curve was calculated in order to measure the QALY gain for each patient. Over the five year period it was found that the incremental QALY gain for the study intervention was 0.07 in comparison with no intervention and when coupled with the associated incremental costs the study authors concluded that the cost effectiveness of an outpatient geriatric assessment with an intervention to increase adherence compared favourably with other interventions.

3.3 Application of generic preference based measures with older people

Although the indirect valuation of health through the utilisation of generic preference based measures has become the most commonly applied method to generate QALYs, specific application in older people remain scant in comparison to applications within the younger adult population. The majority of the studies that have been undertaken to date with older people have been based in community samples and have employed the AQoL [Osbourne et al 2003], the SF-36 [Walters et al, 2001] and the EQ-5D [Holland et al 2004] to assess health status at a population level. Similarly, a variety of instruments have been employed in groups of people living with particular health conditions [Dugan et al 1998; Logsdon et al 2002; Naumann et al 2004]. Comparative evidence relating to the application of two or more generic preference based instruments simultaneously in older people suggests that the EQ-5D is easier to administer and has higher completion rates relative to the AQoL and SF-6D [Brazier et al 1996; Holland et al 2004]. However, it is also important to note that in comparison with the EQ-5D, the SF-6D has been found to be more sensitive particularly for particularly for older adults with milder health problems [Brazier et al 1996]. The instruments were all designed for self-completion but there are strong arguments in favour of interviewer administration to reduce cognitive burden and help in promoting understanding, particularly in frail older people. Coast et al found that the expected probability of requiring interviewer administration of the EQ-5D increased with age and reductions in cognitive functioning [Coast et al, 1998]. Similarly Brazier et al reported that many older women experienced difficulties completing the SF-36 (from which the SF-6D is derived) and recommended interviewer administration as a potential solution [Brazier et al, 1996]. In older people with severe cognitive impairment previous research has indicated that proxy responses may be the only mechanism for obtaining information relating to health status, although there is debate in the literature as to who represents the most appropriate proxy e.g. family carer, other family member or health care professional [Coucil et al, 2001; Sitoh et al, 2003].

4. Advantages and disadvantages of QALYs

The purported advantages of QALYs for the measurement and valuation of health are mainly based upon three important characteristics [Prieto and Sacristan, 2003]. Firstly, QALYs combine changes in the quality of life and changes in the length of life (survival) into a single indicator. Secondly, QALYs are relatively easy to calculate via simple multiplication. However, it is also important to note that the prior step of eliciting utilities for a wide variety of health states is a complicated task, hence the proliferation of indirect methods for valuing health through the utilisation of generic preference based measures with "off the shelf" scoring algorithms. Thirdly, and potentially most importantly for economic evaluation: QALYs provide a common metric for comparing the benefits of disparate health care treatments and programmes relating to very different disease areas and conditions thereby informing resource allocation decision-making across the health care sector.

However, QALYs are not without their critics. Within geriatrics QALYs have been criticised for their focus upon survival. This inevitably means that the life of a younger person with the capacity to survive for a longer duration is more highly valued than that of an older person with a reduced capacity for survival duration [Crotty and Ratcliffe, 2011]. Some commentators have referred to this possibility as reflecting the principle of utilitarian ageism and have argued that QALYs should be weighted in favour of older people to negate this possibility, noting that even small improvements in health related quality of life tends to be highly valued by frail older people and their families when nearing the end of life [Giles et al, 2009]. Others have noted the possibility of the principle of egalitarian ageism encapsulated by the so called "fair- innings" argument. This notion was first proposed in the health economics discipline by Alan Williams [Williams, 1997] and suggests that everyone in society is entitled to some 'normal' span of health and anyone failing to achieve this has been cheated, whilst anyone getting more than this is effectively 'living on borrowed time'. The dilemma for geriatrics is that when questioned in surveys older people themselves have been found to express this view, often more vigorously and with greater frequency than their younger counterparts [Johri et al, 2005]. As the population ages this debate is likely to become even more prominent and it is important that further research is conducted to assess community preferences for priorities in health care expenditures. In particular further research is needed to assess the extent of community support for expenditures which may promote small but highly valued improvements in health related quality of life for frail older people nearing the end of life.

5. Beyond health? The measurement and valuation of quality of life

In addition to being criticised for a focus upon survival, QALYs have also been criticised for their focus upon health alone as many health and aged care services impact upon quality of life more broadly [Higginson and Carr, 2001]. For example, rehabilitation interventions may include education, problem solving and the provision of aids, e.g. electric wheelchairs and walking aids, in order to promote independent living. Whilst the provision of these interventions may have little or no impact upon an individual's health, they may still lead to significant improvements in their quality of life [Hopman and Verner, 2003]. These improvements will not be reflected by the incorporation of QALY's as the main measure of outcome within a cost utility analysis of these types of interventions. A recent innovation in this regard is the newly developed ICECAP index of capability for older people (ICECAP-O) [Coast et al 2008A].

5.1 The ICECAP-O: A capabilities approach to the measurement and valuation of quality of life for older people

The ICECAP-O represents a recent innovation in the measurement and valuation of quality of life for older people [Coast et al 2008A]. It focuses upon quality of life more broadly rather than health alone and therefore has the potential to be utilised in the economic evaluation of health and aged care services in Australia and internationally.

The developers of the ICECAP-O aimed to identify the attributes that were most important to older people in determining their quality of life through a review of the literature and interviews with older people [Grewal et al, 2006]. A set of functioning's that were most important to people were developed, namely; attachment (feelings of love, friendship and companionship), role (having a purpose that is valued), enjoyment (having a sense of pleasure and joy from personal and communal activities), security (feeling safe and secure and not having to worry) and control (being independent and able to make one's own decisions). Coast et al. discovered it was the person's capability to achieve these functioning's, rather than their level of functioning *per se,* which determined their quality of life. Thus, while an individual's state of health impacts on capability, it is not the sole determining factor. The ICECAP-O has the potential for application across the health and aged care sectors in comparing the value of different interventions to older people; including services that may improve quality of life without necessarily improving health (e.g. electric wheelchairs, meals on wheels and carer respite services), and interventions that improve both quality of life and health (e.g. joint arthroplasty and antidepressant medication). The developers of the ICECAP-O have provided early evidence for the construct validity of the ICECAP-O measure [Coast et al., 2008B] based upon the findings from a community based survey of older people in the UK.

5.2 Case study: Application of the ICECAP-O in transition care and rehabilitation programmes for older people

We have recently conducted a study which demonstrates the strong empirical relationships between the concepts of health, disability, hope and capability (as measured by the ICECAP-O) and provides support for the construct validity of the ICECAP-O in a clinical in-patient rehabilitation setting in Australia. The ICECAP-O consists of five attributes (attachment, role, enjoyment, security and control), each with four levels. The respondent is asked to rate themselves for each attribute on the four level scale from 1 (for example, 'I can think about the future without any concern') to 4 (for example, 'I can only think about the future with a lot of concern'). Scores can be summarised as quality of life states, (for example, quality of life state 12112). The combined attributes and levels describe 1024 possible quality of life states. An off the shelf scoring algorithm has been developed for the ICECAP-O which assigns a numerical score to each possible combination of responses ranging from 0 (no capability) to 1 (full capability) [Coast et al 2008A]. In our study a questionnaire containing the ICECAP-O was administered using a face to face interview mode of administration with patients participating in in-patient medical rehabilitation (n=100). The relationships between the ICECAP and other instruments including the EQ-5D [Brooks et al, 2003], Modified Rankin Scale (a measure of disability completed by the health care professional) [Banks and Moratta, 2007] the Herth Hope Index [Herth, 1992], and socio-demographic characteristics were examined.

The EQ-5D is a measure of health related quality of life consisting of five attributes (mobility, self care, usual activities, pain/discomfort and anxiety/depression). Each attribute has three levels and respondents are asked to indicate which level best describes their current health state [Brooks et al, 2003]. The combined attributes and levels describe 243 possible EQ-5D health states Application of the existing UK general population based scoring algorithm to individual responses to the instrument generates EQ-5D values ranging from a minimum of -0.594 (for health state 33333) to a maximum of 1.0 (health state 11111 full health). It was anticipated that there would be a strong positive relationship between capability as measured and valued by the ICECAP-O and health related quality of life as measured and valued by the EQ-5D, supporting the previous findings from studies conducted by the developers of the ICECAP-O [Coast et al, 2008B; Grewal et al, 2006].

In addition to the EQ-5D self-report instrument, we included an instrument which was designed to be completed by a health care professional directly involved in the provision of the participant's care. The Modified Rankin Scale (MRS) was completed by the study occupational therapist following discussion with the participant about their previous and current ability to manage everyday activities. The MRS describes global disability, which includes basic activities of daily living (for example walking, dressing) and instrumental activities of daily living (for example shopping, meal preparation). The MRS is commonly used in rehabilitation settings and clinical trials. The participant is assigned a score ranging from 0 (no symptoms at all) to 5 (severe disability). The MRS has demonstrated construct and convergent validity, and good test-retest reliability [Banks and Moratta, 2007]. Similarly to the EQ-5D, it was predicted that capability would be inversely related to disability as measured by the Modified Rankin Scale implying that as the level of disability increased, overall capability would decrease.

The Herth Hope Index is designed to measure the concept of hope. The tool consists of 12 statements (for example: 'I believe that each day has potential'), each with a 4 point Likert scale (1=strongly disagree, 2=disagree, 3=agree or 4=strongly agree). The tool is scored using a simple summative scoring system ranging from 12 (lowest hope) to 48 (highest hope). The tool has demonstrated good construct validity and internal consistency [Davis 2005; Snyder et al 1991] and has been applied previously in a variety of clinical settings including palliative care and organ transplantation [Benzein and Berg, 2005; Evangelista et al 2003]. Hope can be defined as 'a positive motivational state that is based on an interactively derived sense of successful goal directed energy and planning to meet goals' [Snyder et al, 1991]. Several studies have found a positive correlation between hope and quality of life in a variety of patient populations [Davis, 2005; Evangelista et al, 2003; Sigstad et al, 2005; Yadav, 2010]. It has been found that individuals recovering from major health events including heart failure and stroke report higher levels of hope than healthy individuals from the general population [Laver, 2009; Rustoen et al, 2005]. The concept of hope is thought to play a central role in rehabilitation as individuals with higher levels of hope have been found to perform better in terms of setting and achieving their rehabilitation goals [Snyder et al, 2006]. The relationship between hope and capability has not previously been well documented. However, it is plausible to expect that hope may also impact positively upon capability.

A significant proportion, 50% (n=50), of the study participants had a diagnosis of stroke as their main reason for admission. The second most common reason for admission was a fall (15%, n=15). All of the remaining participants had a variety of diagnoses that could broadly be described as 'de-conditioning' or the effects of decreased physical activity following medical illness or non-surgical fracture. The majority of participants were females (68%, n=68) and the mean age of participants was 75 years (range 27-92) with the vast majority [78%, n=78] being 65 years or older. The distribution of responses to the EQ-5D (Table 1) indicates that the majority of participants reported at least some problems in one or more dimensions of the instrument. Participants generally reported more problems with the physical dimensions (mobility, self- care and usual activities) of the EQ-5D which is

Mobility	
I have no problems in walking about	14 (14%)
I have some problems in walking about	83 (83%)
I am confined to bed	3 (3%)
Self Care	
I have no problems with self care	39 (39%)
I have some problems washing or dressing myself	59 (59%)
I am unable to wash or dress myself	2 (2%)
Usual activities	
I have no problems with performing my usual activities	12 (12%)
I have some problems with performing my usual activities	70 (70%)
I am unable to perform my usual activities	18 (18%)
Pain/Discomfort	
I have no pain or discomfort	46 (46%)
I have moderate pain or discomfort	43 (43%)
I have extreme pain or discomfort	11 (11%)
Anxiety/Depression	
I am not anxious or depressed	49 (49%)
I am moderately anxious or depressed	43 (43%)
I am extremely anxious or depressed	8 (8%)

Table 1. Distribution of individual responses to EQ-5D (n=100)

consistent with what would have been predicted for this population. The mean score for the EQ-5D was found to be 0.53 (SD 0.32) for the total sample and 0.55 (SD 0.28) for the proportion of the sample aged 65 years or over (n=78). The mean scores are well below previously reported norm values from the general population in the UK of 0.78 for adults in the 65-74 years age group and 0.73 in the 75 + years age group [Kind et al, 1999]. The mean scores reflect the significant levels of health impairment in this clinical population relative to community based samples.

The distribution of responses for each dimensions of the ICECAP-O are presented in Table 2. It can be seen that while the majority of participants reported high levels of love and friendship (attachment), many participants expressed some concern about their future (security) and reported limitations in their independence (control) and ability to do things that made them feel valued (role). The mean ICECAP-O score was 0.76 (SD 0.15) for the total sample and 0.77 (SD 0.14) for the proportion of the sample aged 65 years or over (n=78). These mean scores are lower than reported by Coast et al [2008A] who found a mean ICECAP score of 0.814 in a community based general population sample of older people. However the difference in mean values between this clinical population and the community based population is not as pronounced for the ICECAP as was evident for the EQ-5D.

Attachment	
I can have all of the love and friendship that I want	58 (58%)
I can have a lot of the love and friendship that I want	30 (30%)
I can have a little of the love and friendship that I want	9 (9%)
I cannot have any of the love and friendship that I want	0
Security	
I can think about the future without any concern	20 (20%)
I can think about the future with only a little concern	31 (31%)
I can only think about the future with some concern	28 (28%)
I can only think about the future with a lot of concern	20 (20%)
Role	
I am able to do all of the things that make me feel valued	14 (14%)
I am able to do many of the things that make me feel valued	32 (32%)
I am able to do a few of the things that make me feel valued	46 (46%)
I am unable to do any of the things that make me feel valued	6 (6%)
Enjoyment	
I can have all of the enjoyment and pleasure that I want	24 (24%)
I can have a lot of the enjoyment and pleasure that I want	36 (36%)
I can have a little of the enjoyment and pleasure that I want	33 (33%)
I cannot have any of the enjoyment and pleasure that I want	6 (6%)
Control	
I am able to be completely independent	9 (9%)
I am able to be independent in many things	45 (45%)
I am able to be independent in a few things	36 (36%)
I am unable to be at all independent	9 (9%)

Table 2. Distribution of responses to the ICECAP-O (n=100)

Table 3 presents the mean EQ-5D, Herth Hope Index and Modified Rankin Scores according to individual responses to the ICECAP-O. Increases in mean EQ-5D scores were evident with increases in capability levels particularly pertaining to participants' ability to do valued activities (role), and improved levels of enjoyment and attachment. There is a clear pattern of association between disability as classified by the Modified Rankin Scale and levels of

Attribute	Mean EQ-5D (n=100)	Mean HHI (n=100)	Mean MRS (n=100)
Attachment			
I can have all of the love and friendship that I want	0.53	36.25	3.09
I can have a lot of the love and friendship that I want	0.54	36.00	2.90
I can have a little of the love and friendship that I want	0.44	35.13	3.22
I cannot have any of the love and friendship that I want	N/A	N/A	N/A
Security			
I can think about the future without any concern	0.57	37.95	2.95
I can think about the future with only a little concern	0.60	36.97	3.00
I can only think about the future with some concern	0.55	34.96	3.00
I can only think about the future with a lot of concern	0.36	34.28	3.25
Role			
I am able to do all of the things that make me feel valued	0.63	37.64	2.79
I am able to do many of the things that make me feel valued	0.58	36.67	3.00
I am able to do a few of the things that make me feel valued	0.47	35.48	3.20
I am unable to do any of the things that make me feel valued	0.35	34.00	2.83
Enjoyment			
I can have all of the enjoyment and pleasure that I want	0.68	36.68	2.88
I can have a lot of the enjoyment and pleasure that I want	0.54	37.00	2.97
I can have a little of the enjoyment and pleasure that I want	0.46	35.52	3.15
I cannot have any of the enjoyment and pleasure that I want	0.33	32.33	3.50
Control			
I am able to be completely independent	0.69	37.22	2.44
I am able to be independent in many things	0.63	36.64	2.91
I am able to be independent in a few things	0.49	35.45	3.22
I am unable to be at all independent	0.69	33.86	3.56

Table 3. Distribution of mean EQ-5D, Herth Hope Index and Modified Rankin Scale values across levels of capabilities

enjoyment and control with increases in disability being associated with lower levels of enjoyment and control on average. Table 3 also illustrates that there was a clear pattern of increased mean Herth Hope Index scores with higher levels of the ICECAP-O indicating that, in general, individuals with higher levels of hope as measured by the Herth Hope Index, also reported higher levels of capability. However, it is important to note that the range of responses to the Herth Hope Index was relatively small (Inter Quartile Range: 34.5-37) indicating relatively small levels of differentiation in levels of hope across this population.

Table 4 illustrates that the ICECAP-O was found to be inversely correlated with the Modified Rankin Scale (Spearman's r = -0.286; P < 0.01) indicating that as the level of disability increased, capability decreased. The ICECAP was also found to be positively correlated with the EQ5D (Spearman's r = 0.418; P<0.01) indicating that as the level of self-reported health status increased, capability increased. The ICECAP-O scores were also found to be positively correlated with the Herth Hope Index (Spearman's r =0.402; P<0.01)) suggesting higher levels of hope was accompanied by higher levels of capability.

	ICECAP-O
EQ-5D	**0.418****
Herth Hope Index	**0.402****
Modified Rankin Scale	**-0.286****

** correlation is significant at the 0.01 level
* correlation is significant at the 0.05 level

Table 4. Relationship between the ICECAP-O and other measurement tools calculated using Spearman's rho

Overall, the results indicate that whilst health related quality of life and hope were positively associated with capability, the level of disability impacts negatively upon capability.

This is the first study, to our knowledge, which has examined the construct validity of the ICECAP-O in a clinical setting. There are similarities between our findings and the findings of Coast et al. [2008B] who examined the construct validity of the ICECAP-O in a general population sample in the UK. Coast et al. also found strong correlations between capability, disability and health status. Although the sample size for our study was relatively small, our total consent rate for participation of 92% was very high and therefore suggests good representation of older people from the South Australian clinical rehabilitation population. We applied existing general population scoring algorithms for the EQ-5D and ICECAP-O which were generated from values of the UK general population. However, it is important to note that Australian general population specific scoring algorithms are currently being developed for both the EQ-5D [Cronin et al, 2009] and ICECAP-O [Flynn et al, 2010] instruments and future studies applying these instruments in an Australian context should attempt to apply these new country specific scoring algorithms once these become publicly available.

It is also important to highlight that whilst self-report measures of health related quality of life are commonly used in clinical and economic evaluation, there may potentially be compromised validity of these measures in a proportion of this population of older people. Several studies have found that older patients with cognitive impairment may have difficulty understanding the concept of quality of life, and may lack insight into their functional ability [Bryan et al, 2005; Hulme et al, 2004; Novella et al., 2006]. In this study, a total of 19 participants were defined by the occupational therapist [applying the Modified Rankin Scale] as grade 4 – having a moderately severe disability [defined as being unable to walk and attend to own bodily needs without assistance] on the scale of 1 to 5 where 1=no symptoms at all and 5=severe disability. Despite this, one participant [n=1] within this group reported that they had no problems with self care, and, three participants [n=3] reported that they were able to be independent in many things. Further research is required to investigate the relationship between patient's own self report of health status and capability and the assessment of proxy assessors including family carers and/or health care professionals involved in the delivery of care.

Finally, this study was essentially opportunistic, the instruments being presented as part of a wider study to assess patient preferences for alternative rehabilitation programs. Therefore this study was designed to elicit responses at one time point only. Further studies should be conducted in a clinical setting to apply the ICECAP-O with older people at more than one point in time in order to determine it's sensitivity to change over time and to assess the test re-test reliability of the instrument.

In summary, the findings from our study demonstrate the potential for the wider application of the ICECAP-O in clinical populations of older people. By focusing upon quality of life more broadly, the ICECAP-O offers new insights into the benefits of interventions which may be more appropriate than traditional measures of health for the economic evaluation of new innovations in aged care service delivery. The ICECAP-O instrument may be more widely applicable than traditional health focussed instruments in facilitating decision making regarding the allocation of scarce resources across health, social and aged care sectors. Whilst the findings from this study provide support for the construct validity of the ICECAP-O in this particular patient population, further research is required to explore the construct validity of the ICECAP-O in other settings and with older people exhibiting different clinical characteristics.

6. Consumer engagement in the measurement of preferences for geriatric services

Health economists have increasingly recognised that consumers in geriatrics and other areas of medicine typically obtain 'utility' or value from more than just the outcome of the services they are exposed to (regardless of whether outcome is defined in terms of improvements in health or quality of life more broadly). Typically the 'process' by which geriatric services are provided is also highly important, both for older people themselves and for their families. Consumer satisfaction surveys offer one method for consumer engagement which has been and continues to be widely used. However a review of the patient satisfaction literature found that consumer satisfaction surveys in health care are often developed on an adhoc basis with little theoretical development and with insufficient evidence of their psychometric properties [Hawthorne, 2006]. In addition, a well-known problem with consumer satisfaction surveys in health care, particularly where these are conducted in populations of older people is that they tend to suffer from 'gratitude bias'. An extensive review of responses to consumer satisfaction surveys concluded that high levels of satisfaction are typically reported by at least 80% of respondents [Fitzpatrick, 1991].

An alternative approach for systematically engaging older people and their families to elicit their preferences in relation to the process of geriatric service delivery is to employ discrete choice experiment (DCE) methodology. DCE has strong theoretical foundations originating in Lancaster's characteristics approach to micro-economic consumer theory [Lancaster, 1966]. Lancaster hypothesized that rather than deriving utility directly from goods and services themselves, consumers derive utility from the characteristics or attributes of the good or service. Application of Lancaster's theory to health care highlights the potential importance of the characteristics of health care 'process' in addition to health outcomes in determining the overall utility or value to patients of health care. It is possible that there are other characteristics of the commodity health care (in addition to good health) which the patient finds utility or dis-utility bearing. Such characteristics may include factors relating to the provision of information (including reassurance and patient choice), in addition to other process factors such as continuity of staff, waiting time, location of care etc. For example, a change in the provision of out-patient rehabilitation services for older people such that greater continuity of staff is achieved may be highly valued by patients' and their families. However, measuring utility or value from out-patient rehabilitation services purely in terms of the health outcomes achieved by patients receiving this service would overlook this positive influence.

DCE is an economic technique based upon stated preference which is designed to establish the relative importance and impact of individual attributes, or characteristics, upon the overall utility of a good or service [Ryan, 2004]. DCEs are typically administered through a questionnaire in which the respondent is presented with a series of choices between alternative health or rehabilitation programs and asked to choose the program that they would prefer. The alternative programs are described in terms of their attributes and associated levels (for example waiting time, location of treatment, type of treatment and staff providing the treatment). The attributes and levels for inclusion in the DCE can be derived using qualitative methods (e.g. through interviews or focus groups), from a literature review, by consultation with clinical experts or health policy-makers or a combination of these approaches [Ryan et al 2008]. DCEs provide information about the acceptability of different characteristics of programs, the trade-offs that patients are willing to make between these characteristics, and the relative importance of each of these characteristics in determining overall utility or value [Ratcliffe and Buxton, 1999; Ryan, 2004]. Within health care there has been an exponential increase in the number of DCE studies undertaken to assess patient preferences within a wide variety of health care programmes and services within the last decade [9]. However, DCE studies specifically designed for and conducted with older people (aged 65 years and over) remain rare in comparison with those conducted with general adult samples. The authors have recently undertaken several DCE studies to obtain the views of older people as to how services should be provided to best meet their needs in transition care and in rehabilitation following stroke and hip fracture [Laver et al 2011; Ratcliffe et al 2010]. These studies have demonstrated the potential for the wider application of DCE methodology as a valuable tool for engaging with, and eliciting the views and preferences of older people and their families in relation to the provision of health and aged care services.

6.1 Case study: Application of a DCE in measuring patient preferences for liver transplantation

An example of a DCE question from a study conducted to elicit patient preferences for liver transplantation [Ratcliffe and Buxton, 1999] is presented in Figure 1.

Choice 1	Programme A	Programme B
Time spent on waiting list	4 months	2 months
Continuity of care	Low	High
Chance of successful liver transplant	85%	80%
Amount of information received	Some	Lots
Amount of follow up support received	Some	Some
Distance from home	200 miles	50 miles

Fig. 1. Example DCE question liver transplantation

The relevant attributes to present within the DCE and their associated levels were determined following a literature review and qualitative interviews with a small group of patients (n=12) who had recently undergone liver transplantation. The questionnaire contained 9 discrete choice questions in total with differing levels of the attributes presented in each choice. Two of the discrete choice questions represented a situation where one alternative was clearly dominant over another and hence should rationally be the chosen alternative. These questions were included as a test of internal consistency and assumed that, all other things being equal, patients would prefer a shorter waiting time, more continuity of contact with the same medical staff, a greater chance of a successful liver transplant, more information about the transplant, more follow up support and a shorter distance between the transplantation centre and the patient's home. The questionnaire was designed for self-completion and was administered by post to all patients with primary biliary cirrhosis who had undergone liver transplantation at one regional liver transplantation centre during the period January 1987-December 1996 and who were, in the opinion of a clinical research nurse based at the centre, considered well enough to complete the questionnaire (n=213). The reasons for choosing patients who have received a transplant rather than those awaiting transplant were two fold. Firstly, there is evidence to suggest that prospective patients may have difficulty in determining the relative importance of attributes relating to a service they had not yet experienced [Salkeld et al, 2000B]. Secondly, ethical concerns relating to the possibility of patient sensitivity with regard to the questions asked, particularly in relation to the length of the waiting period and chance of success attributes, could lead to increased anxiety amongst some patients awaiting transplantation. The questionnaire was sent by post to the patient's home address and included a covering letter by a physician from the centre involved in administering their care.

The data from the DCE can be analysed within the framework of random utility theory [Hannemann 1984]. Within the random utility framework therefore, an individual will choose Centre B over Centre A (the base alternative) if the measurable component of utility (V_b) plus the unobservable component of utility associated with Centre B (E_b) is greater than the measurable component of utility (V_a) plus the unobservable component of utility associated with Centre A (E_a).

$$\text{Choose B if } (V_b + E_b) > (V_a + E_a) \quad (1)$$

The measurable components of utility for each centre (V_b and V_a) can be estimated empirically. Assuming a linear additive utility function, the utility to be estimated in moving from Centre A to Centre B is:

$$\Delta V = \Delta 1 WAITDIFF + \Delta 2 CONTDIFF + \Delta 3 SUCCDIFF + \Delta 4 INFODIFF + \Delta 5 FOLLDIFF + \Delta 6 DISTDIFF + E \quad (2)$$

where ΔV is the change in utility in moving from Centre A to Centre B and Δ_1-Δ_6 are the parameters of the model to be estimated. 'WAITDIFF' is the difference in waiting time, 'CONTDIFF' is the difference in continuity of care experienced, 'SUCCDIFF' is the difference in the chance of success, 'INFODIFF' is the difference in the amount of information received about the transplantation process, 'FOLLDIFF' is the difference in follow up care received, 'DISTDIFF' is the difference in the distance between the hospital centre and the patient's home and E is the error term representing the unobservable component of utility. The marginal rate of substitution (MRS) between any pair of continuously defined attributes can be estimated by the ratio of the relevant parameters e.g. the MRS between the level of waiting time experienced and continuity of care is equal to Δ_1/Δ_2. The model is estimated without a constant term since the treatment option being considered in the model does not differ across choices. Given that the dependant variable is binary with discrete choice data and also given the repeated measurement aspect of the data (whereby multiple observations are obtained from the same individual), an appropriate model for data analysis is the random effects probit model [Propper, 1995; Ryan 1996]. Hence the random effects probit model was used to analyse the data generated within this study.

A response rate of 89% was achieved based upon 189 usable questionnaires which were returned (6 additional questionnaires were returned but the DCE choice questions were not completed and hence these individuals were excluded from the main data analysis). This response rate is higher than is typically achieved in postal DCE surveys to elicit patient preferences in health care [De Bekker-Grob et al, 2010] and may have been facilitated by the covering letter sent with the questionnaire which was sent from the consultant who was involved in the care of a large number of the patients in the sample. In addition, there is evidence to suggest that patients who have received a transplant are generally very grateful for the care they have received, many of them believing that they have been given a new chance [Tymstra, 1989]. Hence such individuals are potentially more likely than other groups to respond to questionnaires about the care they have received. Respondents were mostly female (90%), and the age range of respondents was 50-79 years. A total of 29 respondents (15%) exhibited a dominant preference for the chance of success attribute. Hence they consistently chose the centre with the higher chance of success regardless of the levels of the other attributes for all 9 discrete choice questions. The tests of internal consistency revealed that a small number of respondents [17 (9%)] answered inconsistently. The responses to the discrete choice questions were analysed using the random effects model in the statistical package STATA. The results from the random effects probit model excluding subjects revealing dominant preferences and inconsistent responders are given in Table 7. For comparison, the results from the random effects probit model including subjects revealing dominant preferences and excluding inconsistent responders only are given in Table 8. It can be seen that although the size of the coefficients differs slightly in Tables 7 and 8, the results are broadly similar. The results indicate that all of the attributes are highly significant in determining the choice of centre. The results also provide some support for the model's theoretical validity since the signs of the coefficients for each of the attributes are all in the expected direction.

Attributes	Coefficient	P	95% CI
WAITDIFF	-0.1537	<0.001	-0.2048 to -0.1026
CONTDIFF	0.6026	<0.001	0.4491 to 0.7561
SUCCDIFF	0.1184	<0.001	0.1010 to 0.1358
INFODIFF	0.4883	<0.001	0.3960 to 0.5805
FOLLDIFF	0.5436	<0.001	0.4521 to 0.6351
DISTDIFF	-0.0049	<0.001	-0.0060 to -0.0037

Number of observations = 1266

Number of groups = 145

Observations per group (min / avg / max) =1 / 8.73 / 9

Chi^2 =418.13 (p=0.000).

Table 7. Random effects probit model excluding subjects revealing dominant preferences and inconsistent responders

Attributes	Coefficient	P	95% CI
WAITDIFF	-0.1663	<0.001	-0.2203 to -0.1139
CONTDIFF	0.7152	<0.001	0.6472 to 0.8516
SUCCDIFF	0.1297	<0.001	0.1135 to 0.1391
INFODIFF	0.4929	<0.001	0.4016 to 0.5722
FOLLDIFF	0.5376	<0.001	0.4436 to 0.6058
DISTDIFF	-0.0052	<0.001	-0.0064 to -0.0040

Number of observations = 1544

Number of groups = 175

Observations per group (min / avg / max) =1 / 8.82 / 9

Chi^2 =538.81 (p=0.000)

Table 8. Random effects probit model including subjects revealing dominant preferences and excluding inconsistent responders

The negative sign on the waiting time and distance attributes suggests that respondents prefer lower levels of these attributes i.e. a shorter waiting time and a shorter distance between the transplantation centre and the patient' home. The positive signs on the chance of success, continuity, information and follow up support attributes suggest that respondents prefer higher levels of these attributes. The marginal rates of substitution between attributes are calculated by dividing the coefficients of the attributes of interest. For example the marginal rate of substitution between chance of success and waiting time for non-dominant respondents (0.77) is estimated by dividing the coefficient of chance of success (0.1184) by the coefficient of waiting time (-0.1537). The estimate indicates that respondents were prepared to exchange an increase in waiting time of 0.77 months for an increase in the probability of a chance of a successful transplant of 1%.

These models can be used to estimate the preference scores for different combinations of levels of the attributes included in the DCE exercise, by inserting the values for the relevant levels into the equation (Table 9). Such preference scores have also been defined in the literature as utility scores [Ryan, 1996]. However, when defined in this way, it is important to note that the scores generated are specific to the study being considered and it is not possible to compare the utility scores across studies in a manner akin to the comparison of the results of cost utility studies. One might move towards comparable utilities by examining more clearly the trade-offs that respondents are prepared to make between the health outcome attribute and the other attributes included in the DCE exercise. For example, if the health outcome attribute were presented in a format whereby an interval scaled utility value lying between 0 (death) and 1 (perfect health) could be assigned to each level presented then it is possible that the overall impact in terms of a reduction or improvement in the utility value of the other attributes included in the exercise could be examined.

Attributes and levels	**Codings**
Waiting time	2, 4, 6 (months)
Continuity	High =1, Low=0
Success	0.80, 0.85, 0.90 (percentage)
Information	Lots=2, some=1, little=0
Follow up support	Lots=2, some=1, little=0
Distance	50, 100, 200 (miles)

Table 9. Coding for levels of attributes included in the DCE

The preference score for Scenario 1 in Table 10 is:

$$V = -0.1537*4 + 0.6026*1 + 0.1184*0.85 + 0.4883*1 + 0.5436*1 - 0.0049*100 \quad (3)$$

Solving this equation gives a total score of 0.63. The combination of attributes can then be ranked in order of preference with a higher score indicating a higher preference. In Table 10, Equation (1) has been used to estimate the preference scores for each of the nineteen scenarios (S) presented in the questionnaire. It is possible, however, to generate such scores for all possible combinations of the levels of the six identified attributes. It can be seen that, of the restricted set of options presented to respondents, the most favoured mode of delivery using the DCE approach i.e. the one that was ranked first, would not be a liver transplantation programme with the highest chance of success.

S	Wait in months	Cont	Success %	Inform	Follow	Distance in miles	CA score	Rank Health Outcome	Rank CA
3	2	0	0.85	2	2	50	1.61	7 =	1
12	6	1	0.9	2	2	100	1.36	1=	2
15	4	1	0.85	2	1	50	1.36	7 =	2
17	4	1	0.8	1	2	100	1.17	14=	4
14	2	1	0.85	1	2	200	0.99	7 =	5
19	2	1	0.9	2	0	100	0.89	1 =	6
1	4	1	0.85	1	1	100	0.63	7 =	7
10	6	1	0.8	0	2	50	0.62	14 =	8
5	6	1	0.9	1	1	50	0.57	1 =	9
9	2	1	0.8	2	0	200	0.39	14 =	10
11	2	0	0.8	1	1	100	0.33	14 =	11
16	2	1	0.8	0	0	50	0.14	14 =	12
18	4	1	0.85	0	1	100	0.14	7 =	13
13	2	1	0.9	0	1	200	-0.03	1 =	14
8	4	0	0.9	1	0	50	-0.26	1 =	15
6	6	0	0.8	2	1	200	-0.29	14 =	16
4	4	0	0.9	0	2	200	-0.40	1 =	17
2	6	1	0.85	1	0	200	-0.71	7 =	18
7	6	0	0.85	0	0	100	-1.31	7 =	19

Table 10. Comparison of health outcome and DCE rankings for alternative service configurations

The scenario ranked first from the restricted DCE subset of possibilities is a centre with the following characteristics: an 85% chance of success, lots of information provided about the transplant process, lots of follow up support received, a short distance from the patient's home to the transplant centre and an average 2 month waiting period for the transplant operation (Scenario 15). The same scenario would be ranked 7th using a "health outcome maximisation" approach (whereby scenarios are ranked according to their chance of success with those scenarios with a 90% chance of success being ranked highest in this particular context). Alternatively, Scenario 17, which is ranked 4th using the DCE approach would be ranked only 14th using the health outcome maximisation approach. A comparison of the scenarios ranked 1st and 2nd using the DCE approach (scenarios 3 and 12 respectively) reveals that a reduction in 5% in the probability of survival at five years post-transplantation is more than compensated for by a reduction in transplant waiting time and a shorter distance between the patient's home and the transplant centre. This result implies that patient's would prefer to attend a centre closer to their home, even if the chance of a successful outcome were reduced, providing that the average waiting time would be no longer than 2 months. Similarly, a comparison of the scenarios ranked equal 2nd using the DCE approach (scenarios 12 and 15 respectively) reveals that a reduction in average waiting time of 2 months coupled with a reduction of 50 miles in the distance between the patient's home and the transplant centre would equally compensate for a reduction of 5% in the probability of survival at five years post-transplantation.

The existence of a 'centre' effect, whereby larger transplantation centres with a relatively high throughput of patients tend to have higher success rates than smaller transplant centres, has been proposed as an argument for retaining a small number of geographically dispersed transplantation centres throughout the UK [Taylor et al, 1985]. A review of evidence from the NHS Centre for Reviews and Dissemination indicated that there is no general relationship between volume of activity and clinical outcome, although this review did not focus upon transplantation specifically [NHS CRD, 1996]. The evidence presented from the findings of the DCE study suggests that patient's may prefer the provision of smaller transplant centres in many geographical locations, even if the chance of success would be reduced.

However, these results must be interpreted with caution due to the nature of the sample upon which the survey was conducted. In addition, as previously highlighted all of the patients in the sample had successfully survived the transplantation process and hence it is possible that respondents did not place as much emphasis on the chance of success attribute as they would have done if they had been awaiting transplantation. Despite these limitations. the results of this comparative exercise illustrate the extent to which factors associated with the 'process' of health care service delivery may influence patient's preferences for the service provided. A utility function, which is defined only in terms of health outcome e.g. QALYs, would overlook these influences. The potential importance of such characteristics is such that many respondents indicated that they would be prepared to sacrifice a reduction in the health outcome expected for an increase in the process characteristics of the service. These findings raise important issues for the organisation and delivery of the liver transplantation service. Whilst the QALY may remain an adequate model for addressing the broader allocative efficiency question 'should we provide a liver transplantation programme in the first instance', the potential for trade-offs between process characteristics and health outcome raises important issues concerning how a liver transplantation service should be provided to best meets the needs and preferences of patients.

6.2 Issues raised in the application of DCE's with older people

Application of DCEs with populations of older people raises a number of important issues. The research we have conducted to date with older patient populations receiving liver transplantation and geriatric rehabilitation services indicates that, although DCEs are often challenging for older people, they are often well received. The majority of older people with good levels of cognitive functioning (defined as a mini-mental score of 24 or above) are able to fully engage with and complete a DCE task [Folstein et al, 2001]. Our previous research also indicates that an interview mode of administration is often preferable to self-completion postal or on-line surveys as this helps to aid respondent understanding and promotes completion rates. The maximum number of attributes and levels respondents can adequately process and the maximum number of discrete choice questions which respondents can be expected to complete reliably are issues of controversy in the DCE literature. In a review of the conduct of DCEs in the health care literature Lancsar and Louviere [2008] indicated that the specification of the number of attributes and levels to be included is context specific. However, DCE applications in health care have included as many as 12 attributes in one scenario and up to 16 choice questions per experiment. For older people our previous research indicates that simpler experiments with a maximum of 6 attributes and 5-6 choice questions are preferable [Laver et al 2011; Ratcliffe et al 2010]. Within this context, our preliminary findings point towards high acceptance levels and good reliability and validity of the technique in older populations. However, further work should be undertaken to more formally investigate the reliability and validity of the DCE approach in older people including: the acceptability of the approach in different elderly populations, the threshold level of cognitive ability required to reliably complete a DCE task and where cognitive impairment precludes completion, who is the most appropriate proxy respondent.

7. Summary and conclusions

This chapter has outlined how health economics methods can be usefully applied in geriatrics and has described some recent innovations in health economics methodology and applications in relation to older people. An ageing population coupled with a desire for greater autonomy and choice are creating new pressures and demands for the aged care sector and health economic techniques can be helpful in facilitating difficult decisions about how scarce resources should best be allocated to ensure benefits are maximised. Firstly, economic evaluation and the methods for assessing the cost effectiveness of new interventions and modes of service delivery have been outlined and practical examples from the literature have been highlighted. The disadvantages of the QALY for the measurement and valuation of the benefits of health care for older people have been highlighted, in particular in terms of the focus upon expected length of survival and in terms of the focus upon health alone as the main indicator of benefit. A case study of the application of a newly developed instrument the ICECAP-O index of capability for older people has demonstrated its potential for application in measuring and valuing the quality of life of older people in the community and clinical based patient populations. Secondly, this chapter has outlined the potential for the wider application of DCEs methods, as a valuable tool for engaging with, and eliciting the views and preferences of older people and their families in relation to the provision of health and aged care services. In summary, it is our belief that the discipline of health economics has much to offer geriatrics. Although many challenges lie ahead, the future potential for health economists and health professionals engaged in geriatrics to work productively together to facilitate decision-making with the aims of promoting both efficiency and responsiveness within health and aged care systems is immense. For many countries, given the current era of an ageing population and demographic change the application of health economics to geriatrics represent an opportunity which should not be missed.

8. References

Australian Government Treasury 2007, Intergenerational Report 2007, Canberra.

Banks J, Marotta C. (2007). Outcomes validity and reliability of the modified rankin scale: implications for stroke clinical trials. *Stroke*; 38:1091-1096.

Brazier J, Walter S, Nicholl J, Kohler B. (1996). Using the SF-36 and Euroqol on an elderly popoulation. *Quality of Life Research*; 5: 195-204.

Brazier J, Roberts J, Deverill M. (2002). The estimation of a preference based measure of health from the SF-36. *Journal of Health Economics*; 21: 271-292.

Brazier J, Ratcliffe J, Salomon J, Tsuchiya A. (Jan 2007). Measuring and valuing health benefits for economic evaluation. *Oxford University Press*, Oxford.

Brooks R, Rabin R, de Charro F, editors. (2003). The measurement and valuation of health status using EQ-5D: a European perspective. *Kluwer Academic Publishers*.

Bryan S, Hardyman W, Bentham P, Buckley A, Laight A. (2005). Proxy completion of EQ-5D in patients with dementia. *Quality of Life Research*; 14:107-118.

Church J, Goodall S, Norman R, Haas M. (June 2011). An economic evaluation of community and residential aged care falls prevention strategies in NSW. New South Wales Public Health Bulletin; 22(3-4):60-8.

Coast J, Peters T, Richards S, Gunnell D. (1998). Use of the EuroQol among elderly acute patients. *Quality of Life Research*; 7: 1-10.

Coast J, Flynn T, Natarajan L, et al. (2008A). Valuing the ICECAP capability index for older people. *Social Science and Medicine*; 67:874-882.

Commonwealth Department of Health, Housing and Community Service. (2002). Guidelines for the pharmaceutical industry on the submission to the Pharmaceutical Benefits Advisory Committee. Australian Government Publishing Service, Canberra.

Colón-Emeric C, Datta S, Matchar D. (Jan 2003). An economic analysis of external hip protector use in ambulatory nursing facility residents. *Age and Ageing*; 32(1):47-52.

Coucill W, Bryan S, Bentham P, Buckley A, Laight A. (2001). EQ-5D in patients with dementia: an investigation of inter-rater agreement. *Medical Care*; 39: 760-771

Cronin P, Norman R, Viney R, et al. (2009). Can time trade off be implemented online? A case study from Australia using the EQ-5D (poster). *iHEA 7th World Congress*. Vol Beijing, China.

Crotty M, Ratcliffe J. (2011). If Mohammed won't come to the mountain, the mountain must go to Mohammed. Editorial *Age and Ageing* published online March 31st.

Davis B. (2005). Mediators of the relationship between hope and well-being in older adults. *Clinical Nursing Research*; 14(3):253-272.

De Bekker-Grob E, Ryan M, Gerard K. (2010). Discrete choice experiments in health economics: a review of the literature. *Health Econ* Dec 19. [Epub ahead of print]

Department of Health. (2001). National service framework for older people. London.

Drummond M, Sculpher M, Torrance G, O'Brien B, Stoddart G. (June 2005). Methods for the Economic Evaluation of Health Care Programmes Third Edition. *Oxford University Press*.

Dugan E, Cohen S, Robinson D et al. (1998). The quality of life of older adults with urinary incontinence: determining generic and condition specific predictors. *Quality of Life Research*; 7: 337-44.

Euroqol.(2004). *Measuring self reported health: an international perspective based on EQ-5D*. Hungary. Springmed publishing.

Evangelista L, Doering L, Dracup K, Vassilakis M, Kobashigawa J. (2003). Hope, mood states and quality of life in female heart transplant recipients. *The Journal of Heart and Lung Transplantation*; 22(6):681-686.

Fitzpatrick R. (2001). Surveys of patients satisfaction: I--Important general considerations. *British Medical Journal*; 302: 887-889.

Flynn T, Huynh E, Terlich F, Louviere J. (2010). What are Australian preferences for quality of life? Results from Best-Worst Scaling studies to value the ICECAP instruments. *AHES*. Vol Sydney.

Giles L, Hawthorne G, Crotty M. (2009). Health related quality of life among hospitalized older people awaiting residential care. *Health and Quality of Life Outcomes*; 7:71.

Glendinning C. (2003). Breaking down barriers: integrating health and social care services for older people in England. *Health Policy;* 65: 139-151.

Grewal I, Lewis J, Flynn T, Brown J, Bond J, Coast J. (2006). Developing attributes for a generic quality of life measur for older people: Preferences or capabilities. *Social Science and Medicine*; 62:1891-1901.

Hamel M, Phillips R, Davis R et al. (2001). Are aggresisve treatment strategies less cost effective for older patients? The case of ventilator support and aggressive care. *Journal of the American Geriatric Society*; 49: 382-390.

Hannemann W. (1984). Welfare evaluations in contingent valuation experiments with discrete responses. Reply. *American Journal of Agricultural Economics*; 69: 332-341.

Hawthorne, G. (2006). Review of Patient Satisfaction Measures, Australian Government Department of Health and Ageing, Canberra.

Herth K. (1992). Abbreviated instrument to measure hope: development and psychometric evaluation. *Journal of Advanced Nursing*; 17:1251-1259.

Higginson I. & Carr A. (2001). Using quality of life measures in the clinical setting. *British Medical Journal*; 322: 1297

Holman A, Sefarty M, Leurent B, King M (2011). Cost effectiveness of cognitive behaviour therapy versus talking and usual care for depressed older people in primary care. *BMC Health Services Research*; 11:33.

Holland R, Smoth R, Swift L, Lenaghan E. (2004). Assessing quality of life in the elderly: a direct comparison of the EQ-5D and AQoL. *Health Economics*; 13: 793-805.

Honkanen L, Mushlin A, Lachs M, Schackman B. (2006). Can hip protector use cost-effectrively prevent hip fractures in community dwelling geriatric populations? *Journal of the American Geriatrics Society*; 54: 1658-1665.

Hopman W, & Verner J. (2003). Quality of life during and after inpatient stroke rehabilitation. *Stroke*; 34: 801-805.

Hulme C, Long A, Kneafsy R, Reid G. (2004). Using the EQ-5D to assess health-related quality of life in older people. *Age and Ageing*; 33(5):504-507.

Johri M, Damschroder L, Zikmund-Fisher B, Ubel P. (2005). The importance of age in allocating health care resources. *Health Economics*;14(7):669-78.

Jowett S, Bryan S, Mant J, Fletcher K, Roalfe A et al. (2011). Cost effectiveness of warfarin versus aspirin in patients older than 75 years with atrial fibrillation. *Stroke*; 42(6): 1717-21.

Keeler E, Robalino D, Frank J et al. (Dec 1999). Cost-effectiveness of outpatient geriatric assessment with an intervention to increase adherence. *Medical Care*; 37(12):1199-206.

Kind P, Hardman G, Macran S. (1999). *UK Population Norms for EQ-5D*. University ofYork.

Kodner D. (2006). Whole-system approaches to health and social care partnerships for the frail elderly: an exploration of North American models and lessons. *Health and Social Care in the Community*; 14: 384-390.

Lancaster K. (1966). A new approach to consumer theory *Journal of Political Economy;* 74: 134-157.

Lanscar E, Louviere J. (2008). Conducting discrete choice experiments to inform healthcare decision making: A user's guide. *Pharmacoeconomics;* 26(8):661-77.

Laver K. (2009). *Goals, hope and response shift: the first six months after stroke* [Masters thesis]. Adelaide: Rehabilitation and Aged Care, Flinders University.

Laver K, Ratcliffe J, George S, Lester L, Walker R, Burgess L, Crotty M (2011). Early rehabilitation management after stroke: what do stroke patients prefer? *Journal of Rehabilitation Medicine;* 43(4):354-8.

Logsdon R, Gibbons L, McCurry S et al. (2002). Assessing quality of life in older adults with cognitive impairment. *Psychosomatic Medicine;* 64: 510-19.

Macadam M. (2009). Moving toward health service integration: Provincial progress in system change for seniors. In Canadian Policy Research Networks [Ed.]. Ontario.

National Health Service Centre for Reviews and Dissemmination, Nuffield Institute for Health. (1996). Hospital volume and health care outcomes, costs and patient access. Effective Health Care Bulletin; 2: 8.

National Institute for Health and Clinical Excellence. (2008). Guide to the Methods of Technology Appraisal, NICE, London.

Naumann V, Bryne G. (2004). WHOQoL-Bref as a measure of quality of life in older patients with depression. *International Psychogeriatrics;* 16: 159-73.

Novella J, Boyer F, Jochum C, et al. (2006). Health status in patients with Alzheimer's disease: An investigation of inter-rater agreement. *Quality of Life Research;* 15:811-819.

Osborne RH, Hawthorne G, Lew EA, Gray LC. (Feb 2003). Quality of life assessment in the community-dwelling elderly: validation of the Assessment of Quality of Life (AQoL) Instrument and comparison with the SF-36. *Journal of Clinical Epidemiology;* 56(2):138-47.

Prieto L, Sacristan J. (2003). Problems and solutions in calculating quality-adjusted life years (QALYs) *Health and Quality of Life Outcomes*: 1: 80

Productivity Commission. (2005). Economic implications of an ageing Australia. Research report. Canberra.

Propper C. (1995). The disutility of time spent on the United Kingdom's National Health Service waiting lists. *The Journal of Human Resources;* 30: 677-700.

Ratcliffe J and Buxton M. (1999). Patient's preferences regarding the process and outcomes of life saving technology: an application of conjoint analysis to liver transplantation. *International Journal of Technology Assessment in Health Care;* 15:340-351.

Ratcliffe J, Milte R, Crotty M, Cameron I, Miller M, Whitehead C. (2010). What are frail older people prepared to endure to achieve improved mobility following a hip fracture? A discrete choice experiment. *Australasian Journal on Ageing;* 29:1.

Rustoen R, Howie J, Eidsmo I, Moum T. (2005). Hope in patients hospitalized with heart failure. *American Journal of Critical Care.;* 14(5):417-425.

Ryan M. (1996). The application of conjoint analysis in health care. OHE publications, London, UK.

Ryan M. (2004). Discrete choice experiments in health care. *British Medical Journal;* 328;360-361.

Ryan M, Gerard K, Amaya-Amaya M (2008). Using discrete choice experiments to value health and health care. Springer, Dordrecht the Netherlands 2008.

Salkeld G, Cameron I, Cumming R et al. (2000A). Quality of life related to fear of falling and hip fracture in older women: a time trade off study. *British Medical Journal*; 320:241–6

Salkeld G, M Ryan and L Short. (2000B). The veil of experience: do consumers prefer what they know best? *Health Economics*; 9:267-270.

Schousboe J, Ensrud K, Nyman J et al. (2005). Universal bone deensitrometry combinedwith alendronate therapy for those diagnosed with osteoporosis is highly cost effective. *Journal of the American Geriatrics Society*; 53: 1697-1704.

Sigstad H, Stray-Pedersen A, Froland S. (2005). Coping, quality of life, and hope in adults with primary antibody deficiencies. *Health and Quality of Life Outcomes*; 3(31).

Sitoh Y, Lau T, Zochling J, Cumming R, Lord S, Schwarz J, March L, Sambrook P, Cameron ID. (2003). Proxy assessment of health related quality of life in the frail elderly. *Age and Ageing*; 32: 459-461.

Snyder C, Irving L, Anderson J. (1991). Hope and health. In: Forsyth D, Snyder C, eds. *Handbook of social and clinical psychology: the health perspective*. New York: Pergamon Press.

Snyder C, Lehman K, Kluck B, Monsson Y. (2006). Hope for rehabilitation and vice versa. *Rehabilitation Psychology*; 51(2):89-112.

Taylor RM, Ting A, Briggs J. (1995). Renal transplantation in the UK and Ireland-the centre effect. *The Lancet*; 1: 798-802.

Tymstra T. (1989). The imperative character of medical technology and the meaning of anticipated decision regret. *International Journal of Technology Assessment in Health Care*; 5: 207-213.

Walters SJ, Munro JF, Brazier JE. (Jul 2001). Using the SF-36 with older adults: a cross-sectional community-based survey. *Age Ageing*; 30(4):337-43.

Weinstein M, Torrance G. & McGuire A. (2009). QALYs: The Basics. *Value in Health;* 12: S5-S9.

Williams A. (1997). Intergenerational equity: an exploration of the 'fair innings' argument *Health Economics*; 6(2):117-32

Yadav S. (2010). Perceived social support, hope, and quality of life of persons living with HIV/AIDS: a case study from Nepal. *Quality of Life Research*; 19:157-166.